D0323885

WITHDRAWN

Recent Developments in
Adolescent Psychiatry

**WILEY SERIES IN CHILD
AND ADOLESCENT MENTAL HEALTH**

Joseph D. Noshpitz, Editor

FATHERLESS CHILDREN
by Paul L. Adams, Judith R. Milner, and Nancy A. Schrepf

**DIAGNOSIS AND PSYCHOPHARMACOLOGY OF CHILDHOOD
AND ADOLESCENT DISORDERS**
edited by Jerry M. Wiener

**INFANT AND CHILDHOOD DEPRESSION:
DEVELOPMENTAL FACTORS**
edited by Paul V. Trad

**TOURETTE'S SYNDROME AND TIC DISORDERS:
CLINICAL UNDERSTANDING AND TREATMENT**
by Donald J. Cohen, Ruth D. Bruun, and James F. Leckman

RECENT DEVELOPMENTS IN ADOLESCENT PSYCHIATRY
edited by L. K. George Hsu and Michel Hersen

Recent Developments in Adolescent Psychiatry

Edited by
L. K. George Hsu
Michel Hersen
University of Pittsburgh Medical Center

WILEY

A Wiley-Interscience Publication
JOHN WILEY & SONS
New York   Chichester   Brisbane   Toronto   Singapore

Library of Congress Cataloging-in-Publication Data:

Recent developments in adolescent psychiatry / edited by L.K. George
  Hsu, Michel Hersen.
    p.   cm.
    "A Wiley-Interscience publication."
    Includes bibliographies and indexes.
    ISBN 0-471-84583-3
    1. Adolescent psychiatry.   I. Hsu, L.K. George (Lee Keung
  George) II. Hersen, Michel.
    [DNLM: 1. Adolescent Psychiatry—trends. 2. Mental Disorders—in
  adolescence. WS 463 R295]
  RJ503.R43 1989
  616.89′022—dc19
  DNLM/DLC
  for Library of Congress   88-5500
                                                  CIP

Printed in the United States of America

10 9 8 7 6 5 4 3 2 1

Contributors

Carol M. Adams, M.S., Graduate Student in Developmental Psychology, Utah State University, Logan, Utah

Gerald R. Adams, Ph.D., Program Director, Laboratory for Research on Adolescence, Utah State University, Logan, Utah

Geary S. Alford, Ph.D., Professor of Psychiatry/Psychology, Department of Psychiatry and Human Behavior, University of Mississippi Medical Center, Jackson, Mississippi

Lorian Baker, Ph.D., Research Psycholinguist, Neuropsychiatric Institute, Center for Health Sciences, University of California, Los Angeles, California

Dennis P. Cantwell, M.D., Joseph Campbell Professor of Psychiatry, Neuropsychiatric Institute, Center for Health Sciences, University of California, Los Angeles, California

Stewart Gabel, M.D., Assistant Professor of Psychiatry, The New York Hospital-Cornell Medical Center, White Plains, New York

Gregory Hanna, M.D., Associate Professor of Psychiatry and Behavioral Sciences, Neuropsychiatric Institute and Hospital, University of California, Los Angeles, California

L.K. George Hsu, M.D., Associate Professor of Psychiatry, Director, Eating Disorders Outpatient Clinic, Department of Psychiatry, Western Psychiatric Institute and Clinic, University of Pittsburgh Medical Center, Pittsburgh, Pennsylvania

043039

Miriam M. Koller, M.D., Assistant Professor of Child Psychiatry, Medical College of Virginia, Medical Director of Adolescent Services, Psychiatric Institute of Richmond, Richmond, Virginia

Melvin Lewis, M.B., B.S., F.R.C.Psych.,D.C.H., Professor of Pediatrics and Psychiatry, Director of Medical Studies, Yale Child Study Center, Yale University, New Haven, Connecticut

Anthony P. Mannarino, Ph.D., Associate Professor of Psychiatry and Psychology, Director, Center for Children and Families, Department of Psychiatry, Western Psychiatric Institute and Clinic, University of Pittsburgh School of Medicine, Pittsburgh, Pennsylvania

Nathaniel McConaghy, M.D., Associate Professor of Psychiatry, Psychiatry Unit, Prince of Wales Hospital, Randwick, New South Wales, Australia

James McCracken, M.D., Assistant Professor of Psychiatry and Biobehavioral Sciences, Neuropsychiatric Institute and Hospital, University of California, Los Angeles, California

Michael McManus, M.D., Associate, Psychiatric Centers at San Diego, Clinical Investigator, Feighner Research Institute, Encinitas, California

Gary B. Melton, Ph.D., Professor of Psychology and Law, Director, Law and Psychology Program, Department of Psychology, University of Nebraska, Lincoln, Nebraska

Debra A. Murphy, Ph.D., Assistant Professor, Attention Deficit Disorders Program, Department of Psychiatry, Western Psychiatric Institute and Clinic, University of Pittsburgh School of Medicine, Pittsburgh, Pennsylvania

William E. Pelham, Jr., Ph.D., Associate Professor of Psychiatry, Director, Attention Deficit Disorders Program, Department of Psychiatry, Western Psychiatric Institute and Clinic, School of Medicine University of Pittsburgh, Pittsburgh, Pennsylvania

Cynthia R. Pfeffer, M.D., Associate Professor of Clinical Psychiatry, Cornell University Medical College, and Chief, Child Psychiatry Inpatient Unit, New York Hospital, White Plains, New York

Linda K. Schmechel, Ph.D., Assistant Professor of Counseling/Psychology, Department of Psychology, Wayne State College, Wayne, Nebraska

S. Charles Schulz, M.D., Chief, Pharmacologic and Somatic Treatments Program, Schizophrenia Research Branch, National Institute of Mental Health, Rockwell, Maryland

Mary E. Schwab-Stone, M.D., Assistant Professor of Psychiatry, Yale Child Study Center, Yale University, New Haven, Connecticut

Arthur M. Small, M.D., Clinical Professor of Psychiatry, Department of Psychiatry, New York University Medical Center, New York, New York

Derek Steinberg, M.B., B.S., M.Phil., F.R.C.Psych., Consultant Psychiatrist, Adolescent Unit, Bethlem Royal Hospital and the Maudsley Hospital, London, England

Michael Strober, Ph.D., Associate Professor of Psychiatry and Biobehavioral Sciences, Neuropsychiatric Institute and Hospital, University of California, Los Angeles, California

Series Preface

This series is intended to serve a number of functions. It includes works on child development; it presents material on child advocacy; it publishes contributions to child psychiatry; and it gives expression to cogent views on child rearing and child management. The mental health of parents and their interaction with their children is a major theme of the series, and emphasis is placed on the child as individual, as family member, and as a part of the larger social surround.

Child development is regarded as the basic science of child mental health, and within that framework research works are included in this series. The many ethical and legal dimensions of the way society relates to its children is the central theme of the child advocacy publications, as well as a primarily demographic approach that highlights the role and status of children within society. The child psychiatry publications span studies that concern the diagnosis, description, therapeutics, rehabilitation, and prevention of the emotional disorders of childhood. And the views of thoughtful and creative contributors to the handling of children under many different circumstances (retardation, acute and chronic illness, hospitalization, handicap, disturbed social conditions, etc.) find expression within the framework of child rearing and child management.

Family studies with a central child mental health perspective are included in the series, and explorations into the nature of parenthood and the parenting process are emphasized. This includes books about divorce, the single parent, the absent parent, parents with physical and emotional illnesses, and other conditions that significantly affect the parent-child relationship.

Finally, the series examines the impact of larger social forces, such as war, famine, migration, and economic failure, on the adaptation of children and families. In the largest sense, the series is devoted to books that illuminate the special needs, status, and history of children and their families within all perspectives that bear on their collective mental health.

Joseph D. Noshpitz

Children's Hospital Medical Center, and
The George Washington University
Washington, D.C.

Preface

Adolescent psychiatry is a growing field that only recently has differentiated itself from child and adult psychiatry. As attested within the chapters of our text, there are some unique developmental, diagnostic, therapeutic, and legal issues that are endemic to adolescent psychiatry. However, it is fair to say that among the various subdivisions of psychiatry, adolescent psychiatry has been the most resistant to change. A perusal of several recent monographs on the topic will confirm that the field is still largely dominated by psychoanalytic viewpoints, and although each monograph does contain several chapters on recent advances in adolescent psychiatry, each still is unreconciled in philosophy and spirit to the empirical body of knowledge that now is available. We therefore believe that our book serves to fill a gap in the extant literature.

Our stand is primarily empirical. The topics that we have chosen to include in the book are those where, we believe, most advances have been made. The book contains relatively little psychodynamic material, not because we are opposed to it, but because empirical data on the psychodynamic aspects of adolescent psychiatry are lacking. Furthermore, we believe that establishing a diagnosis and then developing a treatment plan is clinically useful even for a disturbed youngster going through the storm and stress of an adolescent crisis. With a few exceptions, we have therefore adopted the diagnostic scheme of the DSM-III-R throughout the book. Imperfect though the scheme may be, we believe that it serves at least as a common frame of reference.

The book is divided into three parts. Part I (General Issues) considers the historical context of the field, developmental aspects, diagnostic issues, and medical and psychological evaluations. Part II (Specific Issues) is devoted to examination of management, crises, and legal issues.

The nine chapters in Part III (Specific Disorders) detail how pharmacological, psychodynamic, and behavioral approaches apply in the context of the particular diagnostic, developmental, and clinical considerations for each disorder.

Many individuals have contributed their time and effort to this volume. First and foremost, we thank our respective experts for sharing their views with us. Second, we are most appreciative of the technical assistance of Jenifer Brander, Beth Fryman, Mary Jo Horgan, Mary H. Newell, Robin Santhouse, and Theresa Sobkiewicz. Finally, but hardly least of all, we thank Herb Reich, our editor at John Wiley, for his willingness to publish and for his good cheer and advice throughout the project.

L.K. George Hsu, M.D.
Michel Hersen, Ph.D.

Contents

Part I

General Issues

CHAPTER ONE

Historical, Developmental, and Societal Perspectives on Adolescence

Melvin Lewis

Adolescence as a phase of development existed in some form long before it was recognized and conceptualized in the United States by G. Stanley Hall in 1904. For example, at the time of the Sumerian culture of 4000 to 3000 BC, the first case of juvenile delinquency was recorded on clay tablets (Kramer, 1959). The *Oxford English Dictionary* traces the word itself to the fifteenth century. Rousseau, in his book *Emile* (1762) noted, "We are born, so to speak, twice over; born into existence, and born into life; born a human being and born a man" (pp. 128, 172).

In all cultures and in all times, the period has been marked by rites of passage. In simple cultures where young men and women are needed to do adult work, the period of initiation is short. The initiation rites vary from culture to culture but often involve periods of fasting or other ordeals. The Australian Aborigines and some African peoples circumcize adolescents. Tattooing is used in the South Pacific. Changes in hair style and clothing are common in some Indian tribes of South America. Mixtecan Indians of Mexico begin assuming some parental functions at age 6 or 7 and learn to perform adult tasks quite easily, with full parental approval (Phillips, Phillips, Fixsen, & Wolf, 1973), whereas the Mundugumor adolescents in the South Seas have a far more unpleasant time, with much hostility from parents of the same sex (Paulson & Lin, 1972). The Chewa of Africa and the Lepcha of India cohabit and copulate early (by age 11 or 12), whereas the Aina of Panama remain ignorant of adult sexual information until the last stages of the marriage ceremony (Hauser, 1976).

The concept of individuation and the developmental task of separating from the family, so central in our Western view of adolescence, is not universally accepted. The Chinese, for example, see child and adolescent development differently: "The self does not develop in a process of gradual separation and individuation as is often conceptualized in western psychological theories. We see, instead a 'little me' maintaining its interdependency within the context of the 'big me'—that is, the family, the state and the world, throughout the life-span" (Dien, 1983).

As society becomes more complex, the duration of adolescence lengthens, and the degree of stress for the adolescent increases. The law also becomes confused when dealing with adolescents. Thus the legal ages for marriage, driving, voting, conscription, compulsory education, and alcohol consumption may vary immensely and are subject to change according to the needs of a given society at a given time. Adolescents in poor families often have to start work early and may have a correspondingly shorter adolescence. Adolescents of more prosperous families tend to stay in school and college longer.

What is particularly remarkable about the concept of adolescence is that in essence it is comprised of those psychological processes mobilized to negotiate the change from the biopsychosocial characteristics of childhood to those of adulthood; however, the actual form and intensity of these characteristics and processes is determined by the interaction of social forces and the individuals' genetically programmed potential of capabilities. Thus when tremendous changes occur in society over the course of history, astonishing changes emerge in the complex adaptive psychological mechanism of the individual adolescent. These psychological changes sometimes produce what amounts to a new stage of psychological development. Changes in American society illustrate this point.

The great social changes in American society that took place in the eighteenth century and in the industrial revolution from about the 1880s markedly changed our human social experience. This change in turn brought about different kinds of adaptive mechanisms, which in the aggregate came to be known as the stage of adolescence. Furthermore, changes in society did not stop with the industrial revolution. We are now, for example, in a "high-tech" age, characterized in part by a computer technology that is advancing exponentially. Such social changes make demands on the individual, such as the need for ever more continuing education and the need to solve new problems created by social changes. New issues are being brought into focus by modern technology, for example: How shall we conduct our sexual lives when, on the one hand, contraception is widely available, while on the other hand, AIDS represents a growing threat? Who shall control, and by what means, the immensely violent destructive forces now possible with nuclear energy? The adolescent, acutely sensitive about these and other issues but not in control of them, sometimes reacts with great anxiety and behaves accordingly.

Each epoch in social change brings about the emergence of different characteristics which hitherto had been present only as a potential awaiting the appropriate stimulus. In turn, these new characteristics may undergo change. Substages may be demarcated. Shortly after the descriptions of adolescence began to appear, the subphases of early and late adolescence (Blos, 1962) were described. Subsequently, as the social changes of the 1960s increased in intensity, a whole new stage in development appeared to emerge—the stage of "youth" (Kenniston, 1970). The characteristics of any of these substages or new stages are not necessarily homogeneous and might be found somewhat asynchronously in any of several lines of development, including social behavior, sexual mores, cognitive functioning, and moral reasoning. No doubt more stages and substages will be identified.

Once the stage of adolescence was recognized, described, and subdivided, theories were developed to account for the phenomena described. Hall's (1904) theory, for example, seemed to be influenced by Darwin's evolutionary theory and suggested a kind of recapitulation that paralleled the development of the human race (Weiner, 1970). Freud (1905) conceptualized a psychosexual developmental sequence culminating in genital primacy at the conclusion of adolescence. Recapitulation of early phases became a prominent theme in the psychoanalytic writings of Blos (1962) and others. The idea of a normative crisis, with particular emphasis on the development of "identity" versus "identity diffusion" during adolescence was put forward by Erikson (1950). The stages of cognitive development with the achievement of "formal operations" during adolescence were described by Piaget (1958; 1969). Implications of "normal" disturbance as the adolescent attempted to deal with his or her "developmental tasks" was adumbrated by Anna Freud (1958). Other psychoanalysts sometimes carried this concept of disturbance to extremes. For example, Geleerd (1961), stated that she "would feel great concern for the adolescent who causes no trouble and feels no disturbance" (p. 267).

Still others (e.g., Rutter, Graham, Chadwick, & Yule, 1976) began using the methodological tools of the day to produce epidemiological data that seemed to refute the view of adolescence as a pervasive state of storm, stress, and turmoil. Thus Rutter stated, "alienation from parents is *not* common in 14-year-olds" (p. 40), and most young teenagers in a general population get on rather well with their parents, who in turn continue to have a "substantial influence on their children right through adolescence" (p. 54). Offer (1969), Masterson (1968), and more recently Kaplan, Hong, and Weinhold (1984) have tended to confirm this questioning of the so-called ubiquity of adolescent turmoil.

Once clinical phenomena were described and theories were formulated, learned societies were founded—sometimes to study the questions posed, sometimes to promulgate one or another viewpoint, and sometimes to provide camaraderie for those with similar interests. Sometimes they were formed, it has to be said, to protect professional guild interests. In the case of adolescence, quintessentially a twentieth-century phenomenon, professional societies, clinical services, and research about all of its aspects began to blossom. Numerous journals devoted to the publication of papers on adolescence soon appeared. Different professional disciplines proffered their expertise. Specialized training programs were developed. Soon a worldwide interest in adolescence developed, culminating in international meetings.

Does the emergence, prolongation, and subdivision of a developmental phase such as adolescence bring with it a new range of psychopathology? Few psychiatric illnesses are confined to adolescence, but some, such as depression and attempted suicide, show an increase in prevalence and severity during that stage of development, and others, such as schizophrenia, may have their onset at this time.

What is striking is the increase in social problems that appear as the stage of adolescence is lengthened. These social problems include teenage pregnancy, venereal disease, alcohol and drug abuse, violence, and delinquency. However, the rapidly changing social environment makes prediction hazardous, and it is only safe to say that we do not know what further developmental stages and developmental psychopathology will be identified for those individuals between age 11 and 22 now living in our rapidly advancing society. Much depends on the demands of a given society. Since we cannot predict with any kind of certainty what form our society will take, we cannot predict with accuracy the future of adolescence. Therefore, we need to keep open multidisciplinary pathways to the understanding and treatment of troubled adolescents in the years ahead.

Finally, does adolescence ever really completely end in contemporary society? The phases of development that commonly occupy the years 18 to 23 may include late adolescence (Blos, 1962), youth (Kenniston, 1970), the periods of "Intimacy and Distantiation versus Self-Absorption" and "Generativity versus Stagnation" (Erikson, 1956), and young adulthood (Lidz, 1968). Indeed, the word *adolescence* means becoming an adult and was first used in the English language in 1430, when it referred to age 14 to 21 years in males and 12 to 21 years in females. Adolescents "going on 30" are not uncommon nowadays.

A stabilization of biological maturation occurs as epiphyses close, adult stature is achieved, and drive upheaval settles. At the same time, an increasing stabilization of the personality should take place. Conflict between the self and the changing *milieu interieur* abates and is displaced by conflict within the self and between the self and the external world. Thus consolidation and integration of one's personality and the adaptation to a changing and unfamiliar society become the pivotal developmental tasks at the end of adolescence. Specific developmental tasks include the achievement of gratifying heterosexual relationships, deciding upon a career, and committing oneself to marriage or an alternative lifestyle. Clearly, these are also the tasks of young adults.

Failure to resolve any of these developmental tasks may occur, and the result may be persisting adolescence and adolescent psychopathology. Difficulties arising from unresolved earlier conflicts, can prevent adolescents from resolving developmental tasks. Moreover, current conflicts may be heightened by interaction with the existential anxiety that arises when adolescents are confronted with certain challenges of society. These challenges, at least in Western society, include attitudinal and technological confrontations. Modern technology of instantaneous mass communication, for example, has enabled young people all over the world to realize that they have much in common and that in some societies they constitute the majority.

Another, more immediate, variable is the socioeconomic status of the individual (Esman, 1977). For example, a white, middle-class, professional person has an entirely different experience from a Native American. Additional variables are sex and parenthood. Recent psychoanalytic investigations, however, have continued to focus for the most part only on the affluent individual. For example, Ritvo (1971) has concentrated on college students and those who have dropped out of college, and even among this group there is change. Thus the striking difference in the behavior of students in the late 1960s compared to those seen in the early 1970s seems to reflect both intrapsychic development and the individual's responsiveness to the particular (historical) social context.

By age 18 to 23 years, a sufficient history of personality traits and intellectual development has occurred to enable the individual to observe his or her own behavior in response to internal urges and external demands. This conscious identity, including a new decision-making capability, is now more fully integrated into the ego and should be more or less independent of superego reinforcement. Moreover, decisions can now be made in the context of lengthier commitment rather than immediate wishes or superego sanctions. In addition, a greater degree of intimacy becomes possible as independence from the family is established and a conscious sense of identity is achieved. A new relationship with society emerges as the individual's horizons widen and the inequalities of society are recognized, if not tolerated. In some young adults there is an acute disillusionment with society, reminiscent of the disillusionment with parents that occurs in the post-oedipal phase. Disillusionment with society may be an extension of, or a displacement from, that earlier disillusionment. However, in many, if not most, instances it is a true recognition of human frailty and social reality. Identity is, therefore, a complex achievement, involving a sense of one's personal sameness within a comprehensible social reality and having both conscious and unconscious aspects. Identity emerges within a particular historical moment and is subject to change.

Both males and females who are at the border of adolescence and adulthood are on the threshold of establishing new, long-lasting relationships based primarily on reality considerations. The short-lived relationships based on replication of original objects (part-identification or overidealization) that characterize earlier adolescence are now replaced by a full sense of identification and the need to form realistic and real, lasting relationships that "fit" the now-consolidated identification. The motivations and forces acting on the formation of long-term, heterosexual relationships (including marriage) are the following: early conscious and unconscious need fulfillment, unconscious incestuous fantasy wishes, the need for intellectual stimulation, sexual pleasure, self-esteem and narcissistic gratification, the influences of family and peer relationships, social striving, neurotic role interlocking, the wish to have children, and desire for complementarity. The degree to which any one of these components overrides the others will determine whether the relationship will succeed or fail.

Since few, if any, relationships stay the same, a strong conscious commitment is usually required to resolve difficulties and misunderstandings. Older adolescents and young adults are generally capable of making this strong commitment, particularly as they approach their midtwenties. Failure to make this kind of commitment, overriding and interfering unconscious motivation, or even preconscious motivation that is not allowed recognition or expression is likely to result in a failure or radical change in such relationships. A further complication is that ideas about commitment change as society changes. The recent high rate of divorce among young couples is a vivid example of societal change affecting individual development.

During this intermediate adolescent-adulthood phase, the individual also becomes capable of parenthood, during which the individual's own childhood experiences are reworked (Benedek, 1959). The individual's children act as stimuli and provide opportunities for this development. This, in turn, is a part of the individual's growing capacity for mutuality during what Erikson (1959, p. 97) calls the stage of "Generativity versus Stagnation." Parenthood, however, is more than a single developmental phase. It is a series of interconnected subphases: fantasies of parenthood; the psychological process for man and woman during pregnancy, labor, and childhood (Bibring, Dwyer, Huntington, & Valenstein, 1961); and the identity changes in the parents as they experience change in their relationships to each other and to their children as their children move through developmental phases. Historically, recent societal changes have led to an enormous increase in the number of single adolescent-to-early adult parents, with all the sequelae that affect the child who is being reared by the single young parent.

Parents age 18 to 23 years old often experience being between two generations—one's parents and one's children. While they are emancipated from their parents, these young people are concerned about being pulled back into the family of origin as a child and not as an adult (Gould, 1972). Consequently, there is a tendency nowadays to intensify peer relationships, provided such relationships (especially in the aggregate) do not in turn threaten one's autonomy and individuality.

An individual at this stage is actively involved in mastering a work skill, profession, or lifestyle. Sociocultural and family influences, sex, economic conditions, physical status, cognitive abilities, education, job opportunities, personality type and needs, specific conscious and unconscious motivations, identifications, talents, and skills are some of the factors that determine an individual's work. Sometimes the choice of a particular career provides an environment in which group values can take the place of individually derived moral and ethical values. The individual superego may become dissolved in the group superego or may be reinforced by the group-ego ideal. Repetition compulsion may be another factor in determining not only the individual's choice of work, but the outcome, that is, the degree of success or failure in that work. Work may thus be an end in itself, a means of satisfying old urges, or a force acting upon the young adult—or all three. Adolescence should end, and adulthood should begin. However, our rapidly changing society and job obsolescence may affect this development: Adolescence may be prolonged further—or may have to terminate abruptly.

In overview, the normal individual at the end of adolescence ideally is experiencing for the first time the consolidation of identity, the mastery of drives, the achievement of unfettered, true heterosexual object relationships, and a realistic view of the world as he or she enjoys new heights of intellectual activity. Few achieve this ideal state. Indeed, even if this state were achieved, it would not last; the next phase of development or societal shifts would once again demand change.

REFERENCES

Benedek, T. (1959). Parenthood as a development phase. *Journal of the American Psychoanalytic Association, 7,* 389–407.

Bibring, G. L., Dwyer, T. F., Huntington, D. S., & Valenstein, A. F. (1961). A study of the psychological processes in pregnancy and of the earliest mother-child relationship. *The Psychoanalytic Study of the Child, 16,* 9–44.

Blos, P. (1962). Phases of adolescence. In P. Blos (Ed.), *On adolescence: A psychoanalytic interpretation* (pp. 52–157). New York: Free Press.

Dien, D. S. (1983). Big me and little me: A Chinese perspective on self. *Psychiatry, 46,* 281–286.

Erikson, E. (1950). *Childhood and society.* New York: Norton.

Erikson, E. (1959). Growth and crises of the healthy personality. *Psychological Issues, 1,* 50–100.

Esman, A. H. (1977). Changing values: Their implications for adolescent development and psychoanalytic idea. In S. Feinstein & P. Giovacchini (Eds.), *Adolescent psychiatry* (Vol 5, pp. 18–34). New York: Jason Aronson.

Freud, A. (1958). Adolescence. *The Psychoanalytic Study of the Child, 13,* 255–278.

Freud, S. (1953). Three essays on sexuality. *Standard Edition* 7. London: Hogarth Press. (Original work published 1905)

Geleerd, E. R. (1961). Some aspects of psychoanalytic technique in adolescence. *The Psychoanalytic Study of the Child, 12,* 263–283.

Gould, R. L. (1972). The phases of adult life: A study in developmental psychology. *American Journal of Psychiatry, 129,* 521–531.

Hall, G. S. (1904). *Adolescence: Its psychology and its relations to physiology, anthropology, sociology, sex, crime, religion and education.* New York: Appleton.

Hauser, S. T. (1976). Self-image complexity and identity formation in adolescence. *Journal of Youth and Adolescence, 5,* 161–178.

Kaplan, S., Hong, G. K., & Weinhold, C. (1984). Epidemiology of depressive symptomatology in adolescents. *Journal of the American Academy of Child Psychiatry, 23,* 91–98.

Kenniston, K. (1970). Youth: A new stage in life. *The American Scholar, 39,* 631–653.

Kramer, S. N. (1959). *History begins at sumer.* New York: Garden City.

Lidz, T. (1968). The young adult. In T. Lidz, *The person* (pp. 362–367). New York: Basic Books.

Masterson, J. F. (1968). The Psychiatric significance of adolescent turmoil. *American Journal of Psychiatry, 124,* 1549–1554.

Offer, D. (1969). *The psychological world of the teenager.* New York: Basic Books.

Paulson, M. J., & Lin, T. T. (1972). Family harmony: An etiologic factor in alienation. *Child Development, 43,* 591–604.

Phillips, E. L., Phillips, E. A., Fixsen, D. C., & Wolf, M. M. (1973). Achievement place: Behavior shaping works for delinquents. *Psychology Today, 7,* 75–79.

Piaget, J. (1958). *The growth of logical thinking.* New York: Basic Books.

Piaget, J. (1969). The intellectual development of the adolescent. In G. Caplan & S. Lebovici (Eds.), *Adolescence: Psychosocial perspectives.* New York: Basic Books.

Ritvo, S. (1971). Late adolescence: Developmental and clinical considerations. *The Psychoanalytic Study of the Child, 26,* 241–263.

Rousseau, J. J. (1966). *Emile* (Barbara Foxley, Trans.). New York: Dutton. (Original work published 1762)

Rutter, M., Graham, P., Chadwick, O. F. D., & Yule, W. (1976). Adolescent turmoil: Fact or fiction? *Journal of Child Psychology and Psychiatry, 17,* 35–56.

Weiner, L. B. (1970). *Psychological disturbances in adolescence.* New York: Wiley.

CHAPTER TWO

Developmental Issues

Gerald R. Adams
Carol M. Adams

Adolescent psychiatry has, from its very origins, held a strong developmental perspective. Focusing on individuality in the form of ego and character formation, we can demonstrate this developmental foundation. A reading of Sigmund Freud's *The Interpretation of Dreams* (1900), *Introductory Lectures on Psychoanalysis* (1917), or *The Ego and the Id* (1923) readily reveals a developmental process underpinning the id, ego, and superego constructs of personality. Differentiation, organizational, and maturational processes of normal and psychopathological personalities are foundational to this psychiatric perspective.

Other psychiatric perspectives also hold a developmental foundation. While Harry Stack Sullivan was strongly influenced by S. Freud, he chose to focus on what is called interpersonal or social psychiatry. In a series of published lectures (*Interpersonal Theory of Psychiatry*) Sullivan (1953) argues that individual differences are actually reflections of two or more individuals at different stages of a simple developmental sequence. Based on his "single-genus postulate," Sullivan argues for a developmental view of character formation (individuality) when he states, "everyone is much more simply human than otherwise, and . . . anomalous interpersonal situations, insofar as they do not arise from differences in language or custom, are a function of differences in relative maturity of the persons concerned" (pp. 32–33). Therefore, according to Sullivan, the self-system emerges and develops to meet the needs of interpersonal relations. As such, the ego or self-system's maturing needs are thought to developmentally unfold as new interpersonal situations dictate such change.

Perhaps the developmental perspective of adolescent psychiatry can be seen most vividly in the often-cited writings of Peter Blos, Anna Freud, and Erik H. Erikson. In *On Adolescence: A Psychoanalytic Interpretation*, Blos (1962) delineates the qualitative distinctions between latency, early adolescence, adolescence proper, and late adolescence. Qualitatively distinct ego and superego functions are detailed with considerable attention given to aspects of character formation, individuality, genital primacy, self-representation, and identity. Issues or conditions associated with progressive and regressive development are discussed in detail. Further, in his recent treatise entitled *Son and Father: Before and Beyond the Oedipus Complex,* Blos (1985) elaborates the proposed importance and distinctions between the dyadic and triadic allogender or isogender complexes and the influence that the father complex and its resolution have on male development. Of particular usefulness to students of personality has been Blos's notion of "the second individuation process of adolescence" with its corresponding self-divestiture of infantile dependencies.

Anna Freud's (1965) classic volume on *Normality and Pathology in Childhood* elaborates on several psychoanalytic-based developmental patterns. For example, she discusses the developmental progressions from dependency to emotional self-reliance and adult object relationships; movement toward body independence through outer to inner psychic foci; egocentricity to social and other-focused behavior; topographical, temporal, and formal regression in ego development, and much more. Throughout her writings, she continually strives to understand the developmental nature of intrapsychic structures of personality as they mature from childhood, through adolescence, and into adulthood. Both conflict-free ego processes and ego defense mechanisms were discussed and analyzed indepth through her clinical and research career.

Finally, the developmental perspective within adolescent psychiatry with which we are most involved is the psychosocial theory of Erik H. Erikson. In *Identity: Youth and Crisis,* Erikson (1968) provides an epigenetic portrait of eight central life stages that contribute to ego-identity formation. Each life-stage dilemma has a positive (desirable) pole, which represents progressive social maturity, opposed by a negative (undesirable) pole, which represents a fixated characteristic of that developmental crisis. According to Erikson, with the personal resolution of each new life crisis, the ego incorporates a new quality into the ego-identity. Therefore, a healthy personality (ego-identity) is acquired through the resolution of a series of life crises. With each new resolution, a corresponding personal recognition of a meaningful accomplishment and a growing sense of individuality and personal uniqueness emerge.

Erikson views adolescence as a state of *psychosocial moratorium,* a period wherein adolescents are expected to prepare themselves for adult status through the formation of a self-defined identity. He views adolescence not only in terms of personality development, but as a psychosocial process reflecting life-event transitions between childhood and adulthood. In particular, he has expanded the socialization influences on individual development to include a larger cultural, historical, societal, and social influence. While recognizing the unconscious influences of instincts, he emphasizes the developmental opportunities, defeats, triumphs, and virtues of a universal sequence of life-stage development.

In summary, adolescent psychiatry embodies varying psychiatric theoretical perspectives founded on developmental based constructs. However, further clarification on what is to be considered central developmental issues in adolescent psychiatry is needed. Therefore, in the remainder of this chapter, we will focus on the clarification of what are major dimensions of developmental issues. Focusing on individuality in the form of ego-identity, we will provide illustrations of these developmental issues in our own research program on normality and ego-identity development. From available research literature on identity disorders, we will briefly illustrate several major related developmental considerations for understanding psychopathology. However, given the limitations of available developmental research literature, we are unable to fully examine from an empirical base the full range of developmental issues for adolescent identity disorders. We will conclude with a brief section on developmental issues yet unaddressed by carefully designed systematic clinical research on identity disorders in adolescence.

CHALLENGES TO A SCIENCE OF DEVELOPMENTAL-BASED ADOLESCENT PSYCHIATRY

Having established that the theoretical and conceptual foundation of adolescent psychiatry rests on a broadly defined conception of development, let us turn our attention to the delineation of what are the central foci of this perspective and illustrate how it has been used to study normality and psychopathology in individuality. To begin, we must recognize that the developmental perspective is based on three general research questions: (1) How do individuals differ between groups? (2) What are the major changes in individual behavior over time? and (3) What are the major psychic structures of individuals (and do they change over time)?

Buss (1974) has provided a straightforward general model of development that helps us visualize these three central questions of a developmental perspective. As depicted in Figure 2.1, he proposes that there are three commonly used variables in the study of change. Comparisons are made between individuals, of the same individual over several occasions, and of the same individual across variables. Comparison between individuals is the study of *interindividual differences*—commonly called individual differences. For example, we can compare nonclinical versus clinical groups, males versus females, or different types of psychopathological groups on the

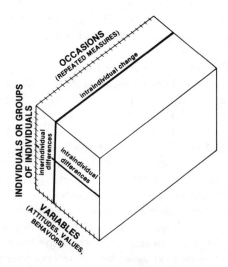

Figure 2.1. An illustration of Buss's general model of development.

same research variable. Comparison of the same individual(s) over repeated occasions on the same variable (behavior) is the study of *intraindividual change*—commonly called individual development. Intraindividual change is illustrated in physical, social, emotional, or cognitive development during adolescence. Likewise, we may be interested in the "within" characteristics of an individual, where we strive to understand what type of psychological profile most accurately reflects the general psychological makeup of the individual. In this case, we study the same individual and compare responses to many different measures to determine the within variability (*intraindividual similarities* and *differences*) between psychological characteristics. For example, is complexity in ego structure reflective of high creativity and low rigidity? Likewise, developmentally oriented scholars are interested in how intraindividual patterns change qualitatively over time.

Each of these three basic developmental foci has its own corresponding research methodologies and central research questions. Most pertinent to our discussion for this book are the central research questions rather than the research methodologies employed. However, as McCall (1977) has concisely noted, if we are truly interested in the study of (1) change within individuals, (2) sequence and timing of developmental transitions, and (3) the specification of social, historical, or environmental factors that permit development to occur, we must utilize the various longitudinal methodologies available for developmental research. Indeed, we refer interested readers to a host of useful publications that highlight and evaluate the many available strategies (e.g., Adams, 1983; Adams & Schvaneveldt, 1985; Baltes, 1968; Nesselroade & Baltes, 1979; Schaie, 1965; Wohlwill, 1973).

What, then, are the central research questions or concepts for the study of interindividual differences, intraindividual change, and intraindividual similarities and differences? Simply put, they are: (1) What are the consistent differences between males and females, between racial or cultural groups, or between groups that have been separated or segregated due to socioeconomic, geographical, political, or segregationist factors (interindividual differences)? (2) What are the progressive and regressive patterns of growth, and when does stability or a plateau in growth emerge (intraindividual change)? (3) What is the qualitative and structural nature of the individual differences or developmental patterns manifested (intraindividual similarities and differences)? and (4) What are potential determinants of individual differences, developmental change, and the structure of psychological profiles?

In the next section of this chapter, we will illustrate aspects of these central developmental research questions through a selective review of studies on normal personality development during adolescence. Through this illustrative effort, we will attempt to demonstrate how various theoretical and research efforts in the study of adolescent psychiatry can be analyzed to find the commonalities and differences in developmental constructs, their definitions, and their basic foundation for understanding adolescent behavior.

NORMALITY AND ADOLESCENT IDENTITY

Two theoretical perspectives of considerable use to the study of ego psychology during adolescence include a focus on identity formation (Erikson, 1968) and ego development (Loevinger, 1976). The ego is thought to synthesize and resynthesize throughout childhood and adolescence the "evolving configuration of identity" (Erikson, 1968) and to provide the structure for meaning, purpose, and direction of behavior (Loevinger, 1976). In its complexity, ego identity is thought to include the integration of such diverse factors as "constitutional givens, idiosyncratic libidinal needs, favored capacities, significant identifications, effective defenses, successful sublimations, and consistent roles" (Erikson, 1956, p. 71). Based on the psychoanalytic notion that the ego organizes a coherent personality with a sameness and continuity perceived by others, Erikson (1968) concludes:

> *Ego identity then, in its subjective aspect, is the awareness of the fact that there is a self-sameness and continuity to the ego's synthesizing methods, the style of one's individuality,* and that this style coincides with the sameness and continuity of *one's meaning for significant others* in the immediate community. (p. 50) . . . The term identity . . . connotes both a persistent sameness within oneself (self-sameness) and a persistent sharing of some kind of essential character with others. (Erikson, 1956, p. 57)

Ego functions as components of individuality have been measured through the operationalization of ego identity and ego stages. Using Marcia's (1966) measure of identity, we have utilized both clinical interviews and self-report scales (Adams, Shea, & Fitch, 1979; Grotevant & Adams, 1984; Bennion & Adams, 1986; Craig-Bray & Adams, 1986) to categorize individuals into identity *diffusion, foreclosure, moratorium,* or *identity achievement* status. Diffusion is defined as the absence of psychosocial crisis or personal commitment to an identity. Foreclosure involves a reported identity commitment based on early primitive childhood identifications only. Moratorium is associated with a crisis and exploration process currently in progress. Identity achievement involves a personal identity based on a successful resolution of the identity crisis.

A broader assessment of ego functions, which is thought to include egoidentity, is the Loevinger system of measuring ego character styles based on a developmental continuum. According to Hauser (1976), the Loevinger measure of ego function assesses the "framework of meaning which one subjectively imposes on experience" (p. 930). Thus ego functions are thought to direct behavior and provide meaning in the form of character. Six basic stages or character types include: the lowest level, consisting of *impulsive* or *self-protective* individuals; middle ego stages, consisting of *conformist* and *conscientious* characters; and higher stages, reflecting *autonomous* and *integrative* characterological ego functioning.

Interindividual Differences

Individual differences in character or ego-identity formation have generally been studied in two ways: Comparisons have been made between genders and among the four identity status or ego stages. Due to a societal focus on socializing males toward independence and encouraging females to be more nurturing and dependent, it has been proposed that males will be more advanced in their identity formation than females—a proposition found in Erikson's (1968) writings. We have, for example, found that males (on the average) are more advanced in their identity formation than are females and that females are, generally, more foreclosed than males (Adams & Fitch, 1982). Other gender-related findings on measures of ego development suggest that during the college-age years males are at greater risk than females for regressive ego functioning, while no consistently observed gender differences have been observed in differential patterns of growth in ego development (Adams & Fitch, 1982; Fitch & Adams, 1983).

Numerous investigations have examined interindividual differences among the four basic identity status types on various behaviors. In our own research, we have examined differences in overt or manifested behaviors reflecting self-consciousness (Adams, Abraham, & Markstrom, 1987), conformity behavior in peer relation contexts (Adams, Ryan, Hoffman, Dobson, & Nielsen, 1985), and social-influence styles in persuasion settings (Read, Adams, & Dobson, 1984). In general, we find that identity achieved males and females are less self-focused in their social behavior, likely to conform only when it serves an achievement need or goal, and likely to have strong and more effective interpersonal skills. Acutely diffused individuals are self-conscious, are highly likely to conform to peer pressure, and are minimally effective in their social-influence behaviors. These investigations and findings are illustrative of the type of directions and research questions that have been explored on individual differences in individuality in the form of identity or ego development.

Intraindividual Change

The study of individual development in individuality has used three related strategies. In the first strategy, cross-sectional methodologies have been used to contrast differences between college-attending and working youth in their rate of growth in ego-identity formation. Because college can be viewed as an extended psychosocial moratorium, we hypothesized that working youth who enter the workforce after high school graduation (the termination of moratoria) should be more advanced in their identity when comparisons are made with college attending peers (Munro & Adams, 1977). The findings confirmed our hypothesis and suggested that sociocultural contingencies of ego-identity development should be considered in understanding normal personality and ego development.

The second, and most notable, form of studying intraindividual change involves the use of cross-sequential longitudinal designs. In such a study, Adams and Fitch (1982) explored (1) potential differential rates in male versus female development, (2) possible cohort differences, and (3) consistency in theoretically predicted patterns of change. Regarding the latter interest, we focused on documenting the approximate percentage of college students who would remain stable, show progressive growth, or regress in ego functioning over a period of 1 to 1 1/2 years. Although a few gender and cohort differences were observed, approximately 50 % of the students remained stable, with about the same proportion of the remaining students showing progressive or regressive ego functioning. These findings confirmed the general notion that ego growth and restructuring is a gradual process and that regressive patterns (possibly in service of the ego) and varying progressive patterns of growth can be documented using a nomothetic research approach.

The third line of research has examined the predictive association between ego functions or between ego functioning and later critical developmental stages or crises. In one line of work, we have asked whether Erikson is correct in assuming that advancement in ego-identity development is predictive of later intimacy formation (e.g., Fitch & Adams, 1983; Kacerguis & Adams, 1980; Adams & Fitch, 1981; Craig-Bray, Adams, & Dobson, in press). Overall, our findings supported the theoretical assumptions of Erikson regarding interstage crisis resolutions. More mature identity was observed to be predictive of higher levels and greater depth of heterosexual and friendship intimacies.

Intraindividual Similarities and Differences

In clinical-developmental perspectives, we are frequently interested in identifying a profile of characteristics that accompanies a central personality construct (such as identity). Typically, correlational strategies are used to identify significant covariations. In our own research program, for example, we have examined the covariation among ego-identity formation, locus of control, ego development, self-concept, rigidity, social desirability behavior, and measures of personal commitment and exploration on identity issues (e.g., see Adams & Shea, 1979; Adams, Shea, & Fitch, 1979; Grotevant & Adams, 1984; Craig-Bray & Adams, 1986). Considerable intercorrelational covariance can be found among these constructs of personality.

However, the most promising strategy of exploring intraindividual pro-files of personality development has emerged in our use of discriminant function analysis techniques. Using a measure of attentional and interper-sonal aspects of personality (Nideffer, 1976; 1977), we have utilized this statistical methodology to identify attentional/interpersonal personality profiles of the four identity statuses. For example, we observed that fore-closed women showed the least capacity for integration of ideas and lim-ited analytic thought, whereas moratorium and achievement women were found to be able to effectively process broad and complex arrays of social information and were comfortable with their own thoughts, feelings, and ideas (Read, Adams, & Dobson, 1984). Further, both diffusion and fore-closure women were inclined to make considerable errors in social judg-ment due to a restriction of gathering social information. Once again, these findings are consistent with Erikson's writings on the personality of acutely diffused persons and the foreclosure of identity.

Potential Determinants of Development

In addition to identifying individual differences, developmental change, and intraindividual psychological profiles, the developmental perspective goes beyond description to explanation and modification. That is, we ask what factors contribute to progressive or regressive patterns of growth. In several cross-sectional and longitudinal studies (e.g., Adams & Jones, 1981a; Adams, 1985; Campbell, Adams, & Dobson, 1984; Adams & Mon-temayor, 1986) we have addressed the identification of family relations and socialization factors that are either predictive of different identity statuses among adolescents or are progressive, stable, and regressive patterns (or trajectories) in ego-identity development. At this time, we can tentatively conclude that (1) rejecting and emotionally distant families have diffused youths; (2) emotionally enmeshed families have foreclosed youths; and (3) families that are emotionally supportive, are highly involved with their ado-lescents, and provide a reasonable range of conflict and discussion, while encouraging independence striving, have identity achieved or moratorium adolescents. Considerably more research is needed, however, before these tentative conclusions can be recognized with complete affirmation.

Let us now turn to a brief discussion of developmental and conceptual issues of identity disorders. We will then conclude with comments on devel-opmental issues needing attention in the form of future research programs.

IDENTITY DISORDERS

In clinical case studies, problems related to establishing a solid sense of identity have been identified as a major psychiatric developmental concern for adolescents. Identity disorders are often discussed in relation to narcissistic and borderline disorders. Indeed, many psychiatrists believe that these disorders share similar commonalities (Evans, 1982). For example, in the *Diagnostic and Statistical Manual of Mental Disorders* (DSM-III), (American Psychiatric Association [APA] 1980), identity disorders are characterized by inner preoccupation and self-doubt, which is suggestive of a narcissistic focus on the self. According to the American Psychiatric Association (1987), in order to be diagnosed as experiencing an identity disorder, an adolescent must be experiencing distress in regard to issues related to the assumption of adult responsibilities and commitments. Severe subjective distress regarding any three of the following is thought to be reflective of identity disorder symptoms: long term goals, career choice, friendship patterns, sexual behavior or orientation, religious identification, moral values, or group loyalties. These issues are parallel to the adolescent developmental tasks first identified by Havighurst (1951) and have been discussed in the psychiatric literature as components of psychosocial maturity of adolescents (Berlin, 1980; Offer & Sabshim, 1984). The failure to accomplish these tasks or to demonstrate psychosocial maturity in these areas is thought to be at the core of identity disorders.

Anna Freud (1971) has defined the period of adolescence as a developmental disturbance because of the many simultaneous changes in development adolescents experience. As a result of such changes, many aspects of normal adolescent behavior resemble characteristics of adult pathological behavior. Although pathology is indeed present in both adolescents and adults, a distinction between what is considered normal and expected behavior in adolescence (as a function of that stage of development) and that which is considered pathological is necessary to continue our discussion.

NORMALITY VERSUS PATHOLOGY IN ADOLESCENCE

The relationship between the failure to establish a sense of identity and narcissistic disorders has been a subject of interest for many practitioners. Self-focusing and self-consciousness of adolescence, as a part of one's search for identity, share many similarities with narcissism (Munich, 1986). However, the term narcissism, which is suggestive of pathology, often is used to refer to what is considered part of a normal developmental process of adolescents.

Blatt (1983), in a cogent presentation, has attempted to clarify the difference between the personality constructs of narcissism and egocentrism by suggesting that the term narcissism be confined to pathological self-focusing, while the term egocentrism be used to refer to a specific type of self-focusing which is part of the normal adolescent developmental process. In regard to the latter, David Elkind (1968, 1979) has written extensively on the development of adolescent egocentrism, in a Piagetian sense. According to Elkind, as a result of the onset of formal operational thought and the resulting confusion between subject and object, the young adolescent is overcome by feelings of self-consciousness, uniqueness, and a sense of indestructibility. Although the behavioral manifestations of the adolescent's focus on the self often are disturbing to adults, Elkind has asserted that such behavior is expected, is normal, and will decline over the course of adolescence. Several recent investigations support this assumption (e.g., Adams & Jones, 1981b, 1982; Elkind & Bowen, 1979; Gossens, 1984; Markstrom & Mullis, 1986; Riley, Adams, & Nielsen, 1984).

In contrast to normal self-focusing at various phases in the developmental process, Blatt (1983) has argued that the term narcissism should be reserved for defensive gestures which protect the self from confronting underlying feelings of being unloved, loneliness, inauthenticity, and emptiness. Thus the individual avoids forming attachments to others in order to protect one's frail sense of self. This type of narcissism cannot be termed just a "phase" of normal adolescence. Without proper treatment, it may be an enduring pathological component of the individual. In contrast, for the adolescent who is exhibiting expected egocentric behaviors, social interaction and the formation of object relations are the facilitating factors which give freedom from self-focused behavior and encourage decentering and perspective taking. The narcissistic adolescent remains trapped by his or her own anxieties and fears, which prevents the formation of attachments to others.

Several writers in the clinical field, drawing on case studies as illustrations of the problem, have addressed how narcissistic tendencies are evident in problems related to identity development in adolescence. For example, Burch (1985) has identified one form of adolescent narcissism, calling it identity foreclosure. The major distinguishing factor is that these adolescents commit themselves to an identity by early adolescence, without engaging in the normal exploratory process in identity formation. This syndrome is believed to occur because identity foreclosed children receive too much independence and decision-making power at a young age, and parents are overly responsive to their children's narcissistic demands. Therefore, by the time these children reach adolescence, they strive to avoid it and are desirous to be treated as peers by adults.

Identity foreclosed adolescents do not engage in the normal adoption and rejection of various roles as part of an exploration of their identities. They present a contradiction of mature and immature behaviors through avoiding involvement with their peers and continually seeking adult company. They demonstrate, among other characteristics, intense mood fluctuations, attempts to manipulate, and inability to tolerate frustration. They have rigid personality structures and are avoidant of any type of vulnerability which might upset their narcissistic equilibrium. Thus they engage in self-focused grandiose fantasies and attempt to present a more mature, yet false, image of themselves to others.

Munich (1986) also has written of the complications that arise in adolescent identity and self-concept formation as a result of the narcissistic or self-conscious tendencies of adolescents. In a delineation of the actual self, the ideal self, and the unacceptable self, Munich has written of the adolescent developmental task of forming a coherent self-representation of these three concepts. Further, he suggests that the formation of coherent object representations is an important parallel task. The narcissistic individual, in particular, demonstrates a confusing blend of these tasks. For example, Munich notes that in the narcissistic individual "the actual self, the ideal self, and the ideal object are fused to form what is referred to as the pathological grandiose self" (p. 89).

Depersonalization is cited by Munich as one example of a form of narcissism seen in both normal and narcissistically pathological adolescents. In normal adolescent development, a form of depersonalization may be present in that the individual, for brief episodes, "feels detached from while at the same time looking at himself" (p. 90). Illustrating an exception to normal adolescent depersonalization through the presentation of a case study, Munich notes that the superego is not well integrated into the personality structure in narcissistic disorders. In this particular case study, Munich relates that an adolescent girl escaped negative feelings about her mother and the guilt associated with such feelings in that her "withdrawal was from the condensed unacceptable self, unacceptable object, and actual object into a pathological grandiose self" (p. 92). The depersonalization in which this particular adolescent engaged was pathological in the sense that it was symptomatic of a deeper disorder of self-object representation.

As it is important to distinguish between the normal developmental process of egocentrism in adolescence and the pathological syndrome of narcissism, Akhtar (1984) has delineated the difference between the adolescent identity crisis (phase specific) and identity diffusion (severe pathology). The identity crisis is a temporary condition in adolescence when the individual demonstrates doubts, regressions in behavior, and a reorganization of identity. Such symptoms are not considered pathological, as the individual still retains feelings of authenticity and the self as a whole is not in total upheaval. In contrast, although the identity crisis and identity diffusion often first appear in adolescence, identity diffusion also appears in adults and is characterized by symptoms of severe pathology.

INDIVIDUAL DIFFERENCES: THE CHARACTER
OF IDENTITY DIFFUSION

Using Erikson's (1956) definition of identity diffusion as a lack of a cohesive identity, Akhtar (1984) has provided a descriptive summary of clinical signs and symptoms of identity diffusion. One clinical characteristic of the diffused individual is the lack of a cohesive self-concept and the presence of contradictory character traits. Not surprisingly, the individual also is unable to acquire a sense of the personality of others. There is a temporary discontinuity in the self because the individual's past, present, and future are unconnected. Consistent with the remarks made by Blatt (1983) about narcissism, Akhtar has also described diffused individuals as those who are lacking in authenticity. They act not according to their own beliefs and feelings, but according to how someone else might act in a given situation. When alone, these individuals feel empty inside and may attempt to escape such feelings through behaviorally manifesting compulsive behaviors and even self-mutilation. Identity diffused individuals are gender dysphoric, in that they have failed to accomplish developmental tasks related to developing a core sense of their gender identity, gender roles, and sexual partner orientation. Akhtar also has identified diffused individuals as lacking an understanding of their ethnic heritage and a sense of inner values and/or morality.

DEVELOPMENTAL ISSUES IN PSYCHOPATHOLOGY:
THE CASE OF IDENTITY DISORDERS

Within the emerging field of developmental psychopathology, there are numerous unanswered questions. Our understanding of identity disorders is reflective of the field in general. To date, most efforts have remained at the level of clinical conceptualization based on a case study approach. However, as the field of adolescent psychiatry expands, the importance of the following unanswered questions will surface with considerable interest and hopefully will be given careful empirical attention.

At the level of individual differences, what identity disorder distinctions will be found to differentiate between male and female adolescents with an identity disorder? Given our growing concern about ideological versus interpersonal identity (e.g., see Grotevant & Adams, 1984), are we likely to find that interpersonal identity disorders are more common for females than males, while ideological identity disorders are more prevalent among males? How can we define and assess identity disorder constructs to make meaningful comparisons across subcultural adolescent groups, assuming that cultural and subcultural ethnic distinctions interact with the definition of ethnic or racial identity? Are individual differences in identities merely a reflection of different adolescents being at different stages of a universal identity development sequence?

Regarding sequencing of identity development, when is diffusion a normal aspect of adolescence, and when does it become pathological? Is a 13-year-old who is identity achieved potentially as pathological as a 35-year-old who is diffused? What are the major developmental trajectories in identity development? Are there clearly discernible developmental trajectories that reflect regressive behavior associated with psychopathology? At what point in the developmental process can we discern regression in service of the ego from negative regressive effects associated with an identity disorder?

Turning to intraindividual similarities and differences, can we discern the major psychological correlates of normal identity and identity disorder growth and development? Are these constructs peripheral or central to a disorder that we should label psychopathological? Is ego-identity a core personality construct that serves the function of integrating and serving as a cohesive force in determining the various psychological aspects of character?

These are but a few major questions that emerge from a brief analysis of the central developmental foci of adolescent psychiatry when directed at the issue of identity—normal and psychopathological. The same basic dimensions of individual differences, intraindividual development, and intraindividual similarities and differences can be applied to the broader field of adolescent psychiatry. Throughout this book, the reader can ask similar questions, as a developmental perspective is applied to the content of the remaining chapters. It will become quickly apparent that much is yet to be learned about the nature and extent of the viability of a developmental psychopathology perspective to adolescent psychiatry.

SUMMARY

Adolescent psychiatry is a developmental science. Focusing on individuality, we have demonstrated its developmental foundation through a brief examination of the work of such notables as S. Freud, H. S. Sullivan, P. Blos, A. Freud, and E. H. Erikson. Given the numerous developmental perspectives with adolescent psychiatry, we have pointed out that certain clarifications are needed as a challenge to a developmental science.

The challenge to a developmental science includes the analysis of individuals, variables, and occasions of observations. At the most basic level, comparisons are made between groups of individuals to establish interindividual differences. Within an individual, comparison across variables (commonly viewed as a psychological profile) involves the study of intraindividual similarities and differences. Comparison of the same individual over repeated occasions is the study of intraindividual change or development. The use of these three basic variables provides the fundamental structure for the study of the three basic developmental questions of individual differences, intraindividual similarities, and intraindividual development.

Through a selective analysis of research on normality and psychopathology of identity during adolescence, we have illustrated the utility of the three basic developmental-based questions presented in this chapter. Our intent is to provide this chapter as a foundation for considering developmental issues in the broader field of adolescent psychiatry and its promotion as a developmental science.

REFERENCES

Adams, G. R. (1983). The study of intraindividual change during early adolescence. *Journal of Early Adolescence, 3,* 37–46.

Adams, G. R. (1985). Family correlates of female adolescents' ego-identity development. *Journal of Adolescence, 8,* 69–82.

Adams, G. R., Abraham, K. G., & Markstrom, C. A. (1987). The relation among identity development, self-consciousness and self-focusing during middle and late adolescence. *Developmental Psychology, 23,* 292–297.

Adams, G. R., & Fitch, S. A. (1981). Ego stage and identity status development: A cross-lag analysis. *Journal of Adolescence, 4,* 163–171.

Adams, G. R., & Fitch, S. A. (1982). Ego stage and identity status development: A cross-sequential analysis. *Journal of Personality and Social Psychology, 43,* 547–583.

Adams, G. R., & Jones, R. M. (1981a). Female adolescents' identity development: Age comparisons and perceived child-rearing experience. *Developmental Psychology, 19,* 249–256.

Adams, G. R., & Jones, R. (1981b). Imaginary audience behavior: A validation study. *Journal of Early Adolescence, 1,* 1–10.

Adams, G. R., & Jones, R. (1982). Adolescent egocentrism: Exploration into possible contributions of parent-child relations. *Journal of Youth and Adolescence, 11,* 25–31.

Adams, G. R., & Montemayor, R. (1986). Patterns of ego identity growth during adolescence. Poster session at the biennial meetings of the Society for Research on Adolescence, Madison, Wisconsin, April.

Adams, G. R., Ryan, J. H., Hoffman, J. J., Dobson, W. R., & Nielsen, E. C. (1985). Ego identity status, conformity behavior and personality in late adolescence. *Journal of Personality and Social Psychology, 47,* 1091–1104.

Adams, G. R., & Schvaneveldt, J. D. (1985). *Understanding research methods.* New York: Longmans.

Adams, G. R., & Shea, J. (1979). The relationship between identity status, locus of control, and ego development. *Journal of Youth and Adolescence, 8,* 81–89.

Adams, G. R., Shea, J., & Fitch, S. A. (1979). Toward the development of an objective assessment of ego-identity status. *Journal of Youth and Adolescence, 8,* 223–237.

Akhtar, S. (1984). The syndrome of identity diffusion. *American Journal of Psychiatry, 141,* 1381–1385.

American Psychiatric Association (1987). *Diagnostic and statistical manual of mental disorders* (3rd ed., rev.). (DSM-III-R). Washington, DC: Author.

Baltes, P. B. (1968). Longitudinal and cross-sectional sequences in the study of age and generation effects. *Human Development, 11,* 145–171.

Bennion, L. D., & Adams, G. R. (1986). A revision of the extended version of the objective measure of ego identity status: An identity instrument for use with late adolescents. *Journal of Adolescent Research, 1,* 183–198

Berlin, I. N. (1980). Opportunities in adolescence to rectify developmental failures. *Adolescent Psychiatry, 8,* 231–243.

Blatt, S. J. (1983). Narcissism and egocentrism as concepts in individual and cultural development. *Psychoanalysis and Contemporary Thought, 6,* 291–303.

Blos, P. (1962). *On adolescence: A psychoanalytic interpretation.* New York: Free Press.

Blos, P. (1985). *Son and father: Before and beyond the Oedipus complex.* New York: Free Press.

Burch, C. A. (1985). Identity foreclosure in early adolescence: A problem of narcissistic equilibrium. *Adolescent Psychiatry, 12,* 145–161.

Buss, A. R. (1974). A general developmental model for interindividual differences and intraindividual change. *Developmental Psychology, 10,* 70–78.

Campbell, E., Adams, G. R., & Dobson, W. R. (1984). Familial correlates of identity formation in late adolescence: A study of the predictive utility of connectedness and individuality in family relations. *Journal of Youth and Adolescence, 13,* 509–525.

Craig-Bray, L., & Adams, G. R. (1986). Different methodologies in the assessment of identity: Congruence between self-report and interview techniques? *Journal of Youth and Adolescence, 15,* 191–204.

Craig-Bray, L., Adams, G. R., & Dobson, W. R. (unpublished). Identity formation and social relations during late adolescence. Submitted for publication.

Elkind, D. (1968). Cognitive structure and adolescent experience. *Adolescence, 2,* 427–434.

Elkind, D. (1979). *The child and society: Essays in applied child development.* New York: Oxford.

Elkind, D., & Bowen, R. (1979). Imaginary audience behavior in children and adolescents. *Developmental Psychology, 15,* 38–44.

Erikson, E. H. (1956). The problem of ego identity. *Journal of the American Psychoanalytic Association, 4,* 56–121.

Erikson, E. H. (1968). *Identity: Youth and crisis.* New York: Norton.

Evans, J. (1982). *Adolescent and pre-adolescent psychiatry.* London: Academic.

Fitch, S. A., & Adams, G. R. (1983). Ego-identity and intimacy status: Replication and extension. *Developmental Psychology, 19,* 839–845.

Freud, A. (1965). *The writings of Anna Freud: Normality and pathology in childhood: Assessments of development* (Vol. 6). New York: International Universities Press.

Freud, A. (1971). *The writings of Anna Freud: Problems of psychoanalytic training, diagnosis and the techniques of therapy* (Vol. 7). New York: International Universities Press.

Freud, S. (1958). *The interpretation of dreams.* Standard Edition, 4. London: Hogarth Press. (Original work published 1900)

Freud, S. (1963). *Introductory lectures on psychoanalysis.* Standard Edition. London: Hogarth Press. (Original work published 1917)

Freud, S. (1961). *The ego and the id.* Standard Edition, 19. London: Hogarth Press. (Original work published 1923)

Gossens, L. (1984). Imaginary audience behavior as a function of age, sex and formal operational thinking. *International Journal of Behavioral Development, 7,* 77–93.

Grotevant, H. D., & Adams, G. R. (1984). Development of an objective measure to assess ego identity in adolescence: Validation and replication. *Journal of Youth and Adolescence, 13,* 419–438.

Hauser, S. T. (1976). Loevinger's model and measure of ego development: A critical review. *Psychological Bulletin, 83,* 928–955.

Havighurst, R. (1951). *Developmental tasks and education.* New York: Longmans.

Kacerguis, M. A., & Adams, G. R. (1980). Erikson stage resolution: The relationship between identity and intimacy. *Journal of Youth and Adolescence, 9,* 117–126.

Loevinger, J. (1976). *Ego development.* San Francisco: Jossey-Bass.

Marcia, J. E. (1966). Development and validation of ego-identity status. *Journal of Personality and Social Psychology, 3,* 551–558.

Markstrom, C. A., & Mullis, R. (1986), Ethnic differences in the imaginary audience. *Journal of Adolescent Research, 1,* 289–301.

McCall, R. B. (1977). Challenges to a science of developmental psychology. *Child Development, 48,* 333–344.

Munich, R. L. (1986). Some forms of narcissism in adolescents and young adults. *Adolescent Psychiatry, 13,* 85–99.

Munro, G., & Adams, G. R. (1977). Ego-identity formation in college students and working youth. *Developmental Psychology, 13,* 523–524.

Nesselroade, J., & Baltes, P. (Eds.). (1979). *Longitudinal research in the study of behavior and development.* New York: Academic.

Nideffer, R. M. (1976). Test of attentional and interpersonal style. *Journal of Personality and Social Psychology, 34,* 394–405.

Nideffer, R. M. (1977). *Test of attentional and interpersonal style: Interpretation manual.* New York: Behavioral Research Applications Group.

Offer, D., & Sabshim, M. (Eds.). (1984). *Normality and the life cycle: A critical integration.* New York: Basic Books.

Read, D., Adams, G. R., & Dobson, W. R. (1984). Ego-identity status, personality and social influence style. *Journal of Personality and Social Psychology, 46,* 169–177.

Riley, T., Adams, G. R., & Nielsen, E. (1984). Adolescent egocentrism: The association between imaginary audience behavior, cognitive development, parental support and rejection. *Journal of Youth and Adolescence, 13,* 401–417.

Schaie, K. W. (1965). A general model for the study of developmental problems. *Psychological Bulletin, 64,* 92–107.

Sullivan, H. S. (1953). *The interpersonal theory of psychiatry.* New York: Norton.

Wohlwill, J. F. (1973). *The study of behavioral development.* New York: Academic.

CHAPTER THREE

Diagnostic Issues: DSM-III and DSM-III-R

Mary E. Schwab-Stone

The identification and diagnosis of psychopathology in the adolescent is complicated by a number of factors. Some are intrinsic to the adolescent and the developmental events of this stage. For example, adolescent "turmoil" and moodiness may be mistaken for more serious symptomatology or, conversely, may obscure it. The adolescent may choose to be extremely private about inner feelings and mood states, leaving parents and clinicians poorly or even mistakenly informed about the youngster's symptomatology. However, some factors contributing to the difficulty of accurate diagnosis are not intrinsic to this stage but relate instead to our level of knowledge about adolescent psychopathology and to the concepts that we as clinicians and researchers bring to the task. For example, the system used to classify disorders and our clinical expectations regarding the occurrence and presentation of psychopathology in this age group are based on incomplete knowledge, which further threatens diagnostic accuracy.

This chapter will focus on a number of issues involving the diagnosis of psychopathology in adolescents. These issues will be illustrated by referring to selected psychiatric syndromes, drawing from both clinical and epidemiologic perspectives. Implicit in this discussion is the view that although the concerns of clinicians and researchers are partially shaped by differing goals, in the area of diagnostic assessment, there is at least as much ground that is commonly shared as not.

TURMOIL VERSUS PSYCHIATRIC DISORDER IN ADOLESCENCE

Adolescence has long been considered a phase of moodiness and brooding, and indeed there is some empirical support for the presence of inner turmoil as well as for the distinction between turmoil and psychiatric disorder (Rutter, Graham, Chadwick, & Yule, 1976; Rutter, 1980). The epidemiologic work of Rutter et al. (1976) with youngsters from the Isle of Wight showed a marked increase in feelings of misery and depression from age 10 to 11 years, when about 12% of the sample were said to have such feelings, to the follow-up at age 14 to 15 years when over 40% gave positive reports (Rutter et al., 1976; Rutter, 1980). In a study by Larson, Csikszentmihalyi, and Graef (1980), mood variability in adults and adolescents was compared using time sampling techniques. The adolescents were found to have lower moods on average than the adults and to show wider and more frequent mood swings.

Looking at psychiatric disorder per se, in the Isle of Wight study, the one-year period prevalence of psychiatric disorder for the 14 to 15 year olds was found to be in the 10 to 15% range—only a little higher than that for 10-year-olds from the same population (about 11%)—and similar to that for a sample of adults from that population (Graham & Rutter, 1985).

The rate for adults probably represents a slight underestimate because of a bias toward health in the selection of that sample. However, a number of 14- to 15-year-olds on direct interview reported psychiatric symptoms and distress, although they had not been identified as disturbed by teachers and parents at the initial screening stage. Adding these to the overall prevalence estimate increased the rate to about 21%. Whether the true rate is closer to this or to the former figure is not clear, but the discrepancy raises interesting methodological and theoretical issues (see section on Informant Source). In addition, the rate can be expected to vary depending on the population studied. For example, using comparable study methods, rates of psychiatric disorder for 10-year-olds living in an inner London borough were twice those found for the Isle of Wight children (Rutter, Cox, Tupling, Berger, & Yule, 1975).

In sum, the rate of disorder per se may increase moderately in adolescence, and some degree of inner turmoil appears to be common for adolescents in comparison to middle school-age children or adults. However, in the Isle of Wight study, half of the sample did *not* report such feelings. These results have provided an empirical basis to counter some traditional views that inner turmoil and disruption are characteristic or necessary features of normal adolescent development (Rutter et al., 1976).

GENERAL TRENDS IN DIAGNOSIS IN ADOLESCENCE

Reviewing the results of general population studies of adolescents, Rutter (1980) cites a rough breakdown by diagnostic type. About two-fifths show emotional disorders, two-fifths conduct disorder, and one-fifth mixed conduct and emotional disturbances. Enuresis, encopresis, hyperactivity, and psychosis are rare. When these are compared to a similar breakdown for middle school-age children, the differences are not striking. In the Isle of Wight study of 10- to 11-year-olds, of those suffering from a psychiatric disorder, about two-fifths showed neurotic conditions, only a slightly smaller proportion had conduct disorders, and about one-fifth showed mixed conduct and neurotic conditions (Rutter, Tizard, & Whitmore, 1970). Thus in adolescence there is a moderate increase in overall frequency of disorders and little change in the distribution among broad diagnostic groupings, although there are increases in rates of specific disorders and behaviors, such as depressive disorders, anorexia, suicide, delinquency, and substance abuse (Rutter, 1980).

It is within the context of specific disorders such as these that the interesting questions about the diagnosis and classification of psychopathology in adolescence arise. In the remainder of this chapter, selected diagnostic issues will be discussed using specific disorders as examples. (However, a systematic examination of developmental psychopathology is clearly beyond the scope of this chapter. The reader is referred to Rutter & Garmezy, 1983; Achenbach, 1974.)

DSM-III AND THE ROLE OF DEVELOPMENT

Two main purposes of a diagnostic classification system are to organize information in a clinically meaningful manner and to provide a common language for workers in the field. To the extent that these goals are well met, the system should facilitate the clinical diagnostic process and the progress of scientific research.

The developers of the DSM-III (APA, 1980) set an ambitious course to accomplish these ends. The new system was designed to be much more comprehensive than its predecessor, to utilize a multiaxial approach, to provide a phenomenologic, non-etiologically based categorization of disorders, and to include well-specified diagnostic criteria that could be applied reliably by clinicians and researchers. Certainly, this was asking a great deal; that the DSM-III was met with some criticism amidst the acclaim was no surprise (Klerman, Vaillant, Spitzer, & Michels, 1984).

The DSM-III system was also intended to accommodate the diagnostic needs of individuals across the life span. Thus its utility in the child and adolescent populations has been a focus of debate, with criticisms involving the validity of various categories, the implementation of the multiaxial approach, and specific disagreements about criteria (Rutter & Shaffer, 1980; Garmezy, 1978; Quay, 1986; Bemporad & Schwab, 1986). Moreover, a fundamental question in applying DSM-III to younger populations is: Does it allow the diagnostician to capture important developmental considerations in the expression of psychopathology? It neither makes sense to construct numerous classifications with fine divisions for different ages nor to have a system that is unified to the point of being static, so that it does not take into account the various manifestations of an abnormality at different ages (Rutter & Gould, 1985).

A fundamental feature of adolescence is the dramatic effect of development in physical, social, emotional, and cognitive spheres. The diagnostician who works with adolescents must identify meaningful symptom patterns against a background of changing behaviors and mood states that, while new for the individual, may not be pathological in their meaning. Some forms of pathology characteristically appear at certain ages, and existing problems may present in apparently new forms, depending on the youngster's developmental stage (Rutter & Gould, 1985). In many respects, accurate diagnosis demands an understanding of the interplay between psychopathology and development. Rutter and Garmezy (1983) and Achenbach (1978) have pointed out that until recently there has been an unfortunate separation of these two orientations, at least in the research community (although the need to consider developmental issues in evaluating psychopathology in children and adolescents has been emphasized in the tradition of clinical writings: e.g., A. Freud, 1965).

A modern classification system of psychopathology should facilitate a developmental orientation where appropriate; for adolescents, this may be particularly important. The extent to which the DSM-III succeeded in this respect is in part a matter of opinion as there have not yet been many studies on the validity of DSM-III disorders in children and adolescents (Shaffer & Gould, 1987). Certainly, the adequacy of the system varies across diagnoses; some areas of concern will be noted later in the discussion of specific diagnostic issues.

DSM-III-R

In 1987, seven years after the introduction of DSM-III, a revised version, DSM-III-R (APA, 1987), was published. The DSM-III-R is truly a revision rather than a new classification system, and thus it adheres to the principles that guided the development of DSM-III. There are, however, some specific changes in the way the diagnostic criteria have been organized. In particular, for a number of diagnoses there is a shift from the monothetic or "Chinese menu" approach to a polythetic or more scale-like approach. In the monothetic approach, symptoms were grouped and a certain number was required from each group. This meant that each criterion had to be met to qualify for the diagnosis. In the polythetic approach, a list or index of symptoms, without groupings, is provided. A specified number is required for diagnosis, but no certain one symptom is necessary. This is a less restrictive strategy for combining symptoms to yield diagnoses, and it is anticipated that the polythetic approach will improve diagnostic reliability (APA, 1987).

Another change that particularly affects the classification of disorders in childhood and adolescence involves the diagnoses of mental retardation and the pervasive developmental disorders, which along with the specific developmental disorders, are to be recorded on Axis II rather than Axis I. This change acknowledges the chronic, handicapping aspect of these conditions, which in this respect resemble the other Axis II disorders, the personality disorders. This change also answers objections involving the likelihood that multiple diagnoses will be less reliably reported when only one axis is allotted (Rutter & Shaffer, 1980).

Unfortunately, there is relatively little research to support or disprove nosological distinctions in DSM-III categories (Shaffer and Gould, 1987) and clearly far less pertaining to DSM-III-R. Providing the empirical basis for the development of an increasingly accurate diagnostic system is a major challenge for the field of child and adolescent psychiatry. Because the diagnostic categories of DSM-III-R have not yet been examined in a variety of research efforts, many of the diagnostic issues discussed in this chapter will use examples from the DSM-III to illustrate diagnostic problems and controversies.

PROBLEMS IN THE DIAGNOSIS OF SEVERE PSYCHIATRIC DISORDERS IN ADOLESCENCE: LOW INDEX OF SUSPICION, DEVELOPMENTAL ISSUES, THE NEED FOR SYSTEMATIC ASSESSMENT

Schizophrenia and Bipolar Disorder

The accurate diagnosis of severe psychiatric disorders presenting in adolescence can be extremely difficult, and there are some indications that schizophrenia and mania are underdiagnosed in this age group (Weiner & DelGaudio, 1976; Gammon, John, Rothblum, Mullen, and Tischler, 1983; Carlson & Strober, 1978a, b). Reasons for this may be a low index of clinical suspicion, confusion generated by a mixture of developmental and pathological features in the presentation, a reluctance to "label" a young person with a diagnosis that carries a connotation of severe disturbance, and the understandable wish to observe clinical course over a period of time before a definitive diagnosis is made (to some extent a requirement for a DSM-III diagnosis of schizophrenia). For these diagnoses, the study of long-term outcome provides the most convincing evidence regarding differential diagnostic features; however, such efforts are complicated. The general conceptualization and classification of the disorder may change between the initial data-gathering and the follow-up stages, and also the actual tracking of a large sample of disturbed young people can be a difficult and costly endeavor.

Weiner and DelGaudio (1976) conducted a follow-up study of a large cohort of treated adolescents identified through the Monroe County, New York, psychiatric case register. Fifty-four percent were identified in the case register over the 10-year follow-up period; of these, 54.1% showed diagnostic stability on most subsequent psychiatric contacts. For schizophrenia, there was complete diagnostic agreement on subsequent contacts in 62.2% of the cases. The authors note that over 10% of those originally diagnosed as having personality disorders, neurosis, and situational disorders, and over 20% of a mixed group termed "other diagnosis" were diagnosed as schizophrenic on all or almost all subsequent occasions. This suggests that a number of adolescents, whose illnesses became severe enough to require future treatment, either presented with a variety of more benign conditions or did not have the psychotic features of their illnesses recognized at the early stages. Of course, a major limitation of this study is the inability to follow up a substantial proportion of the sample through the case register. One cannot tell whether the subjects who were lost to follow-up would have contributed to a pattern of greater or less consistency in the course of the illness over time (although one suspects that the picture of less consistency is more likely).

Steinberg (1985), reporting on Zeitlin's study of the natural history of schizophrenic and affective disorders in adolescence, notes that predictions based on presenting features in adolescence often were not useful. Only acute onset was found to correctly predict manic-depressive illness; however, the small number of cases for comparison precluded any definitive test of this distinction. Creating one broader psychotic group was found to be more useful than forcing differentiations. This strategy is in keeping with trends in British research to use broad, typological diagnoses in the face of unsettled diagnostic and nosological issues. In the United States, the tendency is to attempt specific diagnoses, assuming identical criteria for adolescents and adults in the absence of evidence to the contrary.

Despite a general recognition that bipolar disorder may present with a manic episode in adolescence, recent reports have noted that it may be missed clinically (Carlson & Strober, 1978a, b; Carlson & Strober, 1979; Gammon et al., 1983). Carlson and Strober (1978a) reported on six adolescent patients who had been admitted with the diagnosis of schizophrenia but on later admission were rediagnosed as manic-depressive. Systematic review of case record data revealed that major affective symptomatology had been evident both at the initial and throughout subsequent admissions and that diagnoses of schizophrenia were made in the absence of clear-cut features of that disorder.

Gammon et al. (1983) compared hospital diagnoses with those obtained from semistructured diagnostic interviews (Schedule for Affective Disorders and Schizophrenia for School-Aged Children and Adolescents, Epidemiological Version) [K-SADS-E] of 17 adolescent inpatients and their mothers. While none of these patients had carried a hospital chart diagnosis of bipolar disorder, the systematic assessment revealed that 5 (29%) of the 17 met DSM-III criteria for bipolar disorder. In all cases, the parental interview confirmed the diagnosis based on the interview with the adolescent.

It is not clear at present whether bipolar disorder is truly rare in adolescence (e.g. Weiner & DelGaudio, 1976; Warren, 1965) or whether it is not so rare but is underdiagnosed (Carlson & Strober, 1978a, 1978b, 1979; Gammon et al., 1983). A low index of suspicion for this diagnosis, combined with flagrant presentations that mix atypical and age-specific features, and a readiness on the part of the clinician to think of schizophrenia as a disorder with a potentially dramatic onset in adolescence are factors that may contribute to the misdiagnosis of such youngsters (Gammon et al., 1983; Carlson & Strober, 1978a, 1978b, 1979). In addition, particularly in the

United States, schizophrenia has traditionally been viewed in broad terms so that the diagnosis might be made in the presence of a single psychotic symptom (Hsu & Starzynski, 1986). Because DSM-III was more extensive, phenomenological, and operational than its predecessor, its adoption and subsequent revision should stimulate the practice of more accurate differentiation between schizophrenia and other disorders with psychotic symptomatology. Finally, premorbid mood lability may be ascribed to "adolescent turmoil," and thus relevant diagnostic features may be ignored (Gammon et al., 1983). Carlson and Strober (1978b) note that the normal tendency of the adolescent to exaggerate capabilities and minimize handicaps, combined with a reluctance to allow adults to delve into the world of his or her private inner experiences, leaves the clinician in the position of interpreting surface behavior with limited information about the patient's internal affective state.

Gammon et al. (1983) stress the diagnostic gains afforded by the addition of systematic structured interviews that elicit information in accord with specified criteria such as those of DSM-III and DSM-III-R. They view such assessment as a potentially helpful adjunct to the usual clinical evaluation. For an area of some diagnostic uncertainty, such as adolescent bipolar disorder, comprehensive assessment techniques can insure that relevant symptom areas are not missed. A more subtle advantage to the adjunctive use of these interviews involves the variable capability of the adolescent to formulate and verbalize symptomatology, particularly that involving his or her inner state (Carlson & Strober, 1978b). It is the experience of this author that some youngsters may not be able to describe such symptoms if asked about them in an open-ended way, whereas, if given a very specific symptom description by means of a question (such as in a structured interview) the adolescent may easily recognize and acknowledge the same symptom. While there is no reason this cannot and should not be achieved in a careful clinical interview, the adjunctive use of standard interviews can facilitate comprehensive symptom coverage while providing a data base for clinical studies on diagnostic issues such as these.

AGE-SPECIFIC MANIFESTATIONS: WHAT CRITERIA TO USE AT WHAT AGE

Depression

Until rather recently, adolescents were included in the controversies on childhood depression (Carlson & Garber, 1986). These ranged from doubt as to its existence to the view that the clinical picture of depression in youngsters is the same as that for adults (Carlson & Garber, 1986; Cantwell & Carlson, 1979; Carlson & Strober, 1979). Another strongly debated view was the idea of "masked depression" which held that, for children and adolescents, depression is often not expressed in the same symptomatic form as in adults but through a range of other behaviors, such as conduct problems or somatic complaints (Glaser, 1968; Toolan, 1962; Cytryn & McKnew, 1972). This conceptualization was criticized on various grounds. In particular, it was noted that the diverse masking behaviors were not in some sense specific to the underlying condition of depression (Gittelman-Klein, 1977); that the masking conditions were often no more than presenting complaints that in a depressed adult would be viewed as manifestations of psychological distress, but not as masks for a depression (Kovacs & Beck, 1977); and that when a behavior disorder and depression coexist, the masked depression can be identified by a thorough clinical evaluation (Carlson & Cantwell, 1980). In addition, as instruments for the direct assessment of depressive symptoms in youngsters were introduced, the need for the concept of a mask diminished (Puig-Antich, 1982) and was ultimately retracted (Cytryn, McKnew, & Bunney, 1980).

Current thinking on the diagnosis of depression follows the view that major depressions, such as are seen in adults, are evident in adolescents (Carlson & Garber, 1986). The DSM-III and DSM-III-R have emphasized such continuity in the phenomenology of depression; thus one set of diagnostic criteria is to be applied regardless of age (with some minor qualifications). In contrast, for instance, the DSM-III and DSM-III-R assign separate entities for anxiety disorders in childhood and adolescence, distinct from those for adults. That operational criteria, conforming to the clinical picture of depression in adults, can be applied to adolescents has certainly been demonstrated. For example, Carlson and Cantwell (1982) and Robbins, Alessi, Cook, Poznanski, and Yanchyshyn (1982) systematically diagnosed samples of adolescent patients (child and adolescent in the Carlson and Cantwell study) using DSM-III or Research Diagnostic Criteria (very similar to DSM-III) for depression. Both studies reported 27% of their samples met criteria for a diagnosis of major depressive disorder.

The Cantwell and Carlson study also applied the Weinberg criteria for depression to their sample. These are a modification of adult criteria and are intended to be developmentally appropriate for youngsters. For example, school-related symptoms are specified, and aggressive behavior is considered a counterpart of agitation and irritability. They found that the DSM-III criteria were considerably more restrictive than the Weinberg Criteria, so a number of youngsters meeting the Weinberg Criteria did not meet those of DSM-III. They naturally raise the question: Which criteria are right? Unfortunately, validating information will require additional studies and will take time to gather. Commenting on these results, Puig-Antich (1982) stated, "we should keep open the possibility that the lower limit of DSM-III major depression may be too high and exclude true depressives from their proper diagnosis."

INFORMANT SOURCE

The problem of deciding what informant or combination of informants to rely on for symptom information is one of the challenging methodological issues facing clinical and epidemiological researchers in the area of child-hood psychopathology, and it is certainly one of clinical relevance as well. The development and increasing use of structured diagnostic interviews has made it easy to compare parent and child reports on identical symptom questions. However, while results from research to date are intriguing, they also impress us with the complexity of the problem. Unfortunately, most of the recent studies have used samples that cover a broad age range, despite the possibility that the potential areas of parent-child agreement and disagreement may be different for children and adolescents.

Herjanic and Reich (1982) found that on a structured interview consisting of 168 questions, only 16 produced reasonably good agreement between parent and child (kappas of .50 or higher). These questions concerned objective, concrete matters, such as being suspended from school, wetting the bed at night, and running away from home overnight. Questions on which there was poor agreement involved relationships at home and with peers or required judgment as to the existence or severity of a symptom (e.g., frequent worrying).

In a recent study by Kashani, Orvaschel, Burk, and Reid (1985), 50 children, ages 7 to 17 years, and their parents were interviewed using a highly structured diagnostic interview. Parent-child agreement was quite low for all the Axis I (clinical psychiatric syndrome) diagnoses, with kappas of .31 and lower. Children were more likely than parents to report depression and anxiety, and parents reported more oppositional behavior and attention deficit disorder.

Another study by Moretti, Fine, Haley, and Marriage (1985) assessed parent-child agreement on several structured assessments for depression. These were administered to 60 psychiatric patients, ages 8 to 17. Consistent with the results of other studies, they found only a moderate correlation between child and parent reports. In this study, parent reports failed to distinguish those children with clinical diagnoses of depression from those children with other clinical diagnoses. However, parents' ratings of their own depression correlated with the perception that their children were depressed.

Kohn and Cohen (1986) have recently examined informant effects using data from a large general population sample that contained a substantial number of adolescents (age range of sample was 9 to 19 years). Psycho-pathology was assessed using parallel mother-report and youth self-report structured interviews. In general, the mothers' reports about their sons and daughters yielded higher levels of psychopathology than did the reports of the young people themselves. And parents with histories of treatment for mental illness showed lower levels of agreement with their youngsters than did untreated parents. For oppositional disorder and depression, parent-youth agreement improved with age, but being older did not lead to better agreement on scales of attention deficit disorder, conduct disorder, over-anxious disorder, and separation anxiety. The authors stress the need for information from both parent and child informants, and they sound a note of caution concerning the practice of interviewing mentally ill probands to gain psychiatric information abut family members.

In summary, investigators consistently find poor levels of agreement between child and parent informants, and similar results have been reported for parent-teacher agreement (Rutter et al., 1981). A fairly, but not completely, consistent result is the finding that children are better reporters of internal feeling states, and their parents are better reporters of certain behaviors. There are some suggestions that the mother's own mental state affects her report of her child's symptoms. If this is in fact the case, it speaks very strongly for the need to obtain reports from multiple informants rather than relying on parental reports.

VALIDITY ISSUES

Conduct Disorder Subtypes

While validity is a basic characteristic of an adequate classification system of disorder, there are still relatively few studies that have examined the validity of DSM-III diagnoses in children and adolescents (Shaffer & Gould, 1987) and virtually none for DSM-III-R. Indeed, the inclusion of unvalidated syndromes was a particular focus of criticism of the DSM-III childhood section (Rutter & Shaffer, 1980; Garmezy, 1978). It has been noted (Rutter & Shaffer, 1980; Rutter & Gould, 1985) that there is evidence for the validity of certain broad diagnostic groupings—emotional disorders, conduct disorders, autism, schizophrenia, developmental disorders, and depression. However, the distinctions that make up the finer-grained subdivisions may often not be empirically justified. One example of this that has received a great deal of attention has been the subtyping of conduct disorders in the DSM-III. These are subdivided according to the aggressive/nonaggressive nature of the conduct disturbance and to the presence or absence of evidence of social attachment (socialized/undersocialized).

The most convincing case for the validity of subtypes would be findings demonstrating that the subtypes differed with respect to background factors, etiology, and natural history. For example, Henn, Bardwell, and Jenkins (1980) did a follow-up of adult criminal activity for a sample of delinquent boys diagnosed retrospectively as having: socialized conduct disorder; undersocialized conduct disorder, aggressive type; or undersocialized conduct disorder, nonaggressive type. The undersocialized delinquents were more likely to be incarcerated or convicted over the 10-year follow-up period than the socialized delinquents. While these results would seem to support the DSM-III subtype divisions, Rutter and Giller (1984) have noted that this distinction is based on results from only a small number of studies, some of which carried methodological limitations (e.g., rating of child and family variables by the same person).

Another strategy for investigating the validity of DSM-III disorders and subtypes involves comparing DSM-III groupings to symptom patterns identified by multivariate statistical techniques. Rutter and Giller noted that not all studies of this type show that the behaviors in question fall into clearly differentiated patterns of socialized and unsocialized types and that many delinquents do not fall into either category. They raised the question as to whether there are separate syndromes based on the socialized/undersocialized distinction or whether what is being assessed is really a dimension relevant to all children, not just those with conduct disorder. Quay (1986), after reviewing a large number of studies based on multivariate techniques, concluded that there is very strong support for the undersocialized aggressive and socialized aggressive subgroups but not for the undersocialized, nonaggressive and socialized, nonaggressive subgroups.

In response to the controversy about the validity of conduct disorder subtypes, DSM-III-R has taken a more limited approach to subtypes. In the DSM-III-R there are three subtypes—group type, solitary aggressive type, and undifferentiated type. The solitary aggressive category roughly includes the undersocialized aggressive type of DSM-III and is a categorization for which there is evidence supporting its validity. The group type is said to correspond roughly to the socialized nonaggressive type of DSM-III, although aggressive behavior can be present. This category is intended to further describe conduct disordered youngsters whose behavior problems occur mainly in gang or group contexts. The undifferentiated type is a larger group, intended to serve as a residual category. While considerable work is needed to complete our understanding of the subtypes of conduct disorder, the more conservative approach to subtyping taken in DSM-III-R stays closer to the field's current knowledge base and thus attempts to avoid the classification pitfall of appearing to validate distinctions that in fact have not been adequately demonstrated.

RELIABILITY ISSUES

Interrater reliability refers to the agreement among evaluators about which cases should receive the same diagnosis. It is considered a requisite for a diagnostic classification system (Rutter & Gould, 1985). Without a reasonable level of agreement as to which cases have a particular disorder, one cannot determine the associated features, natural history, response to treatment, and etiology; that is, one cannot assess the validity of the diagnostic category.

The DSM-III reliability studies were reviewed by Shaffer and Gould (1987) and Quay (1986). Most studies used mixed child and adolescent samples and varied in whether the different raters based their diagnostic judgments on written case histories (Cantwell, Russell, Mattison, & Will, 1979; Mattison, Cantwell, Russell, & Will, 1979; Mezzich, Mezzich, & Coffman, 1985), structured joint interview (Strober, Green, & Carlson, 1981), or clinical presentation at ward rounds (Werry, Methven, Fitzpatrick, & Dixon, 1983). Results varied somewhat, probably a reflection, in part, of these methodological differences. Mattison et al. (1979) reported that interrater agreement was fairly high for cases of psychosis, hyperactivity, conduct disorder, and mental retardation and was less adequate for depression, anxiety disorders, and for complex cases. Mezzich et al. (1985) described their reliability findings for Axis I and Axis II diagnoses as rather modest, with the highest reliabilities for mental retardation, schizophrenia and pervasive developmental disorder, conduct disorder, and enuresis; anxiety and adjustment disorders showed particularly low reliabilities. The Werry et al. (1983) study, which used a broad range of diagnoses, found the diagnoses of substance use, eating disorders, enuresis and encopresis, attention deficit disorder, schizophrenia, and adult anxiety disorders to be reliable. The childhood anxiety disorders and mental retardation achieved moderate reliability, while conduct, adjustment, and oppositional disorders were among the unreliable conditions. These authors noted that when subcategories are considered, there is usually one subcategory that shows reliability comparable to the major category, while the other subcategories usually fall way behind. They concluded that in a number of instances there is little to be gained by the use of subcategorizations.

Changes made in the DSM-III-R are interesting in view of the somewhat mixed picture from reliability studies such as these. Attention deficit-hyperactivity disorder, conduct disorder, and oppositional disorder are grouped under the heading Disruptive Behavior Disorders and are structured according to the polythetic (index or scale approach). Some advantages of the new approach include the use of more specific and varied symptoms, so symptoms appropriate to youngsters across an age range are better represented (e.g., behaviors likely to characterize a younger child with conduct disorder are better represented than in DSM-III). The use of a single index, with a variety of symptom combinations qualifying for a diagnosis, is likely to improve diagnostic reliability. On the other hand, youngsters with rather different symptom patterns may qualify for the same diagnosis; that is, a characteristic behavior may not be shared by those with a single diagnosis. The index of symptoms and the threshold for diagnosis are based on the results of a field trial involving a large sample of youngsters; nevertheless, further demonstration of the reliability, validity, and utility of these categories is warranted.

The only study to look at the reliability of DSM-III diagnoses specifically in adolescents is that of Strober et al. (1981). They found high levels of clinician agreement across most of the 13 diagnostic groupings. The anxiety disorders of childhood and socialized conduct disorder were among the disorders rated with somewhat less reliability. Certainly, these results showed generally higher levels of reliability for this adolescent sample than were found in studies that mixed child and adolescent patients (or case descriptions). The authors conclude that their data "dispute the common view that developmental factors necessarily limit the precision and replicability of psychiatric diagnosis in adolescent patients."

While this is perhaps an optimistic note for students of adolescent psychopathology, it is important to couch this conclusion in an understanding of the methodology employed. The researchers themselves comment that the use of two interviewers, rating subjects jointly on the basis of a semi-structured assessment and examination of the same clinical records, is a study procedure that will tend to enhance agreement. It is not clear that agreement would be similarly high using procedures that more closely simulate clinical practice. However, these findings do demonstrate that the combination of certain DSM-III criteria and standardized assessment procedures can yield reliable diagnoses in symptomatic adolescents. This in itself is an important step in the process of investigation, and it is a necessary one for the further refining our understanding of the diagnostic assessment and classification of adolescent psychopathology.

DIAGNOSIS IN CLINICAL PRACTICE

In practice, the diagnostic assessment of the adolescent involves elements of art as well as thorough knowledge of DSM-III-R diagnostic criteria. The diagnostician must combine an empathic interviewing style with probing, systematic inquiry into various areas of psychopathology. Obstacles to accurate information gathering include the adolescent's reluctance to divulge information about inner feelings, moods, and behaviors. This reticence may be motivated by the adolescent's sense that disclosure of such private material would undermine his or her tenuous sense of independence from parental figures, or such reluctance may result from shame, confusion, or fear about the meaning of these feelings and behaviors. Sincere interest in the young person, a conveyed sense of respect, and, of course, patience are vital tools for diagnostic work with the adolescent.

These considerations do not mean that direct inquiry should be avoided or used hesitantly. Indeed, specific questioning concerning symptoms may help the youngster organize and delineate areas of distress and strength and thus reduce anxiety, as well as yield information. Structured and semistructured diagnostic instruments are promising adjuncts to the traditional unstructured clinical interview. These may be particularly valuable as part of the battery of assessments employed for complete data gathering on inpatient units. Their comprehensiveness and potential for reliable assessment make them a necessary part of the research diagnostic evaluation although further developmental work on these techniques is needed. In addition to the growing use of such interview measures, self report (or parent or teacher report) checklists, such as the Child Behavior Checklist and the Youth Self Report (Achenbach & Edelbrock, 1981; 1983; Edelbrock & Achenbach, 1979) have found increasing use in clinical and research settings. These checklists or any of a number of others that target specific types of psychopathology (e.g., depression, anxiety) can serve as useful screening measures for first-stage data gathering. For the clinician, they provide a way to scan for areas of psychopathology, and for the adolescent, they may serve as useful vehicles for acknowledging problems.

In addition to gathering symptom information from the adolescent, one must interview parents and frequently teachers or other school personnel, as each informant offers a distinct perspective. Information regarding developmental history and family history is best obtained from the parent. Teachers are valuable informants on the youngster's peer relations as well as on achievement in school subjects, learning problems, and areas of particular mastery. Diagnostic evaluation of the adolescent requires a synthetic approach in which information from various sources is combined while close attention is paid to phenomenology and to the fit of symptoms with DSM-III-R criteria.

SUMMARY

This chapter has provided a brief review of selected diagnostic issues in the field of adolescent psychopathology. Clearly, this area holds many questions, particularly in relation to the classification of psychiatric disorders in adolescence. Accurate diagnosis of psychiatric disorders in adolescence requires, in addition to clinical skills: (1) an awareness of developmental trends and their potential interplay with various types of symptoms; (2) an appreciation of the different types of information that may be forthcoming from child, parent, and other sources; (3) a comprehensive assessment strategy (whether more clinical or more structured in style); (4) knowledge about the types of disorders likely to present in adolescence, their associated factors, and natural histories; and (5) an understanding of the limits of our knowledge in all these respects.

Criticisms of the DSM-III and DSM-III-R systems, while necessary to a review such as this one, must be understood in a broader context—a context that recognizes the system itself as one of the elements facilitating scientific investigation and the acquisition of new knowledge. In their discussion of classification in childhood psychopathology, Rutter and Gould (1985) emphasize the useful distinction between public and private classifications. Private classifications are those developed for the purpose of investigating new ideas, and thus they should be speculative and hypothetical. Public classifications are those systems that are intended for the day-to-day use of professionals who may have differing theoretical orientations. To be useful, they should not include controversial or unproven concepts but should be organized according to principles that are basic enough to be generally accepted. The rules of these systems should be adhered to rather rigidly, for the value of such a system as a convention for organizing information is lost if the criteria are interpreted variably and applied nonsystematically. Public classifications are necessarily conservative, and one hopes that they will be rewritten as the result of active research and inquiry.

The DSM-III and DSM-III-R are public classification systems, and in a vital, expanding field, it is necessary that such systems will be outgrown and need rethinking and revision. That clinicians found the DSM-III to be clear and useful, at least more so than the DSM-II (Cantwell et al., 1979a; Mezzich & Mezzich, 1985), and that the period after the introduction of DSM-III coincided with a great increase in child psychiatric research (Shaffer & Gould, 1987), are indications of its importance and value to clinicians and researchers in child and adolescent psychopathology.

REFERENCES

Achenbach, T. (1974). *Developmental psychopathology.* New York: Wiley.

Achenbach, T. (1978). Psychopathology of childhood: Research problems and issues. *Journal of Consulting and Clinical Psychology, 46,* 759–776.

Achenbach, T., & Edelbrock, C. (1981). *Youth self report form—for ages 11–18.* Burlington, VT: University of Vermont.

Achenbach, T., & Edelbrock, C. (1983). *Manual for the child behavior checklist and revised child behavior profile.* Burlington, VT: Achenbach.

American Psychiatric Association (1987). *Diagnostic and statistical manual of mental disorders* (3rd ed., rev.). (DSM-III-R). Washington, DC: Author.

American Psychiatric Association (1980). *Diagnostic and statistical manual of mental disorders* (3rd ed.). (DSM-III). Washington, DC: Author.

Bemporad, J. R., & Schwab, M. E. (1986). The DSM-III and clinical child psychiatry. In T. Millon & G. L. Klerman (Eds.), *Contemporary directions in psychopathology: Toward the DSM-IV* (pp. 135–150). New York: Guilford.

Cantwell, D. P., & Carlson, G. (1979). Problems and prospects in the study of childhood depression. *Journal of Nervous and Mental Disease, 167,* 522–529.

Cantwell, D. P., Mattison, R., Russell, A. T., & Will, L. (1979a). A comparison of DSM-II and DSM-III in the diagnosis of childhood psychiatric disorders: IV. Difficulties in use, global comparison, and conclusions. *Archives of General Psychiatry, 36,* 1227–1228.

Cantwell, D. P., Russell, A. T., Mattison, R., & Will, L. (1979b). A comparison of DSM-II and DSM-III in the diagnosis of childhood psychiatric disorders: I. Agreement with expected diagnosis. *Archives of General Psychiatry, 36,* 1208–1213.

Carlson, G. A., & Cantwell, D. P. (1980). Unmasking masked depression in children and adolescents. *American Journal of Psychiatry, 137,* 445–449.

Carlson, G. A., & Cantwell, D. P. (1982). Diagnosis of childhood depression: A comparison of the Weinberg and DSM-III criteria. *Journal of the American Academy of Child Psychiatry, 21,* 247–250.

Carlson, G. A., & Garber, J. (1986). Developmental issues in the classification of depression in children. In M. Rutter, C.E. Izard, & P.B. Read (Eds.), *Depression in young people.* New York: Guilford.

Carlson, G. A., & Strober, M. (1978a). Manic-depressive illness in early adolescence: A study of clinical and diagnostic characteristics in six cases. *Journal of the American Academy of Child Psychiatry, 17,* 138–153.

Carlson, G. A., & Strober, M. (1978b). Affective disorder in adolescence: Issues in misdiagnosis. *Journal of Clinical Psychiatry, 39,* 62–66.

Carlson, G. A., & Strober, M. (1979). Affective disorders in adolescence. *Psychiatric Clinics of North America, 2,* 511–526.

Cytryn, L., & McKnew, D. H. (1972). Proposed classification of childhood depression. *American Journal of Psychiatry, 129,* 149–155.

Cytryn, L., McKnew, D. H., & Bunney, W. (1980). Diagnosis of depression in children: Reassessment. *American Journal of Psychiatry, 137,* 22–25.

Edelbrock, C., & Achenbach, T. (1979). The teacher version of the child behavior profile: I. Boys ages 6–11. *Journal of Consulting and Clinical Psychiatry, 52,* 207–217.

Freud, A. (1965). *Normality and pathology in childhood.* New York: International Universities Press.

Gammon, G. D., John, K., Rothblum, E. D., Mullen, K., Tischler, G. L., & Weissman, M. M. (1983). Use of a structured diagnostic interview to identify bipolar disorder in adolescent inpatients: Frequency and manifestations of the disorder. *American Journal of Psychiatry, 140,* 543–547.

Garmezy, N. (1978). Never mind the psychologists: Is it good for the children? *Clinical Psychologist, 31,* 1–6.

Gittelman-Klein, R. (1977). Definitional and methodological issues concerning depressive illness in children. In J.G. Schulterbrandt & A. Raskin (Eds.), *Depression in childhood: Diagnosis, treatment, and conceptual models* (pp. 69–80). New York: Raven.

Glaser, K. (1968). Masked depression in children and adolescents. *Annual Progress in Child Psychiatry and Child Development, 1,* 345–355.

Graham, P., & Rutter, M. (1985). Adolescent disorders. In M. Rutter & L. Hersov (Eds.), *Child and adolescent psychiatry: Modern approaches* (2nd ed.) (pp. 351–367). Oxford: Blackwell.

Henn, F. A., Bardwell, R., & Jenkins, R. L. (1980). Juvenile delinquents revisited. *Archives of General Psychiatry, 37,* 1160–1163.

Herjanic, B., & Reich, W. (1982). Development of a structured psychiatric interview for children: Agreement between child and parent on individual symptoms. *Journal of Abnormal Child Psychology, 10,* 307–324.

Hsu, L. K. G., & Starzynski, J. M. (1986). Mania in adolescence. *Journal of Clinical Psychiatry, 47,* 596–599.

Kashani, J. H., Orvaschel, H., Burk, J. P., & Reid, J. C. (1985). Informant variance: The issue of parent-child disagreement. *Journal of the American Academy of Child Psychiatry, 24,* 437–441.

Klerman, G. L., Vaillant, G. E., Spitzer, R. L., & Michels, R. (1984). A debate on DSM-III. *American Journal of Psychiatry, 141,* 539–553.

Kohn, M., & Cohen, P. (1986). *Familial risk and informant effects.* Manuscript submitted for publication.

Kovacs, M., & Beck, A. T. (1977). An empirical-clinical approach toward a definition of childhood depression. In J.G. Schulterbrandt & A. Raskin (Eds.), *Depression in childhood: Diagnosis, treatment, and conceptual models* (pp. 1–25). New York: Raven.

Larson, R., Csikszentmihalyi, M., & Graef, R. (1980). Mood variability and the psychosocial adjustment of adolescents. *Journal of Youth and Adolescence, 9,* 469–490.

Mattison, R., Cantwell, D. P., Russell, A. T., & Will, L. (1979). A comparison of DSM-II and DSM-III in the diagnosis of childhood psychiatric disorders: II. Interrater agreement. *Archives of General Psychiatry, 36,* 1217–1222.

Mezzich, A. C., & Mezzich, J. E. (1985). Perceived suitability and usefulness of DSM-III vs. DSM-II in child psychopathology. *Journal of the American Academy of Child Psychiatry, 24,* 281–285.

Mezzich, A. C., Mezzich, J. E., & Coffman, G. A. (1985). Reliability of DSM-III vs. DSM-II in child psychopathology. *Journal of the American Academy of Child Psychiatry, 24,* 273–280.

Moretti, M. M., Fine, S., Haley, G., & Marriage, K. (1985). Childhood and adolescent depression: Child-report versus parent-report information. *Journal of the American Academy of Child Psychiatry, 24,* 273–280.

Puig-Antich, J. (1982). The use of RDC criteria for major depressive disorder in children and adolescents. *Journal of the American Academy of Child Psychiatry, 21,* 291–293.

Quay, H. C. (1986). A critical analysis of DSM-III as a taxonomy of psychopathology on childhood and adolescence. In T. Millon & G. L. Klerman (Eds.), *Contemporary directions in psychopathology: Toward the DSM-IV* (pp. 151–165). New York: Guilford.

Robbins, D. R., Alessi, N. E., Cook, S. C., Poznanski, E. O., & Yanchyshyn, G. W. (1982). The use of the research diagnostic criteria (RDC) for depression in adolescent psychiatric inpatients. *Journal of the American Academy of Child Psychiatry, 21,* 251–255.

Rutter, M. (1980). *Changing youth in a changing society: Patterns of adolescent development and disorder.* Cambridge, MA: Harvard University Press.

Rutter, M., Cox, A., Tupling, C., Berger, M., & Yule, W. (1975). Attainment and adjustment in two geographical areas: I. The prevalence of psychiatric disorder. *British Journal of Psychiatry, 126,* 493–509.

Rutter, M., & Garmezy, N. (1983). Developmental psychopathology. In E. M. Hetherington (Ed.), *Handbook of child psychology: Vol. 4* (pp. 775–911). New York: Wiley.

Rutter, M., & Giller, H. (1984). *Juvenile delinquency: Trends and perspectives.* New York: Guilford.

Rutter, M., & Gould, M. (1985). Classification. In M. Rutter & L. Hersov (Eds.), *Child and adolescent psychiatry: Modern approaches* (2nd ed.) (pp. 304–321). Oxford: Blackwell.

Rutter, M., Graham, P., Chadwick, O. F. D., & Yule, W. (1976). Adolescent turmoil: Fact or fiction? *Journal of Child Psychology and Psychiatry, 17,* 35–56.

Rutter, M., & Shaffer, D. (1980). DSM-III: A step forward or back in terms of the classification of child psychiatric disorders? *Journal of the American Academy of Child Psychiatry, 19,* 371–394.

Rutter, M., Tizard, J., & Whitmore, K. (Eds.). (1981). *Education, health and behavior.* Huntington, NY: Krieger. (Original work published in 1970)

Shaffer, D., & Gould, M. S. (1987). Issues in the use of DSM-III. J. Noshpitz & R. Cohen (Eds.), *The basic handbook of child psychiatry: Vol. V* (Section III). New York: Basic Books.

Steinberg, D. (1985). Psychotic and other severe disorders in adolescence. In M. Rutter & L. Hersov (Eds.), *Child and adolescent psychiatry: Modern approaches* (2nd Ed.) (pp. 567–583). Oxford: Blackwell.

Strober, M., Green, J., & Carlson, G. (1981). Reliability of psychiatric diagnosis in hospitalized adolescents: Interrater agreement using DSM-III. *Archives of General Psychiatry, 38,* 141–145.

Toolan, J. H. (1962). Depression in children and adolescents. *American Journal of Orthopsychiatry, 32,* 404–414.

Warren, W. (1965). A study of adolescent psychiatric in-patients and the outcome six or more years later: I. Clinical histories and hospital findings. *Journal of Child Psychology and Psychiatry, 6,* 1–17.

Weiner, I. B., & DelGaudio, A. C. (1976). Psychopathology in adolescence: An epidemiological study. *Archives of General Psychiatry, 33,* 187–193.

Werry, J. S., Methven, R. J., Fitzpatrick, J., & Dixon, H. (1983). The interrater reliability of DSM-III in children. *Journal of Abnormal Child Psychology, 11,* 341–354.

CHAPTER FOUR

Medical Evaluation

Stewart Gabel

The potential value of a complete medical evaluation for psychiatric patients is twofold. First, there is the possibility of detecting contributory or causative factors for the presenting mental or behavioral problem. Second, there is the possibility of detecting medical problems which may be unrelated or only peripherally related to the presenting psychiatric problem but which nonetheless merit additional medical attention.

Indeed, studies have shown that psychiatric patients have a high rate of medical problems and physical illnesses that often go undiagnosed (Maguire & Granville-Grossman, 1968; Hollender & Wells, 1980; Muecke & Krueger, 1981); that medical disorders may present with behavioral or emotional problems and be mistaken for primary psychiatric disorders (Reed & Bland, 1977; Penick & Carrier, 1967); that medical problems may also cause new psychiatric problems or exacerbate preexisting psychiatric disorders (Hall, Popkin, Devaul, Faillace, & Stickney, 1978; Gardner & Hall, 1980; Hall, Gardner, Popkin, Lecann, & Stickney, 1981); and that physical complaints thought to be psychological in origin may later be shown to have medical basis (Watson & Buranen, 1979; Koranyi, 1979).

It therefore seems almost axiomatic that the clinician must be aware of and evaluate for medical problems in any patient seeking help for what are believed to be psychological problems (Fogel & Slaby, 1986). The real issues to be addressed have to do with determining which medical examinations and procedures are most effective in evaluating the psychiatric patient and which medical procedures or practices are ineffective and should be eliminated or replaced.

The situation is complicated because different groups of psychiatric patients (e.g., inpatients versus outpatients, chronic versus acute) may have different needs from the standpoint of the medical evaluation. In addition, adult and geriatric patients (who comprised the majority of subjects in the studies previously cited) may have different medical and psychiatric disorders than other groups, such as children and adolescents, and therefore require different medical evaluations.

Several issues will be discussed in this chapter on the medical evaluation of the adolescent psychiatric patient. These issues will include:

1. the utility of the routine medical history and physical examination
2. the utility of screening with routine laboratory tests in detecting psychiatric disorders in the adolescent
3. the utility of screening with routine laboratory tests in detecting medical disorders in the adolescent psychiatric patient
4. the frequency of medical problems in the hospitalized psychiatric adolescent
5. medical or neurologic problems that may be misdiagnosed or confused with psychiatric disorders in the adolescent

An additional important concern, the use of medical or laboratory procedures such as the dexamethasone suppression test or obtaining serum levels of antidepressant medication in the psychiatric evaluation of the adolescent, will be addressed in chapters on specific psychiatric disorders. Since there is so little research available to address several of the questions just noted, clinical experience as well as the literature available will be used in making recommendations.

THE ROUTINE MEDICAL HISTORY AND PHYSICAL EXAMINATION

Johnson (1968) performed full physical examinations on 250 consecutive admissions to a psychiatric hospital. Thirty of these patients (12%) had a physical illness diagnosed or strongly suspected from the routine medical history and physical examination at the time of admission. Twenty-four of the 30 cases were misdiagnosed prior to admission. Eighteen of the 30 cases were over 60 years of age, and therefore in the geriatric age range. None of the cases the author cites (the ages of two were not given) were in the adolescent or young adult age range, however.

The frequency of the full physical examination determining that presenting psychological symptoms are caused by medical problems in the adolescent is probably less than in the adult or geriatric patient, but this possibility does exist. Such a finding may not actually alter the treatment plan for the presenting problem, but the increased understanding of its nature may help involve the patient and family in treatment and, in the longer run, perhaps improve upon existing treatment techniques. This is illustrated by the following two case histories:

Case 1. A well-functioning six-year-old boy sustained a head injury in an automobile accident and was unconscious for three days. He subsequently developed hyperactivity, distractibility, and short attention span. When he was hospitalized at age 14, he was abusing drugs and was truant frequently from school. His diagnosis, according to the DSM-III (APA, 1980) was Attention Deficit Disorder with Hyperactivity (ADD-H).* With further assessment and additional history, the etiology of his disorder was felt most likely to have been the head injury several years earlier. This information was helpful in telling the parents and youngster of the problem and gaining their support in working out a treatment plan, although the actual treatment would not have changed if the youngster's ADD-H had been due (as is usually the case) to unknown causes.

---

* In the revision of the third edition, DSM-III-R (APA, 1987), this disorder has been renamed Attention-deficit Hyperactivity Disorder.

Case 2. A 16-year-old mentally retarded youngster presented with behavior problems of two years' duration. The medical history indicated severe perinatal asphyxia as the likely cause for the mild mental retardation. Additional assessment indicated the behavior problems were the maladaptive response of this retarded youngster to the social and physical pressures of adolescence. A more complete picture, although again not altering treatment, was provided by the medical history.

Information from the medical history and physical examination is, at other times, helpful in contributing to both etiologic information and medical treatment of adolescent psychiatric patients. These cases are often acute in nature and frequently related to head trauma, drug abuse, medication effect, drug toxicity, and/or drug interaction where physical signs (e.g., pupillary dilation, fever, tachycardia of anticholinergic toxicity) are helpful in establishing a diagnosis and treatment plan.

For the majority of cases, however, as noted earlier, the medical history and physical examination alone do not provide conclusive information specifically about the ongoing psychiatric problems of the adolescent psychiatric patient. This is especially true if the symptoms have been relatively stable, long-standing, and not very severe. The medical history and physical examination may be of more help in providing information about the medical needs of the psychiatric patient that are unrelated or marginally related to the presenting psychiatric problems.

In a study done on 100 cases of adolescent psychiatric patients admitted to the adolescent inpatient unit of the Western Psychiatric Institute and Clinic (WPIC), in Pittsburgh, Pennsylvania, Gabel and Hsu (1986) found numerous medical diagnoses based on an initial brief medical assessment of their adolescent psychiatric patients. This assessment was recorded on Axis III of the DSM-III's multiaxial system which was completed on admission, usually before any laboratory studies had been done. These conditions are noted in Table 4.1. Most of the conditions noted in Table 4.1 were probably based solely on medical history, since the physical examination was often completed shortly after admission and after an initial DSM-III multiaxial diagnosis had been made.

The authors found that there were 39 patients who had an Axis III condition noted on admission. These 39 patients had a total of 64 conditions listed. As can be seen from Table 4.1, numerous types of conditions were found. Many would apparently require further medical evaluation or follow-up, but, as will be discussed next, the medical conditions were not felt to be the cause of the patient's psychiatric problems except possibly in one instance of a girl who had an organic brain syndrome and known brain dysfunction reflected in her initial Axis III diagnosis.

It seems desirable for all adolescent psychiatric patients to have a medical history and physical examination at the time of admission to psychiatric hospitalization. The benefits, in terms of psychiatric diagnosis, especially

Table 4.1.   Medical Conditions or Diagnoses Noted on Axis III on Admission

High blood pressure	Seizure disorder
Hemorrhoids	Rule out substance-induced mental
Asthma, in remission	status change
Hypertension	Deafness, right ear
Rule out seizure disorder	Tremors left leg
Right hearing loss	Jaundice
Rule out pseudo seizures	Epilepsy with grand mal seizures
Amenorrhea	Severe facial acne
Bone disorder—exostosis	Rule out temporal lobe epilepsy
Dolichocephaly	Rule out infertility
Milk allergy	Injury to eye
Status/post overdose of Pine-Sol®	Injury to patella
and Sine-Aid tablets	Rule out Hodgkin's disease
Migraine headaches	Diarrhea
Obesity	Status/post Lysol® and ammonia
Abnormal E.E.G.	ingestion
Poor visual acuity	Cardiac arrhythmia
Osgood Schlatter disease	History of syncope
Multiple allergies	History of back pain
Allergies	Rule out hypertension
Arthritis	Exophoria
? Hypothyroidism	Exogenous obesity
"Stomach problems," rule out	Thalassemia minor
gastric ulcer	One functioning kidney
Rule out hyperthyroidism	Tuberous sclerosis
Gastritis	Generalized seizure disorder
Alopecia areata	Frontal glioma, S/P partial resection
Rule out pregnancy	in 1975
Status/post overdose with Doriden,	Sore throat
Benadryl and Erythromycin	Iron deficiency anemia
Fracture T_{12}; subluxation T_{11-12}	Seasonal allergies
Short stature	Chronic sinusitis
Rule out partial complex seizures	Mild right sensorineural hearing loss

of the physical examination, will often be relatively slight in and of themselves but will serve to further evaluate suspicions (e.g., drug intoxication) already raised by the mental status exam and presentation of the patient. The benefits, in terms of detecting or defining medical disorders that need further evaluation and that may not have been known before, will probably be somewhat greater. It should be remembered that chronic medical disorders such as diabetes mellitus, epilepsy, and chronic neurological conditions are more common in adolescence than is generally realized (Steinberg, 1983).

For the less severely psychiatrically disturbed adolescent who has had ongoing medical care and who presently is an outpatient with emotional or behavioral problems that are not severe, not associated with signs and suggestions of organicity on mental status exam, and which have had a stable, ongoing and relatively unfluctuating course, continued routine medical care is indicated. A general medical history should be part of the overall psychiatric assessment. A specific physical and neurologic exam, in these cases, is not usually indicated as part of the overall psychiatric assessment. In general, psychiatric disorders that have a neurological etiology should be suspected when there is a decrease in previous level of intellectual or social functioning, severe or atypical psychiatric problems with relatively rapid or abrupt onset, and when there has been failure to respond to treatment.

ROUTINE LABORATORY SCREENING IN DETECTING PSYCHIATRIC DISORDERS

Certain studies noted at the beginning of this chapter (e.g., Hall et al., 1981) recommend laboratory screening for psychiatric patients as a means of detecting causative factors for a patient's psychological problem. As noted, however, studies of this type have often been done on populations heavily weighted toward the adult and geriatric age range, and while several studies do suggest various screening procedures, there continues to be some dispute about the value of laboratory screening. Willet and King (1977) found a low incidence (3.0%) of unexpected abnormal laboratory tests and a low incidence of new disease (2.2 to 8.5%) that was detected through laboratory screening procedures in 636 patients admitted to a short-term adult psychiatric ward. There was no instance in which a medical cause for a patient's admitting psychiatric problems was detected by the screening procedures.

In a study already mentioned, Gabel and Hsu (1986) evaluated the value of routine laboratory screening specifically in adolescent psychiatric inpatients. The authors reviewed the charts of 100 consecutive admissions to WPIC. All admissions were evaluated by at least two clinicians, one of whom was a psychiatrist or psychiatric resident, in the Diagnostic and Evaluation Center (DEC) prior to the patient's being taken to the inpatient unit. An initial multiaxial diagnosis according to DSM-III criteria was made, and admission orders were written. After admission, orders might be revised by the psychiatric resident or attending psychiatrist. Within one to two days, a more complete medical history and physical exam were done and additional medical needs were then discussed and implemented.

The charts were reviewed to determine initial diagnoses, final diagnoses, the pattern of ordering routine laboratory tests, and the results of these admission laboratory tests that included: thyroid function tests (T_4 [serum thyroxine], T_3U [T_3 uptake], and FTI [free T_4 index]), electroencephalogram (EEG), chest X ray, chemistry panel (i.e., electrolytes, blood urea nitrogen, calcium, glucose), routine urinalysis, complete blood count (only hemoglobin, hematocrit, and white blood cell count were considered in this study), electrocardiogram (EKG), and rapid plasma reagin (RPR). Exactly which and how many of the eight routine tests were ordered on admission was not predetermined. Sometimes one or more of the eight tests were not ordered by choice (e.g., chest X ray, perhaps to avoid radiation exposure) or by chance (forgetting to order a test).

The study showed that 25 patients had all 8 of the routine admission laboratory tests done; 42 patients had 7 tests done; 18 patients had 6 tests done; 9 patients had 5 tests done; 2 patients had 4 tests done; 3 patients had 3 tests done; and 1 patient had no test done.

Gabel and Hsu were particularly interested to learn whether any of the screening test results would result in a change in thinking about a patient's diagnosis so that a functional disorder diagnosis on admission would be changed to an organic disorder diagnosis on discharge or vice versa. The authors somewhat arbitrarily considered only DSM-III category 2 (Organic Mental Disorders) as reflecting organic mental disorders (i.e., disorders with a known or definite organic or physical etiology) and the mental disorders in all the other categories as functional disorders, but this was consistent with the classification of disorders in DSM-III. Category 3 disorders (Substance Use Disorders), for example, were not considered organic mental disorders.

The authors found only one youngster who had an initial diagnosis in Category 2 (i.e., of an Organic Mental Disorder). The final diagnosis of this youngster was also an organic mental disorder (Mixed Organic Brain Syndrome). Therefore, no patient's diagnosis changed from an initial organic diagnosis to a final diagnosis of functional disorder. Five cases had "rule outs" for organic mental disorders on admission. Four of the five related to substance induced disorders; none of these diagnoses remained in Category 2 at discharge (i.e., the "rule-out" diagnosis was ruled out). Importantly, none of the eight routine laboratory screening tests appeared to be instrumental in making this decision. It is probable that drug screening tests were more helpful here. In the one patient of the five with a rule-out not related to substance abuse, routine laboratory tests such as the EEG and thyroid tests were normal, but it is not certain whether these normal results actually helped in ruling out an organic diagnosis.

The authors also found only one case in which an initial diagnosis of a functional disorder changed to a final diagnosis of an organic mental disorder. This was the case of a 17-year-old male who was given an initial diagnosis of adjustment disorder and borderline intellectual functioning. During the course of the hospitalization, a vague history of "brain damage

. . . possibly secondary to perinatal difficulties" was noted in the record although primary records were not available to confirm this. This patient had a Grade I generalized dysrhythmia on his EEG, a "possible area of low density" on a computerized axial tomography (CT) scan that he would not allow repeated, a glucose level of 51 mg/dl that was also not repeated, and neuropsychological testing indicating "mild, diffuse organic involvement" and a Wechsler Adult Intelligence Scale-Revised (WAIS-R) IQ of 65. The patient's final diagnoses were organic personality syndrome with episodic explosive temper and mild mental retardation on Axis I, and static encephalopathy on Axis III. This patient's severe behavior problems may or may not have been on an organic basis. The change in diagnostic thinking from admission to discharge may or may not have been significantly enhanced by any of the eight routine tests since the EEG was only mildly abnormal (not uncommon in this sample) and the low glucose was not repeated. The diagnosis seems to have been based in large part on the history, mental status exam, mental retardation, and neuropsychological test findings.

Overall then, it can be said that in this rather small group of adolescents admitted for short-term hospitalization, routine laboratory screening of the type described in this study was not generally effective in clarifying psychiatric diagnoses or in detecting psychiatric disorders that were caused by unknown organic factors. It may be, however, that particular screening tests specifically designed for the needs of particular populations might have greater efficacy. Routine screening for illicit drugs, for example, might yield a higher percentage of substance induced mental disorders in adolescent populations than would otherwise be found.

ROUTINE LABORATORY SCREENING IN DETECTING MEDICAL DISORDERS

Another purpose of the study of Gabel and Hsu (1986) was to determine if the routine laboratory screening during psychiatric hospitalization was helpful in detecting new or unknown medical disorders in this adolescent psychiatric population, even if the medical disorder was not causative of the psychiatric problem. Table 4.2 provides information on the adolescents who had routine EEGs on admission. In 63 of these patients, the EEG was normal; 5 EEGs were definitely abnormal; 14 EEGs were of the mild, diffusely abnormal, borderline types. None of the patients was given a new medical diagnosis of seizure disorder based on this evaluation during hospitalization.

Table 4.3 provides information on the remaining routine laboratory screening tests used on admission in the group of adolescent inpatients. In order to assess the medical problems in their population and to determine

Table 4.2. Results of "Routine" E.E.G.s in 100 Cases

Number of Patients on Whom E.E.G.s Not Done	Number of Patients with Normal E.E.G.s	Number of Patients with "Abnormal" E.E.G.s*
18	63	19

*Five of these 19 E.E.G.s were definitely abnormal, showing findings such as spikes, focal, and paroxysmal features. One of these five definitely abnormal E.E.G.s was in a patient who had a known seizure disorder at admission. Fourteen of the 19 "abnormal" E.E.G.s were of "mildly abnormal," "diffusely abnormal," or "borderline abnormal" types. One of these 14 patients had a known seizure disorder on admission. In one patient (as discussed in the text), E.E.G. findings of "dysrhythmia, Grade I generalized" may have contributed to a change from an initial functional to a final "organic mental disorder" diagnosis.

Table 4.3. Initial Results of "Routine" Laboratory Studies in 100 Cases

	Number Not Done	Normal	Abnormal or Possibly Abnormal
Thyroid function tests (T4, T3U, F.T.I.)[a]	7	71	22
Chemistry panel (Na, K, Cl, CO_2, Glucose, BUN, Calcium, Creatinine)[b]	9	47	44
C.B.C. (only WBC, Hemoglobin, Hematocrit considered)[c]	5	66	29
R.P.R.[a]	16	84	
Routine urinalysis[a]	7	62	31
E.K.G.[a]	18	68	9
Chest X-ray[d]	56	40	4

Note: Reprinted from Gabel, S., Hus, L. K. G.: "Routine laboratory tests in adolescent psychiatric inpatients: Their value in making psychiatric diagnoses and in detecting medical disorders" *Journal of American Academy of Child Psychiatry 25*, 1:113–119, 1986. Copyright © 1986 American Academy of Child Psychiatry. Reprinted by permission.

[a] See text for discussion.

[b] In 18 of the 44 abnormal results, the glucose level was one of, or the sole, abnormality.

[c] In two of these patients, there was a medical indication (e.g., iron deficiency anemia) to get the test, and it was not therefore strictly "routine." Three others were on anticonvulsant medication known to cause hematologic abnormalities and the tests may not have been "routine" here either.

[d] In three of these patients, there was a medical indication (e.g., complaints of shortness of breath) to get the X-ray, and it was not therefore strictly "routine." All of these X-rays turned out to be normal. See text.

whether the large number of abnormal or possibly abnormal initial laboratory results (Table 4.3) was helpful in detecting medical disorders, the
authors reviewed all the Axis III diagnoses and conditions on admission
and on discharge, particularly those that were present on discharge that
were not present on admission.

DSM-III states, "Axis III permits the clinician to indicate any current
physical disorder or condition that is potentially relevant to the understanding or management of the individual" (page 26).* In actual practice
on the adolescent inpatient unit at the time, physical problems felt to be
of *any* importance to the individual generally were listed on Axis III on
discharge.

As indicated earlier, Gabel and Hsu (1986) found that 39 patients had an
Axis III diagnosis or condition on admission. Sixty-four actual diagnoses or
conditions had been listed on Axis III on admission, as indicated in Table
4.1. By discharge, 50 patients had an Axis III diagnosis or condition, and
there were 69 diagnoses or conditions listed. There were 37 diagnoses or
conditions listed on Axis III on discharge that were not present on admission. These are listed in Table 4.4. It seems clear from Table 4.4 that while
some important conditions were listed, many minor findings were also
noted. Of the conditions newly listed on discharge, only seven resulted from
a screening laboratory test. The other 30 seem to have been the result of
further information from the initial history and physical examination, later
medical history, or medical illnesses that occurred during the hospitalization itself.

Some discussion of the seven Axis III discharge conditions or diagnoses
based on the routine screening laboratory tests may be helpful. In one of
the seven instances, a 17-year-old male with a history of attention deficit
disorder with hyperactivity, substance abuse, and conduct disorder, screening thyroid function tests (T_4, T_3U, FTI) were all elevated initially and on
repeat determination. A pediatrician evaluated the patient in consultation
and found no clinical evidence of hyperthyroidism but suggested following
the youngster and repeating the tests in one month. Abnormal thyroid function tests in adults admitted to psychiatric hospitalization are known to
occur frequently, although the reasons for this are not fully clear (Spratt et
al., 1982). In this study also, numerous adolescents had abnormal thyroid
tests on screening examination, although with this one possible exception,
none was felt to have thyroid disease on clinical grounds.

Three patients had abnormal EEGs noted on Axis III on discharge
that were the result of the routine EEG screening. None of these patients
had clinical findings indicative of a seizure disorder. As previously
noted, all three had discharge diagnoses of nonorganic (i.e., functional)

* DSM-III-R (APA, 1987) contains virtually the same statement, substituting "of the case"
(page 18) for "of the individual."

Table 4.4. Medical Conditions or Diagnoses Noted on Discharge but Not on Admission

Exogenous obesity	Monilial vaginitis
Elevated thyroid studies*	History of head trauma
Mildly and diffusely abnormal E.E.G. with no clinical symptoms*	Static encephalopathy
	History of mastoiditis
Premature ventricular contractions on E.K.G.*	Status/post laceration of left forearm
History of abnormal E.E.G. and blackout spells	Status/post gastric obstruction with dilatation
Impacted third molars	Severe acne
Recurrent epistaxis	Superficial scratches to wrist
Strabismus	Lymphadenopathy (resolving)
Rule out temporal seizures (patient eloped from hospital and work-up not completed)	Hemarthrosis (right knee)
	History of functional heart murmur
Allergies	Moderately abnormal E.E.G. with no clinical symptoms
Obesity	Viral syndrome during hospital-ization
Secondary amenorrhea	
Nerve injury to right lower extremity	Constipation
Esotropia	Myopia
Rule out seizure disorder (patient transferred to another hospital; work-up not done prior to transfer)	Dizzy spells, unknown etiology
	Abnormal E.E.G.*
	Rule out subclinical asthma
Rule out hypoglycemia (patient trans-ferred to another hospital; work-up not done prior to transfer)*	Sebaceous cyst of the axilla
	Questionable abnormality on chest X-ray

Note. Reprinted from Gabel, S., Hsu, L. K. G.: "Routine laboratory tests in adolescent psychiatric inpatients: Their value in making psychiatric diagnoses and in detecting medical disorders", *Journal of American Academy of Child Psychiatry 25*, pp. 1:113–119, 1986. Copyright © 1986 American Academy of Child Psychiatry. Reprinted by permission.
*See text for explanation.

psychiatric illness. Routine EEGs in children and adolescents with isolated behavior and learning problems and without specific neurological complaints or signs of seizure disorder are probably of relatively little value clinically.

One patient had "premature ventricular contractions on EKG" as an Axis III final diagnosis. This 17-year-old, obese male had a history of hypertension, and an EKG may or may not have been considered routine in the light of the history of hypertension itself. The EKG revealed premature ventricular contractions, probably unifocal, and possible incomplete right bundle branch block, or normal variant. No further cardiac evaluation was done.

Another patient, a 17-year-old male with a diagnosis of chronic paranoid schizophrenia, had a final Axis III diagnosis of "rule out hypoglycemia." In the hospital, the patient had a serum glucose level of 54 mg/dl. He was transferred on a commitment to another hospital, and further workup was not done. Numerous adolescents in this study had low serum glucose levels by reference standards of 75–110 mg/dl, but were not thought to have symptoms based on hypoglycemia or medical conditions referable to hypoglycemia. Most authors diagnose hypoglycemia at serum glucose levels of below 45–50 mg/dl (Freinkel, 1979; Haymond, 1982) which no patient in this study had. It does seem, however, that the reason for frequent low glucose levels in adolescent patients needs further evaluation if these findings are confirmed by others.

Another patient, an 18-year-old female with a diagnosis of bipolar disorder on Axis I, received a final Axis III diagnosis of "questionable abnormality on chest X ray." Screening chest X ray showed a questionable soft tissue density which was felt due to either lung infiltrate or breast tissue. This was not followed up during the hospitalization, perhaps on clinical grounds.

In addition to these seven patients, numerous patients had initial abnormalities on hemoglobin, hematocrit, or total leukocyte count even when corrected values based on age appropriate norms were used. None of the abnormalities was in the anemic range, however. Many laboratory results showed mild elevations of hemoglobin or hematocrit or mild total leukocyte depression of uncertain significance and were often not repeated.

Numerous patients also had seemingly mild abnormalities on initial routine urinalysis (e.g., slight pyuria of 5–8 white blood cells per high-powered field; minimal hematuria indicated by reports of "rare RBC," "2–5 RBC"; "trace to one plus proteinuria"). Most of these also were not followed up, and therefore it was not possible to say if there would have been a productive yield of true medical pathology by screening urinalysis in this population.

Nine EKGs in this group were possibly abnormal. Seven of these had minor or questionable changes and were not repeated. One of these was discussed earlier. Another patient's EKG had a probable coronary sinus rhythm and questionable repolarization and was not repeated. One anorexia nervosa patient had an EKG with a junctional rhythm and a rate of 32 beats per minute. When repeated 12 days later, an EKG showed normal conduction time and a rate of 58 beats per minute. EKGs in patients with anorexia nervosa may at times be indicated on clinical grounds and not necessarily considered a screening procedure.

Numerous patients had seemingly minor abnormalities on the chemistry panel, often in electrolyte levels, apart from the serum glucose levels just discussed. Often these were very minor and were not repeated.

Overall, Gabel and Hsu (1986) found a high rate of abnormalities noted on the various screening tests done. Except possibly for the few instances previously noted in which discharge Axis III listings resulted from a routine screening test, however, there was no indication of benefit to patients from the variety of screening tests performed and no definite evidence of undetected medical disorder being newly discovered through the use of screening tests. Furthermore, it is uncertain if the seven conditions resulting from the screening procedures and listed on Axis III resulted in any medical benefit because of that listing. The large number of abnormal results on screening tests that were often minor but had no follow-up leaves open the question of whether some medical screening tests in psychiatrically hospitalized adolescents might be of value.

Gabel and Hsu point out that more research is clearly needed to determine whether thyroid function test abnormalities and low serum glucose levels are frequent in adolescent psychiatric patients. They also point out that routine urinalysis may have a place in screening, and CBCs also may have a place in screening selected adolescent populations (although this was not demonstrated in their population of relatively small sample size). However, such conclusions were not possible in this population because there was no follow-up on seemingly minor abnormal results, making it impossible to establish their importance. Gabel and Hsu found no apparent medical benefit from screening with the rapid plasma reagin (RPR) chest X ray, or EKG, although, again, their sample size was fairly small.

Gabel and Hsu emphasize that the question of whether the routine ordering of laboratory tests has value in a screening sense in detecting medical disorders can be answered only by careful evaluation of each test that is ordered, the needs of the population to be screened, the goals of the screening program, and a variety of other factors related to established guidelines for the development and maintenance of a good screening program (Frankenburg & Camp, 1975). Finally, as Gabel and Hsu (1986) repeatedly pointed out, it is crucial to carefully follow up on abnormal results.

FREQUENCY OF MEDICAL PROBLEMS IN THE PSYCHIATRICALLY HOSPITALIZED ADOLESCENT

Numerous studies cited earlier have emphasized that medical problems are frequent in psychiatric patients. As noted, however, most of the patients in these studies except for that of Gabel and Hsu (1986) seem to have been in the adult and geriatric age ranges. As discussed earlier, the study of Gabel and Hsu found that screening for medical problems using eight laboratory tests was rather ineffective in detecting new medical problems in their group. They did note, however, based on initial Axis III diagnoses or conditions (see Table 4.1) and final Axis III diagnoses or conditions that were not listed on admission (see Table 4.4), that numerous medical conditions were given emphasis or detected during the hospitalization, although not because of the screening tests employed.

Some of these conditions were minor, but some would merit additional medical intervention. It does seem, however, based on this study, that adolescent psychiatric inpatients may have fewer severe medical problems than their adult and geriatric counterparts. To determine whether adolescent psychiatric inpatients had more medical problems than a comparable group of nonpsychiatric patient adolescents would have required a psychiatrically normal adolescent control group which the study of Gabel and Hsu did not have. Nonetheless, it may be stated, based on the numerous problems noted in Tables 4.1 and 4.4, that careful attention to medical problems in adolescent psychiatric inpatients is warranted. Furthermore, careful attention and possible screening for likely sources of medical disorders in the adolescent psychiatric group, such as vaginal infection, pelvic inflammatory disease, hepatitis, and other sequelae of illicit drug use may yield more instances of medical problems in this age group than were found in the Gabel and Hsu study.

Medical Disorders with Early Psychiatric Manifestations

Many medical or neurological disorders and abnormal metabolic states are associated with behavioral or emotional problems at some point in their course and may be confused with primary psychiatric (functional) disorders. The medical physician or neurologist may, in these cases, call on the psychiatrist to help diagnose or treat the psychiatric manifestations of the medical or neurological illness.

On the other hand, as repeatedly pointed out in this chapter, it is well-known that many patients initially felt to have purely psychological problems, conversion disorders, or "hysteria" subsequently demonstrated organic disease (Trimble, 1981). This is notable with disorders of the central nervous system. Rivinus, Jamison, and Graham (1975) reported on 12 children referred to a pediatric neurology service who had had psychiatric disorders diagnosed initially. Later, neurological disorders were diagnosed. The psychiatric diagnoses included anxiety state, child psychosis, hysterical reaction, behavior disorder, and conduct disorder. The neurological disorders diagnosed included tumors, Friedrich's ataxia, subacute sclerosing panencephalitis, metachromatic leukodystrophy, and dystonia musculorum deformans. Characteristic features in the symptomatology of these patients included deteriorating school performance, visual loss, and postural disturbance.

This section will discuss certain medical conditions or problems that may first be present in late childhood or adolescence which have early or prominent psychological symptoms to the degree that the causative medical problem may be overlooked or the problem misdiagnosed as psychiatric or functional. In some cases, there are initially few or no abnormal signs on a physical examination to suggest the underlying medical problem.

Hepatolenticular degeneration (Wilson's disease) is a disorder of copper metabolism that is transmitted on an autosomal recessive basis (Trimble, 1981; Solomon, 1985). The liver and brain are commonly involved, with symptoms related to the deposition of unbound copper in the liver, basal ganglia, and elsewhere. Presenting problems may be neurologic, psychiatric, or related to liver dysfunction. Symptoms of neurologic disorder include rigidity, tremor, dystonia, and athetosis. School phobia, behavior problems, mood swings, depressive, hypomanic, and schizophrenic-like psychiatric symptoms have been reported. Diagnostic aids include presence of the Kayser Fleischer ring, an area of brown coloration along the outer zone of the cornea seen on slit-lamp examination, low blood cerruloplasmin level, increased urinary copper levels, and aminoaciduria. Liver biopsy is sometimes performed. Untreated, death usually occurs in a few years, but penicillamine treatment to decrease copper absorption is usually beneficial.

Huntington's chorea (Steinberg, 1983; Solomon, 1985) is an inherited disorder affecting predominantly the cerebral cortex and basal ganglia. It is inherited as an autosomal dominant. The onset is usually between ages 30 to 50, but earlier onset occurs. Personality change is the first sign of the illness in many cases, and psychosis is present during the illness in half the patients. Dementia develops slowly, often associated with the psychological symptoms, the chorea being later in onset. Sometimes, however, dementia and chorea begin together, and less often the chorea precedes the dementia. There is a high suicide rate. Neuronal loss with atrophy of the caudate, putamen, and cerebral cortex may be found at autopsy.

Metachromatic leukodystrophy (Steinberg, 1983) is one of a group of genetically determined neurological disorders in which progressive degeneration occurs, primarily because of abnormal metabolism of myelin constituents. The mode of inheritance is autosomal recessive. Several forms have been described. In the juvenile form, the onset of symptoms may be in early to later childhood. The initial symptoms may be emotional disturbances or intellectual deterioration, neurological signs becoming prominent later.

Adrenoleukodystrophy (Steinberg, 1983; Solomon, 1985) is an X-linked leukodystrophy with usual onset in middle childhood, but which can occur in late childhood. Neurological manifestations generally precede symptoms of adrenal involvement. Behavioral changes, such as aggression, withdrawal, and decreased school performance (with progressive dementia) are common presenting features.

Complex partial seizures may be a difficult diagnosis. It is well known that there is an increased prevalence of psychiatric disorder among patients with epilepsy. This is especially true for patients with complex partial seizure disorders (psychmotor or temporal lobe epilepsy). In addition, patients with complex partial seizure disorders may be mistakenly diagnosed as having primary psychiatric illnesses because of the patient's behavior during the peri-ictal state (Allen, 1981).

Complex partial seizures may be associated with only a period of altered consciousness, although they characteristically include stereotyped and repetitive movements (automatisms), such as facial grimacing, chewing, lip smacking, hand and finger movements, walking in a circle, and so on. The motor acts appear similar to normal motor activity but are performed repetitively and inappropriately. During the seizure, various emotional states, hallucinations, and sensory experiences may occur. Uncontrollable laughter, fear, or anxiety may also be present. Irrelevant, repetitive, and odd speech patterns may occur. There may be aphasia. The episodes usually last less than 15 minutes. Consciousness is altered, and there is often, but not always, amnesia for the event (Trimble, 1981). Violence is unusual unless the individual is interfered with during the automatism, when conflict can be provoked. Even at those times the behavior is poorly directed and not likely to be harmful to others. When the partial complex seizures are continuous, the prolonged states of confusion with automatisms may resemble psychosis. During these attacks, however, continuous epileptiform activity from the temporal lobes is characteristic on the EEG.

At times the manifestation of the complex partial seizure may be difficult to distinguish from generalized petit mal attacks (Allen, 1981). This is especially true when the former shows alteration in consciousness with only very subtle automatisms. Petit mal seizures (absence attacks or staring spells) are generalized seizures usually beginning between 4 and 10 years of age. They often cease before the age of 20. Seizures last from a few to 30 seconds. During the attacks, the patient loses awareness and has a staring spell or absence; involuntary rhythmic movements of eyelids, mouth, and arms also may occur. There is no aura or post-ictal confusion in petit mal seizures. After an attack, the patient immediately regains consciousness and resumes his or her preseizure activity.

Petit mal seizures generally occur many times a day, where the usual complex partial seizure is less frequent and lasts for minutes, not seconds, as in petit mal attacks. Occasionally, however, the characteristic EEG pattern of petit mal epilepsy, the 2.5–3 Hz spike and wave pattern, may last for hours or days, resulting in petit mal status. During these prolonged periods, the youngster appears like an automaton, interacts poorly with the environment, appears distant and vague, and then suddenly and unexplainably returns to the usual conscious state. Careful evaluation, including EEG recordings, may be necessary to clarify the clinical picture.

Juvenile Thyrotoxicosis. Thyrotoxicosis in childhood occurs almost always as a result of diffuse thyroid hyperplasia (Graves' disease) (Fisher, 1982). While in adult hyperthyroidism, eye manifestations and dermopathy are characteristic of Graves' disease, in childhood, eye manifestations and dermopathy are absent or mild. The disease is not uncommon in preschoolers, but there is a sharp increase in incidence as children approach adolescence. Females are affected about six times as often as males. A high proportion of patients have a family history positive for goiter or thyroid dysfunction. The onset is usually insidious, with a period of increasing nervousness, palpitation, appetite increase, and weakness of the muscles. Some patients experience weight loss, but a voracious appetite may prevent this. Except for the eye findings (e.g., exophthalmos), the symptoms of thyrotoxicosis are nonspecific and may be mistaken for another disorder for prolonged periods. Behavior problems, decline in school performance, and "nervousness" frequently dominate the clinical picture. In other patients, cardiovascular signs are more prominent, and symptoms of decreased exercise tolerance are found. Fatigability and muscle weakness are also common. Diagnosis is made by laboratory evaluation of thyroid function. Treatment may involve radioactive iodine, surgery, medication with antithyroid agents or a combination of approaches.

SUMMARY

Numerous studies indicate that patients with psychiatric disorders have high rates of medical or organic problems either causing or associated with their psychiatric disorders. Such studies generally have based their findings on populations heavily weighted toward the adult and geriatric age ranges and have sometimes recommended laboratory screening procedures as part of an overall attempt to detect these medical problems. Adolescent psychiatric inpatients also have numerous medical problems, but it does not seem that these medical problems are as likely to be causally related to the psychiatric disorder with which they present as is true with older psychiatric patients.

A complete medical history and physical examination, with attention to the neurological evaluation, should be part of initial admission procedures for adolescent psychiatric hospitalization. Subsequent laboratory tests should be based on specific clinical indications in that patient or based on a reasonable likelihood of positive findings that will be clinically useful, given a knowledge of the adolescent population.

REFERENCES

Allen, R. J. (1981). Neurological evaluation of children with behavioral disturbances. In S. Gabel (Ed.), *Behavioral problems in childhood: A primary care approach* (pp. 243–257). New York: Grune & Stratton, Inc.

American Psychiatric Association (1987). *Diagnostic and statistical manual of mental disorders* (3rd ed., rev.). (DSM-III-R). Washington, DC.

American Psychiatric Association (1980). *Diagnostic and statistical manual of mental disorders* (3rd ed.). (DSM-III). Washington, DC.

Fisher, D. A. (1982). The thyroid gland. In A. M. Rudolph (Ed.), *Pediatrics* (17th ed.) (pp. 1517–1534). Norwalk, CT: Appleton-Century-Crofts.

Frankenburg, W. K., & Camp, B. W. (1975). *Pediatric screening tests.* Springfield, IL: Thomas.

Freinkel, N. (1979). Hypoglycemic disorders. In P. B. Beeson, W. McDermot, & J. B. Syngarden (Eds.), *Cecil textbook of medicine* (15th ed.) (Vol. 2, pp. 1989–1997). Philadelphia: Saunders.

Fogel, B. S., & Slaby, A. E. (1986). Neurological screening of psychiatric patients. In I. Extein & M. S. Gold (Eds.), *Medical mimics of psychiatric disorders* (pp. 13–32). Washington, DC: American Psychiatric Press.

Gabel, S., & Hsu, L. K. G. (1986). Routine laboratory tests in adolescent psychiatric inpatients: Their value in making psychiatric diagnoses and in detecting medical disorders. *Journal American Academy of Child Psychiatry, 25,* 113–119.

Gardner, E. R., & Hall, R. C. W. (1980). Medical screening of psychiatric patients. *Journal of Orthomolecular Psychiatry, 9,* 207–211.

Hall, R. C. W., Gardner, E. R., Popkin, M. K., Lecann, A. F., & Stickney, S. K. (1981). Unrecognized physical illness prompting psychiatric admission: A prospective study. *American Journal of Psychiatry, 138,* 629–635.

Hall, R. C. W., Popkin, M. K., Devaul, R. A., Faillace, L. A., & Stickney, S. K. (1978). Physical illness presenting as psychiatric disease. *Archives of General Psychiatry, 35,* 1315–1320.

Haymond, M. W. (1982). Hypoglycemia. In A. M. Rudolph (Ed.), *Pediatrics,* (17th Ed.) (pp. 283–291). Norwalk, CT: Appleton-Century-Crofts.

Hollender, M. H. & Wells, C. E. (1982). Medical assessment in psychiatric practice. In H. I. Kaplan, A. M. Freedmen, & B. J. Sadock (Eds.), *Comprehensive Textbook of Psychiatry, Vol. I.* (pp. 987–989). Baltimore: Williams & Wilkins.

Johnson, D. A. W. (1968). The evaluation of routine physical examination in psychiatric cases. *Practitioner, 200,* 686–691.

Koranyi, E. K. (1979). Morbidity and rate of undiagnosed physical illness in a psychiatric clinic population. *Archives of General Psychiatry, 36,* 414–419.

Maguire, C. P., & Granville-Grossman, K. L. (1968). Physical illness in psychiatric patients. *British Journal of Psychiatry, 115,* 1365–1369.

Muecke, L. N., & Krueger, D. W. (1981). Physical findings in a psychiatric outpatient clinic. *American Journal of Psychiatry, 138,* 1241–1242.

Penick, S. B., & Carrier, R. N. (1967). Serious medical illness in an acute psychiatric hospital. *Journal of the Medial Society of New Jersey, 64,* 651–653.

Reed, K., & Bland, R. C. (1977). Masked "myxedema madness." *Acta Psychiatrica Scandanavico, 56,* 421–426.

Rivinus, T. M., Jamison, J. L., & Graham, P. J. (1975). Childhood organic neurological disease presenting as psychiatric disorder. *Archives of Disease in Childhood, 50,* 115–119.

Solomon, S. (1985). Neurology. In H. I. Kaplan and B. J. Sadock (Eds.), *Comprehensive textbook of psychiatry,* (4th Ed.) (pp. 78–156). Baltimore, MD: Williams & Wilkins.

Spratt, D. I., Pont, A., Miller, M. D., McDougall, I. R., Bayer, M. F., & McLaughlin, W. T. (1982). Hyperthyroxinemia in patients with acute psychiatric disorders. *American Journal of Medicine, 73,* 41–48.

Steinberg, D. (1983). *The clinical psychiatry of adolescence.* New York: Wiley.

Trimble, M. R. (1981). *Neuropsychiatry.* New York: Wiley.

Watson, C. G., & Buranen, C. (1979). The frequency and identification of false positive conversion reactions. *Journal of Nervous and Mental Disease, 167,* 243–247.

Willett, A. B., & King, T. (1977). Implementation of laboratory screening procedures on a short-term psychiatric unit. *Disease of the Nervous System, 38* 867–870.

CHAPTER FIVE

Psychological Evaluation

Anthony P. Mannarino

Reference books in child psychiatry have typically encompassed the areas of child, adolescent, and family psychiatry. The focus of the vast majority of these works has been on prepubertal children. The period of adolescence has not been commonly treated as a separate developmental era with its unique psychiatric problems. This neglect of adolescence also occurs in adult psychiatry, as reference works on adults seldom include sections specifically relevant to adolescents. Thus adolescent psychiatry has been lost between the boundaries of childhood and adulthood, being considered part of each period but often treated as peripheral to both.

Fortunately, this situation is changing. At least part of the change can be attributed to two factors. First, specific psychiatric disorders have been identified that commonly originate during adolescence and often extend into the adult years. For example, it is widely recognized that eating disorders such as anorexia nervosa and bulimia typically arise during the teenage years. Especially if untreated, both disorders can devastate the psychological and physical well-being of afflicted adolescents and make the transition into adulthood highly problematic. In addition, there are other psychiatric disorders, although not unique to adolescence, that are extremely prevalent during this time. In this regard, both the professional literature and mass media have extensively addressed such serious teenage problems as suicide, alcohol and substance abuse, and delinquency. Because of these developments, adolescent psychiatry no longer can be considered an insignificant component of either child or adult psychiatry. The psychiatric problems of adolescence merit special attention. This notion is increasingly being accepted; witness the eight chapters devoted solely to the "problems of adolescence" in a major reference work in clinical child psychology (Walker & Roberts, 1983).

As adolescent psychiatry gains prominence, psychological assessment and evaluation are reemerging as important and valued functions of psychologists. During the post-World War II era, psychological assessment, largely testing, was the major role of clinical psychologists. However, as the field expanded and with the professional enhancement provided by state licensing laws in psychology, clinical psychologists began to devote a much greater percentage of their time to therapy and consultation activities. Assessment became a less valued function, partly due to this professional growth but also because psychologists sought the recognition and status accorded to psychiatry.

Over the past decade, psychological assessment and evaluation have become much more sophisticate and refined. Major advances in such areas as behavioral assessment, neuropsychological assessment, family assessment, and psychophysiological assessment have occurred. All of these areas are highly specialized and require extensive training. These advances have broadened the assessment field and have given it increased value and importance. Few of these advances, however, pertain specifically or only to adolescents. The majority focus on children or adults and have either upward or downward extensions to include adolescents. A major clinical task, therefore, is deciding which among the multitude of new and innovative assessment techniques can adequately tap the unique problems of adolescence.

There are two major areas that will be discussed in this chapter. First, the critical developmental issues of adolescence and how they impact on the process of psychological evaluation will be addressed. Second, a general but not all-inclusive survey of available assessment methods will be presented.

DEVELOPMENTAL CONSIDERATIONS

A comprehensive psychological evaluation of a child cannot be conducted without careful consideration of the issues associated with that child's developmental stage. These issues will vary according to the age of the child. They serve as the "context" within which the child must be assessed. No less is true for the adolescent. The unique social, psychological, cognitive, and physiological changes of this period also serve as the context for a reliable and valid psychological evaluation. Although the developmental issues of adolescence are addressed extensively in another chapter of this volume, they will be highlighted here as they relate specifically to psychological evaluation.

Physiological Changes

The physiological changes for boys and girls associated with puberty are well documented (Tanner, 1962). The adolescent growth spurt, maturation of sexual organs, and development of secondary sex characteristics (Marshall & Tanner, 1969) are now widely recognized phenomena. A comprehensive psychological assessment of a teenager must consider how these physiological changes impact on psychological functioning. For example, these changes may be perceived as a source of embarrassment and could make the adolescent very self-conscious with his or her peer group. This would have implications for self-concept development. In a different light, some research has documented that "early maturers" have higher self-esteem, are more popular, and are better adjusted than "later maturers" (Jones, 1958; Jones & Bayley, 1950). This kind of research underscores the importance of assessing how the physiological changes associated with puberty are perceived by the adolescent and of evaluating how this perception contributes to successful adjustment or development of psychiatric difficulties.

Cognitive Development

According to Piaget (1962), adolescents enter a more advanced cognitive stage called formal operations. Hallmarks of this stage are the capacity to think in an abstract manner and to engage in hypothesis testing. These advances are the cognitive foundation for the idealism that permeates this period, as the adolescent is able to consider the world of possibilities in addition to what already exists. Such "idealism" can easily become alienation when the adolescent faces the "hard reality" of family, friends, and school. Thus the very same cognitive mechanism that permits the adolescent to imagine all the wonderful possibilities of life can also trigger the sense of frustration and disappointment associated with unfulfilled hopes and expectations.

The psychological evaluation of an adolescent must address this issue in at least two ways. First, there must be an assessment of his or her intellectual functioning as it is moderately well correlated with Piaget's hypothesized cognitive changes (Mussen, Conger, & Kagan, 1979). (For example, a retarded adolescent would be less likely to engage in abstract thinking and is more focused on concrete, here-and-now issues. This would have definite implications for ongoing treatment.) This intellectual assessment could take the form of an intelligence test or could be a clinical or global estimation based on the psychologist's experience. Second, the impact of these cognitive changes must be evaluated to determine if they are contributing to unfulfilled expectations, frustration, and alienation.

Identity Formation

A major developmental task of adolescence is identity formation. As Erikson (1950) has stated, a failure to formulate a solid sense of self during this time can result in emotional instability and role diffusion. Clinically speaking, this may mean poor self-esteem, lack of clearly defined goals, inadequate motivation, and excessive susceptibility to negative peer group influence. All of these difficulties can make the adolescent at risk for depressive symptoms or peer-influenced problems such as drug and alcohol abuse and delinquency. Accordingly, a comprehensive psychological evaluation must address the adolescent's sense of self and whether a solid foundation for an organized and systematic identity is being formulated. This information will allow the psychologist to better understand the adolescent's most unique qualities and can be used in diagnostic decisions and treatment planning.

Emancipation-Independence

Another significant developmental task of adolescence is emancipation from the family (Conger, 1977). Although this is a gradual process, it is not always achieved easily. There are many influences, including parent expectations, peer group involvement, and the adolescent's own psychological makeup. The degree to which independence is achieved and the manner in which it is pursued can often provide diagnostic data regarding the adolescent's adjustment and struggles with parents over this issue. A critical variable in the psychological assessment of any adolescent, therefore, is evaluating his or her level of independence, whether the level is appropriate to the age-period, and the impact and influence of parents and peers on the attainment of this goal.

Peer Relations

Greater independence from the family inevitably results in wider peer group participation. This is a healthy step during adolescence. With increased peer activities, the adolescent is able to better establish his or her sense of self and begin preparation for the transition into adulthood. Extreme peer group identification or involvement, though, can be a sign that the adolescent is struggling with his or her parents over issues of emancipation. Furthermore, a peer group can have both a positive and negative impact. For example, the peer group can be a constructive testing group for new behaviors such as dating, leadership roles, and career-oriented activities. It also provides increased opportunity, however, for the development of serious problems such as drug and alcohol abuse and delinquency.

Unfortunately, psychological evaluations have often focused on the internal psychology of the adolescent and his or her relations to family members, especially parents. It is the contention here that peer relations need to be given greater attention because of their impact on the achievement of other developmental tasks of adolescence. Moreover, longitudinal research (Kohlberg, LaCrosse, & Ricks, 1972) has documented that solid peer relations during preadolescence and adolescence are highly predictive of stable adult functioning, while poor peer relations during these periods can lead to an array of adult psychopathologies. Thus an assessment of the adolescent's peer group involvement and its influence may have both short- and long-term predictive value.

Other Context Factors

At the beginning of this section, it was suggested that the developmental issues associated with adolescence must serve as the context for a psychological assessment. There are two additional context factors that must be considered in all evaluations: family and school. The scope of this chapter does not permit a comprehensive discussion of either factor. However, a few comments about each are indicated.

Although the adolescent is beginning to become independent and peer oriented, the impact of the family on his or her development remains significant. The growth of family therapy certainly underscores the notion that parents, siblings, and extended family members contribute to both healthy development and psychopathology. In addition, evidence is accumulating that the family plays a unique role in the development of specific psychiatric problems commonly originating during adolescence, such as eating disorders (Leon & Phelan, 1985). A comprehensive evaluation of an adolescent, therefore, must include an assessment of family interaction and the expectations and perceptions of individual family members.

A decline in school performance is frequently associated with a variety of child and adolescent psychiatric disorders. This decline may apply either to academic performance, behavior in the classroom, or both. In fact, the most serious problems that the child/adolescent presents may be school related, and the school is often the referral source for children/adolescents to psychiatric clinics. For these reasons, a comprehensive psychological evaluation of an adolescent must include school information. Some of this data can be obtained from the teenager and the parents. However, it is important that the psychologist contact the school directly, as classroom teachers, administrators, and counselors may have quite different perceptions of the problem. Of course, this can only be done if the adolescent and his or her parents authorize in writing that the psychologist can obtain the desired information.

To reiterate, a consideration of contextual factors must be a basic component of all psychological evaluations of adolescents. As outlined earlier, these factors include developmental issues, the family, and the school. Regardless of the nature of the referral complaint, these factors cannot be ignored. They are the essential context within which the adolescent must be evaluated.

ASSESSMENT METHODS

Few assessment techniques have been developed which pertain solely to adolescents. They typically focus on children or adults and have either upward or downward extensions to include adolescents. This chapter is far too limited in scope to consider the broad range of evaluation procedures applicable to the adolescent period. The following discussion will concentrate on traditional techniques that are still widely used plus innovative methods that have recently been developed. Issues pertinent to adolescent assessment will be the major emphasis. (Table 5.1 contains a more complete listing of assessment instruments, many of which are not discussed in this chapter.)

Interview

The interview remains the most extensively utilized evaluation procedure with all age groups. Some unique issues arise when it is used to acquire

Table 5.1. Assessment Methods Applicable to Adolescents

Instrument	Reference
A. *Intelligence tests*	
Stanford-Binet Intelligence Scale	Terman & Merrill (1973)
Wechsler Intelligence Scale for Children-Revised	Wechsler (1974)
Peabody Picture Vocabulary Test	Dunn (1965)
Cattell Culture Fair Intelligence Tests	Cattell & Cattell (1973)
Leiter International Performance Scale	Leiter (1969)
B. *Achievement tests*	
Peabody Individual Achievement Test	Dunn & Markwardt (1970)
Wide Range Achievement Test	Jastek & Jastek (1978)
Metropolitan Achievement Tests	Prescott, Balow, Hogan & Farr (1978)
Woodcock-Johnson Psycho-Educational Battery	Woodcock & Johnson (1977)
C. *Personality testing*	
Minnesota Multiphasic Personality Inventory	Marks, Seeman, & Haller (1974)
Thematic Apperception Test	Ames, Metraux, & Walker (1971)
Rorschach	Ames, Metraux, & Walker (1971)
Children's Personality Questionnaire	Porter & Cattell (1972)
Rotter Incomplete Sentences Blank	Rotter, Rafferty, & Lotsof (1954)
D. *Behaviorally-based rating scales*	
Behavior Problem Checklist	Quay & Peterson (1975)
Child Behavior Checklist	Achenbach (1979)
Eyberg Child Behavior Inventory	Eyberg & Ross (1978)
Louisville Behavior Checklist	Miller (1977)
Personality Inventory for Children	Wirt, Lachar, Klinedinst, & Seat (1977)
Devereux Adolescent Behavior Rating Scale	Spivack, Spotts, & Haines (1967)
E. *Self-report, empirically-based instruments*	
Children's Depression Inventory	Kovacs (1981)
Children's Manifest Anxiety Scale	Castenada, McCandless, & Palermo (1956)
State-Trait Anxiety Inventory for Children	Spielberger (1973)
Piers-Harris Children's Self-Concept Scale	Piers-Harris (1969)
F. *Neuropsychological assessment*	
Halstead-Reitan Neuropsychological Battery	Reitan & Davison (1974)
Luria-Nebraska Battery	Golden, Hammeke, & Purisch (1978)

information from adolescents. First, teenagers may be wary of responding to a psychologist's questions because they likely have been extensively criticized before by parents or other authority figures. Accordingly, they need to know that their opinions will be respected and that they will have input into the decision-making process (Goldman, L'Engle-Stein, & Guerry, 1983). If treated without respect or as if they are younger children, they will probably reveal little about themselves.

A second issue is confidentiality. This is of particular concern if questions are being asked regarding sexual involvement, drug or alcohol usage, or extralegal activities (Mannarino, 1986). At the outset of the interview, the psychologist must clarify the limits of confidentiality with the adolescent. Although this discussion may result in some reticence on the adolescent's part to reveal critical information, it is likely to be perceived as honest and forthright and may in fact lead to greater candor.

Since adolescents are usually much more verbally adept than younger children, they may more easily participate in family assessments. Family interviews can provide the psychologist with important data regarding family psychopathology, family interaction, and parental perceptions of problem areas. Some adolescents may be reluctant to reveal information in such an evaluation format, however, because of long-standing conflicts with parents or a general distrust of adult authority figures. If this is so, the adolescent's privacy should be respected. Parents also may request a separate interview because they experience anxiety in discussing information about their son or daughter in the adolescent's presence. In addition, parental interviews can be used to obtain background material and a developmental history. However, it must be remembered that parents have been shown to be unreliable reporters of historical material (Wenar, 1961; Wenar & Coulter, 1962).

Psychological Testing

Volumes have been devoted to psychological testing; however, the author is unaware of any book devoted solely to testing with adolescents. A brief survey of testing methods relevant to adolescents will be presented here. Again, the emphasis will be on special issues that apply when these techniques are used with this age group.

Intelligence Testing. The individual intelligence tests most widely used with adolescents are the Stanford-Binet Intelligence Scale (Terman & Merrill, 1973) and the Wechsler Intelligence Scale for Children-Revised (WISC-R) (Wechsler, 1974). Both offer excellent norms and are supported by numerous reliability and validity studies. Because it is highly weighted toward verbal skills when administered to adolescents, the Binet is particularly useful for youngsters with visual or motor handicaps. The

WISC-R is balanced more evenly between verbal and nonverbal abilities and allows the examiner to develop a profile of skills for each adolescent.

Either test is reliable for ruling out mental retardation in adolescents. It is worth noting, however, that since many adolescents referred for evaluation may have been tested several times previously, practice effects can artificially enhance scores. On the other hand, because of their emotional sensitivity and self-consciousness, adolescents may be more prone to performance anxiety. The psychologist must also clarify with the adolescent who will receive information about test results and other issues pertinent to confidentiality.

Achievement Testing. Two individual achievement tests commonly administered by psychologists are the Peabody Individual Achievement Test (PIAT) (Dunn & Markwardt, 1970) and the Wide Range Achievement Test (WRAT) (Jastek & Jastek, 1978). Both can be used with children and adolescents and include reading, spelling, and mathematics subtests. The PIAT also has reading comprehension and general information subtests and has better standardization than the WRAT (Goldman et al., 1983). Neither test has strongly supportive validity data, however.

As is the case with intelligence testing, the psychologist must be sensitive to practice effects, performance anxiety, and issues of confidentiality when administering achievement tests to teenagers. Moreover, because significant numbers of adolescents referred for psychological evaluation have experienced many years of academic failure, they may be very threatened by achievement testing which, in many ways, is similar to school tasks. This can exacerbate performance anxiety or even result in a lackluster effort by teenagers convinced that they will have little success on such a test.

Personality Testing

The Minnesota Multiphasic Personality Inventory (MMPI) was developed based on data provided by adult psychiatric patients. Marks, Seeman, and Haller (1974) presented tables for adolescents. Their standardization sample included 1800 normal and 3000 emotionally disturbed teenagers. Marks et al. (1974) demonstrated that adult MMPI norms have to be adjusted to be appropriate for an adolescent population. Nonetheless, these adolescent norms are not entirely satisfactory because the standardization sample included only white adolescents living at home. Accordingly, a clinical psychologist using an MMPI with a teenager must be cautious about interpretation of test results.

The Thematic Apperception Test (TAT) and Rorschach continue to be used extensively by many clinical psychologists. They are probably the best examples of the practice of projective testing which assumes that a person's perceptions are determined by underlying psychological processes. Both the TAT and Rorschach have been criticized severely because of their lack of predictive validity and inattention to psychometric properties. However, Ames, Metraux, and Walker (1971) did establish norms for children and adolescents ages 10 to 16. The standardization sample was quite skewed, though, as most of the children had above-average IQ and were from professional families.

Compared to younger children, adolescents referred for psychological evaluation may be much more highly suspicious of projective testing. Because of their greater capacity for introspection, they might feel that such testing is an invasion of privacy. For example, an adolescent who is discovering his or her own sexual impulses may believe that a projective test will reveal innermost thoughts and fantasies. Since such feelings may be new and perhaps discomforting, there can be a concern that the psychologist will perceive the adolescent as being "crazy." Particularly during an initial assessment session, it may be more appropriate to employ more direct, straightforward evaluation methods, such as interviewing and IQ or achievement testing, to lessen these concerns.

Behaviorally Based Rating Scales

Behaviorally based instruments have recently achieved greater prominence. This is consistent with the rise of behavioral interventions and decline of traditional psychodynamic therapies (Goldman et al., 1983). Behavior rating scales typically use either parents or teachers as respondents. Quay and Peterson (1975) developed the 55-item Behavior Problem Checklist which uses parents as raters. It is simple to administer and provides a good descriptive analysis of a youngster's behavior problems. Most of the items are appropriate for adolescents.

The Child Behavior Checklist (CBCL) (Achenbach & Edelbrock, 1979) has a number of distinct advantages over other behavior rating scales. First, it has separate profiles based on sex and age. (For example, there are profiles for both teenage boys and girls ages 12 to 16.) In addition, there are social competence scales to rate adaptive behavior. Finally, three versions of the CBCL (parent, teacher, and self-report) permit comparisons among different respondents. Other commonly used scales appropriate for young adolescents are the Eyberg Child Behavior Inventory (Eyberg & Ross, 1978) and the Louisville Behavior Checklist (Miller, 1977).

All of these instruments are easily administered and provide quantifiable data. However, they also are subject to respondent bias. There is always the possibility that teachers or parents will respond to specific items based on inaccurate observations, poor recall, or simply what they assume the psychologist expects (Goldman et al., 1983).

Self-Report Scales

The Children's Depression Inventory (CDI) (Kovacs, 1981) was designed to assess depression in children aged 6 to 17. There are 27 items geared toward commonly accepted symptoms of depression such as sleep disturbance, sadness, poor self-image, and so on. The CDI is easy to score and administer, and some reasonably good reliability and validity data have been collected to support its use. Other widely known self-report instruments include the Children's Manifest Anxiety Scale (Castenada, McCandless, & Palermo, 1956), State-Trait Anxiety Inventory for Children (Spielberger, 1973), and the Piers-Harris Children's Self-Concept Scale (Piers & Harris, 1969). All of these scales are appropriate for adolescents.

Like the behavior rating scales, self-report instruments are subject to respondent bias. This can be caused by a wish to obtain approval from the examiner, poor recall, or an inability to accurately report symptoms or other personal characteristics. In addition, as mentioned during the discussion on personality testing, adolescents may be quite reticent about responding to items which reflect emotional or behavioral difficulties because of a fear of being perceived as "crazy."

SPECIAL DIAGNOSTIC CONSIDERATIONS

Regardless of assessment methods, psychologists evaluating adolescents need to pay attention to certain diagnostic categories that have special relevance to this age period. Specifically, they are suicide, substance abuse, antisocial behavior, and eating disorders. Each of these areas will be discussed in detail in separate chapters of this book. It needs to be pointed out here, however, that the risk of facing these psychiatric problems is much greater for teenagers than for children. This is at least partly true because the developmental changes of adolescence increase the likelihood that these psychiatric difficulties will arise. For example, the strong influence of a peer group can make an adolescent susceptible to drug or alcohol abuse or antisocial behavior. In addition, some authors have clearly suggested that an inability to cope with the developmental issue of emancipation-independence contributes to the onset of eating disorders (Leon & Phelan, 1985). Finally, the ability to think abstractly during adolescence, although normally a positive cognitive change, can also set the foundation for the hopelessness often associated with severe depression and suicide.

Thus the normal developmental tasks of adolescence and how they are dealt with have special significance for these diagnostic categories. Psychologists must focus their attention to some extent on these developmental issues to insure that important diagnoses are not overlooked and to increase their understanding of the etiology of these psychiatric difficulties.

SUMMARY

This chapter has attempted to accomplish two major tasks. First, the critical developmental issues of adolescence and how they impact on the process of psychological evaluation have been addressed. Then a general but not all-inclusive survey of available assessment methods applicable to adolescents has been presented. The major thrust throughout the chapter has been on developmental considerations and other unique aspects of adolescence that serve as the context for any psychological evaluation.

REFERENCES

Achenbach, T. M., & Edelbrock C. S. (1979). The child behavior profile II: Boys aged 12–16 and girls aged 6–11 and 12–16. *Journal of Consulting and Clinical Psychology, 47,* 223–233.

Ames, L. B., Metraux, R. W., & Walker, R. N. (1971). *Adolescent Rorschach responses: Developmental trends from ten to sixteen years.* New York: Brunner/Mazel.

Castenada, A., McCandless, B., & Palermo, D. (1956). The children's form of the manifest anxiety scale. *Child Development, 27,* 317–326.

Cattell, R. B., & Cattell, A. K. S. (1973). *The culture fair series.* Scale 1, 1950; Scale 2, 1973; Scale 3, 1973. Champaign, IL: Institute for Personality and Ability Testing.

Conger, J. J. (1977). *Adolescence and youth: Psychological development in a changing world.* New York: Harper & Row.

Dunn, L. M. (1965). *Expanded manual for the Peabody picture vocabulary test.* Circle Pines, MN: American Guidance Service.

Dunn, L. M., & Markwardt, F. C., Jr. (1970). *The Peabody individual achievement test.* Circle Press, MN: American Guidance Service.

Erikson, E. H. (1950). *Childhood and society.* New York: Norton.

Eyberg, S. M., & Ross, A. W. (1978). Assessment of child behavior problems: The validation of a new inventory. *Journal of Clinical Child Psychology, 7,* 113–116.

Golden, C. J., Hammeke, T., & Purisch, A. (1978). Diagnostic validity of a standardized battery derived from Luria's neuropsychological tests. *Journal of Consulting and Clinical Psychology, 46,* 1258–1265.

Goldman, J., L'Engle-Stein, C., & Guerry, S. (1983). *Psychological methods of child assessment.* New York: Brunner/Mazel.

Jastek, J. F., & Jastek, S. (1978). *Wide range achievement test* (4th ed.). Wilmington, DE: Jastek Associates.

Jones, M. C. (1958). A study of socialization patterns at the high school level. *Journal of Genetic Psychology, 92,* 87–111.

Jones, M. C., & Bayley, N. (1950). Physical maturing among boys as related to behavior. *Journal of Educational Psychology, 41,* 129–148.

Kohlberg, L., LaCrosse, J., & Ricks, D. (1972). The predictability of adult mental health from childhood behavior. In B. Wolman (Ed.), *Manual of child psychopathology* (pp. 1217–1287). New York: McGraw-Hill.

Kovacs, M. (1981). Rating scales to assess depression in school-aged children. *Acta Paedopsychiatrica, 46,* 305–315.

Leiter, R. G. (1969). *Examiner's manual for the Leiter international performance scale.* Chicago: Stoelting.

Leon, G. R., & Phelan, P. W. (1985). Anorexia nervosa. In B. Lahey & A. Kazdin (Eds.), *Advances in clinical child psychology* (Vol. 8, pp. 81–111). New York: Plenum.

Mannarino, M. B. (1986). Confidentiality and the minor-aged therapy client. Unpublished doctoral dissertation, University of Louisville, Louisville, KY.

Marks, P. A., Seeman, W., & Haller, D. L. (1974). *The actual use of the MMPI with adolescents and adults.* Baltimore: Williams and Wilkins.

Marshall, W. A., & Tanner, J. M. (1969). Growth and physiological development during adolescence. *Annual Review of Medicine, 19,* 283–301.

Miller, L. C. (1977). *Louisville behavior checklist manual.* Los Angeles: Western Psychological Services.

Mussen, P., Conger, J. J., & Kagan, J. (1979). *Child development and personality.* New York: Harper & Row.

Piaget, J. (1962). *Play, dreams, and imitation in childhood.* New York: Norton.

Piers, E. V., & Harris, D. B. (1969). *The Piers-Harris children's self-concept scale.* Nashville: Counselor Recordings and Tests.

Porter, R. B., & Cattell, R. B. (1972). *Woodcock-Johnson psycho-educational battery, part II: Tests of achievement.* Hingham, MA: Teaching Resources Corporation.

Prescott, G. A., Balow, I. H., Hogan, T. P., & Farr, R. C. (1978). *The Metropolitan achievement tests, fifth edition.* New York: Psychological Corporation.

Quay, H. C., & Peterson, D. R. (1975). *Manual for the behavior problem checklist.* Miami, FL: Program in Applied Social Sciences, University of Miami.

Reitan, R. M., & Davison, L. A. (1974). *Clinical neuropsychology: Current status and applications.* Washington, DC: Winston.

Rotter, J. B., Rafferty, J. E., & Lotsof, A. B. (1954). The validity of the Rotter incomplete sentences blank, high school form. *Journal of Consulting Psychology, 18,* 105–111.

Spielberger, C. (1973). *Manual for the state-trait inventory for children.* Palo Alto, CA: Consulting Psychologists Press.

Spivack, G., Spotts, J., & Haines, P. E. (1967). *The Devereux adolescent rating scale manual.* Devon, PA: Devereux Foundation Press.

Tanner, J. M. (1962). *Growth at adolescence* (2nd ed.). Oxford: Blackwell.

Terman, L. M., & Merrill, M. A. (1973). *Stanford-Binet intelligence scale* (3rd ed.). Boston: Houghton-Mifflin.

Walker, C. E. & Roberts, M. C. (1983). *Handbook of clinical child psychology.* New York: Wiley.

Wechsler, D. (1974). *Manual for the Wechsler intelligence scale for children-revised.* New York: Psychological Corporation.

Wenar, C. (1961). The reliability of mothers' histories. *Child Development, 32,* 419–500.

Wenar, C., & Coulter, J. B. (1962). A reliability study of developmental histories. *Child Development, 33,* 453–462.

Wirt, R. D., Lachar, D., Klinedinst, J. K., & Seat, P. D. (1977). *Multidimensional description of child personality: A manual for the personality inventory for children.* Los Angeles: Western Psychological Services.

Woodcock, R. W., & Johnson, M. B. (1977). *Woodcock-Johnson psycho-educational battery, part II: Tests of achievement.* Hingham, MA: Teaching Resources Corporation.

Part II

Specific Issues

CHAPTER SIX

Management of Crises and Emergencies

Derek Steinberg

Emergencies in adolescent psychiatry fall broadly into two groups: those where specifically medical action is urgently indicated, for example, diagnosis of an acute and unusual clinical state, sedation, or attention to self-injury or an overdose of drugs; and those where the urgent need is for containing distress and protecting the adolescent or other people. Clearly there is some overlap in that the first type of emergency is likely to involve distress and danger, too. However, the second type of emergency can present with all the anxiety, chaos, and fear of loss of control of a major crisis, but without any specifically psychiatric solution, nor for that matter with a psychiatric diagnosis at the heart of the matter.

The first task for the clinician in an emergency in adolescent psychiatry is to swiftly sort out what the psychiatrist (and clinical colleagues) can contribute to its resolution and what others looking after the adolescent can contribute. Most emergencies will be resolved along these lines: clarifying what is going on in circumstances which may be confusing, identifying clinical disorder if such exists, and sorting out who has the responsibility, authority, and capacity to do whatever needs to be done.

Elsewhere I have described this approach as "consultative-diagnostic" (Steinberg, 1983) in that it has characteristics of the traditional individual clinical assessment on the one hand and features of a consultative, crisis-intervention strategy on the other (e.g., Brandon, 1970; Bruggen, Byng-Hall, & Pitt-Aikens, 1973). This is not essentially different from sorting out the complexities of *any* referral in adolescent psychiatry, whether presenting urgently or not. This points out the second important task of the clinician in emergencies in this field. With important but unusual exceptions, most are crises of authority and confidence on the part of the adults responsible for the child (Steinberg, 1981; Steinberg, Galhenage, & Robinson, 1981) and the task of the clinician is to restore authority, confidence, and competence.

In this chapter, I will outline the common components of emergencies and discuss those features of work with adolescents that make it problematic. Then I will offer some guidelines about general principles of management.

The first two principles may be stated as follows: First, clarify the presented problems in terms of problems for the clinician and problems for others looking after the boy or girl; second, remember that most will be crises concerning the young person's care and control, with anxiety clouding the picture and undermining those involved.

COMMON CRISES AND EMERGENCIES

Common crises and emergencies are marked by their infinite variety, but most will fall into one or other of the following broad categories:

1. Familiar clinical emergencies involving acute depressive, manic, schizophrenic, or anxiety states; aggression or self-neglect with a

psychiatric cause; or physical disorder presenting with psychiatric features

2. Concern for an adolescent at risk due to feared or threatened self-injury, absconding, or social withdrawal, promiscuity or other forms of potentially dangerous behavior
3. Concern because of an adolescent's threatening, disruptive or aggressive behavior toward others
4. Organizational crises (external) involving an adolescent thought to be in the wrong place, with an imperative wish for a move elsewhere; or requiring other urgent administrative action, for example, a report for a court
5. Organizational crises (internal) involving an acute problem in working relationships for the clinician and his or her colleagues

Before considering the practical management of such emergencies, we should review the factors that tend to complicate adolescent crises.

COMPLICATING FACTORS IN ADOLESCENT PSYCHIATRY

In summary these are:

1. The direct involvement of people other than the patient
2. Questions of consent to medical treatment
3. Diagnostic difficulty in this age group
4. The emotional maturity of the adolescent
5. The adolescent's physical health and maturity
6. The prevailing cultural attitudes toward adolescents

Confirmation of Who Is Involved

In adult emergencies, there may be only one or two people directly involved and concerned, and quite often there is agreement that something has gone wrong with or for the prospective patient, who is distressed and wants help. In emergencies involving adolescents, there are commonly several people with varying degrees of involvement (family members, voluntary and professional helpers, school staff) with a range of concerns and interpretations about the problem, and the adolescent may deny there is a problem and refuse help.

Deciding whom to see at the outset can be a problem. In the heat of a crisis involving several people, too many may wish to be included in the first interview. All of these people want to tell their story about what the adolescent is doing, how they and their colleagues are affected, and how imperative it is for the psychiatrist to take decisive action. Alternatively, making urgent arrangements can result in key people being absent.

There is much said on both sides about family versus individual assessment, especially in emergencies. It can be said that an emergency involving a younger adolescent is always a family issue, while Dare (1985), reviewing the historical development of assessment methods in child psychiatry, points out that it is generally easier to move from a family assessment to individual work later than vice versa. A family-oriented worker is also likely to argue that the logistic problems a family may put forward for not all being present on short notice (father busy, sibling involved with exams, etc.) may well be not only part of the problem, but also part of the crisis. On the other hand, family therapists, perhaps in the flush of their specialty's dramatic development, sometimes seem to play down the fact that individual diagnostic formulations have their place, too, and that people have a right to have their individual needs and wishes considered.

My own procedure is to arrange to see: (1) those people who have the essential information about the facts of the crisis and (2) those who are in a position to do something about it or to give others permission to do so. In practice, this means that a necessary minimum will be the adolescent and both parents and any key community worker (e.g., social worker) who is already involved. I usually see everyone together first, to clarify who is concerned about what, and then spend a varying amount of time with the boy or girl alone. Conclusions about how to proceed are then put to all who have attended.

Consent to Medical Treatment

In the United Kingdom, 16 is the age of consent to medical intervention. Up to this age, the young person must accept parental decisions about medical intervention; however, from the date of the 16th birthday, this decision belongs to the adolescent. The dilemmas which may arise are clear: on the one hand, there is the quite mature and responsible 15-year-old who must do as the parents wish in this respect, however unwise it may seem and perhaps against the adolescent's own judgment; on the other hand, there is the immature, irresponsible 16-year-old who has every legal right to refuse help. This dilemma is currently the subject of much debate.

It hardly needs to be said that, whatever the age of consent, the psychiatrist has a responsibility to attend carefully to the adolescent's point of view, but in emergencies there are many times when the clinician has to act. As Eisenberg (1975) has reminded us, even *not* to act is a decision, with consequences. When the clinician does act, it is worth remembering the five primary bases for legitimate medical intervention:

1. Having the adolescent's own authority, that is, informed consent.
2. Having the parents' informed consent.

3. Using legal action, urgently if necessary, to bring the adolescent under the protection and control of a court of law (e.g., made a ward of court in the United Kingdom) or local authority (e.g., taken into the care of the local authority by the Department of Social Services under the Children's and Young Person's Act in the United Kingdom). The requirements of the latter are complex; the provisions of most relevance to psychiatrists are that the adolescent is at risk or beyond parental control or that normal development is being avoidably impeded.

4. Using in the United Kingdom the Mental Health Act (1983), again with many complex provisions, but primarily to provide assessment and treatment without consent if the patient is mentally disordered (meaning mentally ill), if the patient is suffering from "arrested or incomplete development of mind" or from psychopathic disorder, and if the patient's or others' health or safety is at risk.

5. Using the clinician's professional authority, that combination of personal, technical, and culturally determined "weight" that (rightly or wrongly) leads others to accept his or her recommendations. This is probably the least well-defined but most powerful source of authority in day-to-day medical practice.

Whichever authority the clinician or others use, in work with adolescents they must remember that the proper use of authority is not merely a precondition of therapeutic action; it is integral to it (e.g., see Winnicott, 1971; Bruce, 1978; Lampen, 1978; Bruggen et al., 1973; Bruggen, 1979). Someone must sometimes say "no" (or "yes") to the adolescent; but some battles the adolescent must be allowed to win.

Diagnostic Difficulty

Diagnosis can be difficult in adolescent psychiatry for several reasons. First, there are phenomenological and maturational reasons. Second, disentangling the individual from social and family problems can be less straightforward than perhaps it once seemed, in the light of recent developments in social and family-focused approaches. Third, the adolescent may be, or choose to be, inaccessible.

Clinical signs may be variable, transient, or of uncertain significance in this age group. Thus Rutter, Graham, Chadwick, & Yule, (1976) showed that such symptoms as early waking, sad feelings, self-deprecation, ideas of reference, and (though to a lesser extent) thoughts about suicide are by no means uncommon in the general, nonpatient adolescent population. The expression of mood varies with maturation in adolescence (e.g., see Golombek & Garfinkel, 1983; Graham & Rutter, 1985), and feelings that lead to suicide seem often to be associated with disturbed conduct and do not necessarily present as depression alone (e.g., see Shaffer, 1974; Brooksbank, 1985). Moreover, denial is characteristic of younger people (A. Freud, 1966), and this also adds to the problems of appraisal. Denial does not, of course, mean only that problems are denied to the clinician; adolescents may hide them from themselves, too, and it is possible for young persons to be quite seriously distressed who also seem at times active, excitable, and sociable.

Psychoses may be hard to identify with accuracy in children and adolescents. Hallucinations do not only occur in psychoses in childhood (Garralda, 1985). In emotionally immature or intellectually handicapped young people, it can be very difficult to distinguish vivid, frightening fantasies, paranoid ideas, and anxiety-laden, muddled thinking from a truly psychotic state. (Steinberg, 1983, 1985). It has also been shown that, particularly in younger adolescents, an illness which appears schizophrenic may be followed by a later episode that is manic-depressive, and vice versa (Zeitlin, 1986). Furthermore, in an emergency, it is not always easy to distinguish an acute psychotic illness from distress in an adolescent with one of the pervasive disorders of personality development such as the relatively milder variants of autism.

The problem of distinguishing individual from family problems is as much one of professional approach and intellectual politics as of the facts of our clients' lives. There is no doubt that the family model is currently in ascendance, but any conceptual model can be presented in convincing terms (Tyrer & Steinberg, 1987), and the undoubted persuasiveness of the family approach needs to be set against the other reality that people, including adolescents, are also individuals and have a right to be listened to as individuals.

This is not an ideological argument which will go away nor be readily resolved. For the purposes of this chapter, I will simply describe my own practice, which is to be as sure as one can that crucial people (i.e., those with information, responsibility, and at least nominal authority) are present at the emergency interview. This means taking a consultative approach (Steinberg & Yule, 1985; Steinberg, 1987) with the referrer and making arrangements for key people to be present, rather than accepting the traditional medical approach of having someone "bring" the patient, which is an outmoded way of working in adolescent psychiatry and can lead to major misunderstandings and worse in emergencies. The people needed in most emergencies are both parents, unless the adolescent lives primarily with only one, and the boy or girl. If the youngster is in care, the social worker is needed, too.

One can move later from this part-family assessment to an individual or family assessment if this seems appropriate. I recommend that a dual consultative-diagnostic approach (Steinberg, 1983) should also inform the first assessment at which problems are (as it were) sorted into those for the parents, adolescent, or social worker, and problems (i.e., clinical work) for the psychiatrist. This approach allows appropriate sharing of the components of the emergency and aids clarification of the diagnosis. The emergency can then be formulated in terms of (1) a problem list, in plain language; (2) clinical diagnosis, if any, based on one of the multiaxial schemes of the DSM-III-R (APA, 1987) or ICD-91 (Rutter, Shaffer, & Shepherd, 1975); and (3) an individual or family dynamic formulation.

Inaccessibility may be because of the adolescent's illness or occasionally due to mental retardation, but it may also be due to the putative patient simply refusing to attend the interview, refusing to speak beyond perhaps the occasional "don't know," or retreating to a locked bedroom or bathroom or out the back door.

The psychiatrist will, of course, use all his or her skills to try to engage the reluctant adolescent in conversation, remembering that the cause is fear, however it looks on the surface. Progress can also be made in establishing the nature of the problem by carefully taking a history from the parents; furthermore, work with the parents may enable them to make a more confident, concerted effort to bring their teenager along. Certainly, a proportion of such emergencies amount to a crisis of parental confidence and authority about a child who has been misbehaving for some time and who does not appear to be at immediate risk. In such circumstances, working with the parents about how they will reestablish appropriate relationships with the adolescent may be the best way of starting. Indeed, a message may be conveyed to the teenager that for the time being he or she is not invited to join in.

Having said all this, however, occasions will arise where an adolescent is a cause for serious concern but refuses to be seen, and one of the forms of legal compulsion as outlined earlier in this chapter may be necessary. Indeed, for a wildly aggressive teenager who refuses help or control, it can be quite appropriate for the psychiatrist to advise the parents to seek the help of the police in a dangerous emergency.

Emotional Maturity.   Ethics, courtesy, and common sense, as well as the requirements of the law must be prominent in psychiatric decisions. In this respect, the balance of the child's rights and the parents' rights can be a matter of fine judgment, as can the question of how much autonomy to allow a young person. An important example in English law concerns the prescription of contraceptives to girls under the age of 16 "in emergency." After much controversy, it was ruled that a doctor may prescribe contraceptives for a girl under 16 without her parents' knowledge, provided that the doctor feels she is sufficiently mature. A substantial body of opinion held that the qualification of maturity was an unnecessary one.

There are two sorts of situations in which an adolescent's maturity is of particular significance. First, a 16-year-old is legally entitled to make a decision about accepting or rejecting medical intervention and yet may be an unreflective, irresponsible, impulsive young person who depends on adults to keep or get him or her out of trouble. An emergency may not be the right time to deal with the issue of the adolescent's responsibility (though it could be). Usually it will make more sense to emphasize adult opinion in making a decision. This does not mean that the teenager's legal rights may be overridden, but it does acknowledge that most decisions are reached informally by persuasion and by the weight of adult (parental and professional) opinion; for a relatively immature adolescent, in an emergency, it is reasonable to let the adults' views carry more weight. (The same point can be made more concisely: As a trainee in the Bethlem unit, I asked my distinguished teacher, Wilfrid Warren, about the policy to follow if a 16-year-old demanded to leave the hospital at an unreasonable hour. His advice: "You just tell them to shut up.")

Conversely, a 14-year-old may have no legal right to decide about medical intervention or hospitalization, and yet this adolescent's capacity for thoughtful reflection and discussion of the pros and cons of the proposed move could make it important that his or her views are given special consideration, even if the parents do not agree with this approach.

In general, the clinician will not find the situation clear-cut one way or the other. Rather, it will be a matter of judging how much in each case the views of the adolescent, the parents, and the clinician ought really to prevail in the interests of humanity and good sense.

Physical Health and Maturity. Practitioners sometimes feel bad about taking physical size and strength into account when deciding how to handle a potentially combative adolescent—as if it were a matter of unreasonable prejudice or physical cowardice on the part of the professional worker. However, in adolescent psychiatry and particularly in emergencies, it is absolutely essential to be pragmatic and realistic. The height, strength, and physical skill of an adult is a crucial issue if that adult might be expected to physically restrain an angry, active young person. It can be extremely dangerous for the patient as well as for the clinical workers if instead of firm, calm restraint a struggle or a fight develops.

Medication can be a problem in an emergency. Sedative medication may be needed to calm a seriously disturbed adolescent when all else has failed. However, the clinician may not have the time or opportunity to find out enough about the patient's past health or response to previous medication, or the young person may never have been exposed to sedative medicine before. The clinician may be faced with an adolescent whose weight may range from that of a rather small child to that of a very hefty adult—the weight range of an adolescent psychiatrist's clients will be something like 30 to 80 kilograms (about 65 to 175 lbs) or more. Emergency sedation by injection can cause more distress and difficulty than it relieves if an insufficient dose is given. On the other hand, the clinician may be anxious about giving a smaller adolescent too much.

In an emergency, information about physical health and past reactions to drugs may be scanty. It can be dangerous to prescribe medication if little is known in this respect. Even in an emergency room presentation, there will usually be someone who knows something about the young patient's past. The clinician also will consider the evidence for an acute physical cause for an agitated, aggressive presentation (e.g., metabolic or neurological disorder). Having made what appraisal can be made about the adolescent's physical health and likely diagnosis, the clinician must then make the decision based on the risk of emergency sedation against the risk of not sedating. I have certainly had occasion to sedate extremely disturbed children in whom I suspected a physical cause when their agitated, disruptive state made it quite impossible to give them the physical examination or care that was urgently needed. I must emphasize, however, that this situation is undesirable, rarely indicated, and only justified after carefully balancing one set of risks against the other and after discussing the decision with the child's parent or guardian.

The drug to use is the one with whose effects, side effects, and hazards the clinician is most familiar. Two useful drugs are chlorpromazine (Thorazine; Largactil) and haloperidol (Haldol; Serenace). As a guide to the daily dose, chlorpromazine may be given in the range 1.5 to 3.5 mg per kilogram (1 kilogram = 2.2 lbs), and haloperidol 0.1 to 0.5 mg per kilogram. A reasonable first dose in the case, for example, of a severely agitated adolescent with an acute schizophrenic psychosis, who weighs 50 kilograms (110 lbs), would be 50 mg of chlorpromazine orally or intramuscularly, repeated after an interval if necessary, or 5 mg haloperidol, similarly repeated. If this dose makes a disturbed young person restrainable and manageable, any further dose should be guided by the effects of the first on arousal, respiration, pulse, and blood pressure as monitored over the next 1 or 2 hours. In effect, the doses of sedative should be titrated against the results of such charting, and the dose should be adjusted as necessary. A much higher dose than that just indicated may be needed to calm an acutely manic adolescent. Furthermore, if the clinician does embark on a high dose regime, blood, liver function, and renal function tests should be performed.

For acute extrapyramidal reactions, procyclidine (Kemadrine) 5 mg may be given intravenously or intramuscularly, repeated if necessary after 20 minutes.

These can only be guidelines, and the psychiatrist must use his or her own judgment in assessing the physical and mental state of the adolescent and the risks of undersedation as well as oversedation. It also must be remembered, especially in an emergency, that those giving permission for medication should be informed that drugs can have ill effects as well as helpful effects.

Cultural Attitudes toward Adolescents

Adolescents can generate great depths of feeling, and the psychiatrist acting in an emergency needs to be aware of how the crisis brings a whole range of complex emotional, ethical, and even political dilemmas into sharp focus. Indeed, the focus can feel particularly sharp for the psychiatrist called upon to adjudicate within the hour on dilemmas which others have not resolved to anyone's comfort over many years. The adolescent is variously seen as tyrant and victim, as needing hauling into line on the one hand, or on the other, as needing urgent counsel about not going along with the wishes of dominating adults like doctors and nurses.

About the tumultuous different opinions offered from every angle in any open society, nothing very helpful can be said here to the clinician faced with an emergency, except that one's duty is to the patient and the family, not to this or that pressure group or faction. All the clinician can do is remember this, act in good faith, and if matters become heated, keep a clear head.

MANAGING EMERGENCIES

A General Strategy

The practioner faced with an emergency needs the following: key people who can provide information about the crisis and help in resolving it; clarification of the presenting problem; time and space to initiate management; and medium-term planning to see the emergency through to a time when matters can be handled on a less urgent basis.

Information

There are two main aspects to mustering the necessary facts: *first,* the clinician's own knowledge and experience, not only in terms of therapeutic skill but in the crucial matter of prediction; and *second,* the patient sorting out of precise details of the presenting problem.

Prediction is generally difficult in psychiatry, but a few general points can be made about emergencies in adolescent psychiatry.

1. First, my own experience is that the crises of adolescent psychiatry do not just "blow over" or put themselves right in the way that individual life or health problems can. This is due to the involvement of other people in the lives of adolescents. Dealing with such emergencies is not always difficult, however. On the contrary, it can take remarkably little (of the right thing) to put major crises right. However, once an emergency has developed, it does need attention. If a mother telephones in desperation

that she can no longer cope with a misbehaving teenager, or a parent or family doctor believes that an adolescent with a so-far well-controlled psychotic illness is about to relapse, that person is often right.

2. In the right relationship, one in which the patient knows he or she is being listened to and taken seriously by the clinician, there is a very good chance that the adolescent will tell the clinician what he or she is (or is not) going to do, at least between now and a specified time in the near future: for example, whether there will be a suicide attempt. (Steinberg, 1979).

3. It is a useful medical truism that common things commonly occur. There is evidence of a climbing suicide rate for older adolescents (age 15 to early 20s) throughout the world (Brook, 1974), in European countries (Sainsbury, Jenkins, & Levey, 1980), and in the United States (Holinger, 1978, 1979, 1986; Shaffer & Fisher, 1981). In the United States, it is the third most common cause of death in adolescence (Holinger, 1979). In a useful review of the rising suicide rate in England and Wales, McClure (1986) pointed out that the ratio between male and female suicides (approximately 2:1) is increasing and listed as possible causes of pressure on all adolescents the concurrent increase in family disruption, drug abuse, alcoholism, delinquency, and unemployment.

The suicide rate in younger children is lower. In his study during a 7-year period of suicide among boys and girls age 10 to 14, Shaffer (1974) identified two stereotypes of the children who died. The first type was highly intelligent, socially isolated children, culturally distant from their parents who were less well educated and where the mother was mentally ill. Depressive symptoms may not have been prominent, although these children might have been stealing or avoiding school. The second type was impetuous, aggressive teenagers, especially girls, who were suspicious, sensitive, and resentful of criticism and who were in trouble at school. These factors do not constitute a checklist, however, and Shaffer's numbers were small (30).

Putting together what we know about completed suicide, a threat of suicide in a socially isolated adolescent should be taken seriously. This is especially true if the adolescent is bright and male and is impulsive, angry, or aggressive. Moreover, if there is a history of death or loss and a more recent story of school or social problems, and especially if the adolescent is in the late teens or early 20s, the threat should be taken seriously.

4. Attempted suicide and deliberate self-injury and self-poisoning occupy an uncertain relationship with suicide. Major differences exist in this group, particularly in the preponderance of girls. For example, Hawton, Cole, O'Grady, and Osborn (1982a, 1982b, 1982c) found in studies of this group in England that 90% of the 13- to 18-year-olds were girls.

In the Hawton et al. studies, one-quarter of those adolescents had contact with a family doctor in the previous week, and one-third had physical health problems such as asthma or juvenile arthritis. In addition, most of those studied showed that problems in the family, at school, or with friends were common. Of the whole group, 14% had been in the care of the social service department. In most cases, the problems were transient, but the outlook was bleak (in terms of further overdoses and other problems) for young people whose self-poisoning seemed to be part of a range of behavior disturbance that included habitual drunkenness, stealing, and fighting. In these studies, and also in studies by Leese (1969) and Lumsden-Walker (1980), self-injury seemed to be part of a continuum of behavioral and family problems, which included poor communication with parents, absent parents (especially fathers), impulsive self-injurious attempts, and lack of a clear-cut diagnostic category.

5. The whole issue of dangerousness, in general, has a vast literature (see review by Prins, 1986) but contains little in the way of reliable and reassuring guidance, beyond the old standby that the best predictor of future behavior is past behavior. The questions worth asking are: (1) To what extent is the possible dangerous behavior under the patient's control? (For example, delusions or hallucinatory instructions are not.) (2) To what extent are past stressors or precipitants still operating? (3) What is the patient's impulsiveness or, on the contrary, his or her capacity to reflect on or discuss risk-laden behavior? (4) What is the influence of drugs or alcohol?

Information Gathering. The clinician dealing with an emergency will want the same historical and current information on which one bases routine work, and, in most urgent cases, there will be time to make a comprehensive assessment. However, the situation may be chaotic, the patient may be too disturbed or otherwise inaccessible for a full examination, or the clinician may have less time available than usual. The handling of most emergencies will be helped if the following key areas of information are highlighted:

1. Patient's and relatives' addresses and phone numbers and patient's birth date
2. Referring and other key professionals' names and telephone numbers as well as those of any other workers who may be currently involved
3. Legal status of relevance (e.g., on a care order, on probation, awaiting court appearance)
4. History of past problems or crises: psychiatric, physical (illness, accidents, operations, disabilities, allergies, drug reactions), legal, or social
5. Precise nature of the problem and reason for the *sense of crisis.*

The latter information, though it may seem naive and can cause annoyance to the patient, family, and referrer (who take it for granted that the nature of the emergency is obvious), nonetheless requires calm pursuit, and a willingness to deal with facts and realities rather than assumptions. Even in the best regulated circles, "emergencies," with all the danger of rushed assessment and rushed decisions, sometimes happen. Some of the reasons are as follows:

- A key supporting worker is about to leave the job or go on holiday.
- The professional currently involved does not have time to deal with the present run of events.
- Administrative rather than clinical situations arise. For example, a different sort of crisis (between staff) may develop if a particular adolescent is not moved from A to B at once.
- Anxiety on the part of relatives or workers may be out of proportion to any actual danger.
- Anger or frustration with the adolescent, again on the part of family or professional, gets in the way of adequate care and control.

The clinician who looks for such difficulties and tries to respond to them, however tactfully and sympathetically, will not be popular. Nonetheless, the task is to deal competently with the crisis, which requires facing all the facts rather than attempting to court popularity. In any case, in the heat of a crisis involving children and adolescents, there very often is a great deal of free-floating anxiety and anger, and the clinician who is perceived as big enough and strong enough to help is as likely to be on the receiving end of irrational rage as to receive grateful thanks. The thanks may come later.

Information gathering, then, is best pursued by involving the adolescent's family since it is usually in the family that the relevant information, fears, capacity for future care, and responsibility for future action are found. Bruggen and his colleagues (Bruggen et al., 1973) also involve referring professionals in the assessment process, which, in the light of the nature of most adolescent emergencies and other problems, has much to commend it (Steinberg et al., 1981; Steinberg & Hughes, 1987).

Finally, information is provided by the clinician's assessment of the situation and by the mental state examination of the adolescent, partly in terms of the treatment indicated but also in terms of prediction, as previously discussed. While some practitioners recommend an approach to crises based on understanding the family or social system and while more traditional practitioners recommend basing it on the individual state of health (physical and mental) of the putative patient, I am firmly recommending an assessment that incorporates both.

The patient's state of physical health is important. A full physical examination may not be immediately practicable in an emergency, but it is crucial for the clinician to reach an opinion on the adolescent's physical health. For example, if the clinician believes that infection, intoxication, or another physically pathological process is a factor in the emergency or is even coexistent, appropriate action must be taken. Neurological examination and investigation, computerized axial tomography (CT) scanning or other radiological examination may be needed, or blood or urine biochemical assay if there is the possibility of ingested drugs.

The need for physical assessment of an acutely confused or psychotic young person who is uncooperative may itself be an indication for hospital admission. The opinion of an appropriate specialist may be needed on whether physical pathology is indicated and how best to proceed. It is vital to make a rational and balanced decision on the basis of the risks of proceeding with physical investigation (e.g., damaging distraction from psychosocial issues) against the risks of not proceeding (danger to physical health). Remember that mishandling the former can be life threatening, too.

Information Sharing. The acquisition of information about the emergency is a two-way and sometimes three-way process. *First,* the clinician needs a full picture not only of what has happened, but also of what the people involved fear may happen next. The latter is a guide to the anxieties of those involved, and it is the anxieties that for good or ill fuel the crisis. *Second,* the patient and family need information from the clinician, such as how it looks to the practitioner, what he or she thinks could happen next, and what the options are for management, including their side effects. The *third* arm of information sharing is with other workers who may be able to help. Remember to respect privacy as well as confidentiality in seeking and giving information about the patient and family.

People. It is important, then, to try to include key people in the first meeting. If this is not feasible, the clinician should be pragmatic rather than dogmatic and do the best he or she can. If the clinician thinks that the help of an educational psychologist, social worker, or psychiatric nurse is needed, it is a good idea to involve such people in the assessment from the start. Of course, they will contribute helpfully to the assessment, including their views about their own involvement. In addition, their presence represents the involvement from the start of key therapists, rather than making a rereferral later. For example, if the issue is the admission to residential care of a violent adolescent, then discussion about the patient's containment and the authority to do whatever is needed to minimize the risk of people getting hurt should all be part of the agenda for the emergency meeting; so nursing or other residential staff should be present.

The emergency meeting is an occasion for clarifying authority and responsibility as well as sharing information. An ambivalent adolescent's commitment to whatever is agreed upon may need to be affirmed by a verbal or written contract. The clinician should also explain his or her role. To reiterate, I believe the clinician should not begin with either the view that the problem "must be" in the family or that it "must be" in the adolescent; rather, one should realize that there is often coexistent difficulty in the family system and in the adolescent's internal psychological or psychophysical system. In taking an approach that is partly consultative (Caplan, 1970; Steinberg & Yule, 1985) and partly diagnostic, the clinician differentiates tasks and responsibilities for the parents and other family members from tasks and responsibilities for the clinicians (Steinberg, 1983, 1987).

Remember, however, that the clinician is never *totally* responsible; even compulsory treatment is undertaken, finally, at the request of the patient's relatives, legal guardians, or a court of law. (For a fuller discussion of issues of authority and responsibility see Steinberg, 1983; Hughes & Wilson, 1986.)

Problem Clarification. The process of identifying key people involved and finding out from them in detail the causes for concern will contribute much toward problem-clarification. However, it will sometimes further emerge that what has presented as a crisis is not new, but rather a new development in a long-standing problem in the family or in the adolescent's development. For example, the acute distress parents feel about a new, disabling development in their child's depression, phobia, or obsessional behavior may be based on long-standing guilt feelings or anxiety they had about an earlier problem, such as a physical problem in pregnancy or infancy. I have often found that current mixed feelings and distress about a child seem to be a reenactment of a bad experience with doctors when the child had an epileptic fit, a bad attack of asthma, or serious abdominal symptoms, and the parents found themselves having to rely totally on professionals they did not wholly trust. The problem "our daughter now spends 3 hours in the bathroom performing compulsive rituals and it's getting worse" is actually the problem just stated *plus* the unstated problem: "And we don't really trust any expert to be able to help; she doesn't trust us; and we're not sure we trust each other or ourselves." This is a real problem, one which is serious but not an emergency; therefore, it presents as a panic-stricken, despair-laden crisis.

In this girl's case the personal and shared crisis of confidence is one problem; the girl's as yet untreated disorder is another; and her actual handicaps, inability to meet her friends, go to school, and have a normal relationship with her parents, constitute three more. Defining the problems in terms of clinical disorder, disabilities, and family feelings or assumptions helps distinguish what needs to be done immediately (gain the family's confidence and help them understand the breakdown in confidence within the family) from what will take a little longer (set up a behavioral and family treatment program (e.g., as in Bolton, Collins, & Steinberg, 1983).

To recapitulate, pursuing thoroughly and with precision and asking the right people the question "Who is concerned about what, and why?" will provide much relief for the clinician, who will begin to see what needs to be done. In addition, such action will bring relief to the other people involved.

Making Space and Time. The differentiation of the various components of the crisis helps defuse it. The immediate cause of the urgency and anxiety becomes the focus of the work, and other important but less critical issues can be dealt with in due course. Indeed, it will be helpful to make a timetable with the adolescent and family, deciding when, where, and with whom to meet next, and what priorities to give the various urgent matters identified. In effect, breathing space has been created while dealing with those things that really needed immediate attention.

It should not be assumed, however, that the first responsibility of the clinician is to reduce anxiety at all costs. The primary aim is not to give reassurance for its own sake but to enable family and clinician to deal first with whatever needs immediate attention. There is much that is positive about a crisis, providing that the prevailing arousal permits concentration on the task and high motivation to put things right. On the other hand, anxiety can become overwhelming and undermining. The clinician's responsibility is to manage this anxiety appropriately and humanely. Remember, it is just as unskilled and unkind to have a policy of letting people "sweat it out" as it is to be prematurely reassuring when there can be no grounds for reassurance. Unfortunately, some clinicians prefer to see every emergency as illustrating a general dynamic theory of crisis, each needing much the same approach, when the only common psychodynamic feature of each crisis in fact lies within the therapist concerned.

Planning. Timetabling the urgent matters can then merge with planning how and when to consider those less urgent matters which the clinician recognizes as important, but from which the emergency has successfully diverted attention. For example, a common crisis in adolescence, apparently concerned with a problem "today," arises when parents of a child who is chronically troubled in some way suddenly become anxious about the trouble the youngster will have in becoming independent, such as when he or she leaves school in a year. Drawing attention to how this problem can be helped is not only necessary in its own right, but it will help the family come to a fuller understanding of their present distress and will remove some of the immediate sense of panic. The planning process should also include ways of monitoring progress, for example, by a behavior chart if this seems appropriate and by building into the management program specified occasions when progress can be reviewed. Tasks set or agreed upon can then be considered and modified if necessary. The result is that a confusing, anxiety-laden, and chaotic situation (in which the patient and family hoped for a magical solution from an omniscient expert) is transformed into a shared and orderly piece of practical and understandable work.

This result is not achieved simply by being cool and logical; nor is planning neat programs enough. Devising a workable plan requires a grasp of the dynamics of the situation (i.e., of the emergency itself and a feel for getting the balance right between being overprotective and underprotective, between being too open and too inscrutable, and between being too concerned and too laid back). A useful guide to holding and containing crises sufficiently for the patient and family to feel cared for, but not so much that they feel dependent and enfeebled, is provided by aspects of attachment theory (see, for example, Heard, 1974; Steinberg, 1983).

Planning also implies record keeping. It is essential to make a note of what happened in handling the emergency, including, of course, what advice was given. Having created breathing space (and perhaps a few days for everyone to reflect about what happens next), it is crucial to bring into the picture the people who will have to pick up the pieces if things fall apart prematurely, such as the clinician's immediate colleagues, the family physician, and if appropriate, other community services.

General Strategy: Outline and Aide-Mémoire

1. Basic data, including the date:
   Adolescent and family: names, address, telephone number
   Referring agent(s):   names, addresses, telephone numbers
   Other professionals: names, addresses, telephone numbers
2. The referrer's problems
3. The adolescent's problems
4. The problems as others involved perceive them
5. Who is in charge of the adolescent? (age issues, custody issues, care and legal factors)
6. History A:
   What precisely is going on now?
   Who is concerned about what?
   What do people fear may happen?
   What have people tried?
   What has been helpful/unhelpful?
   History B: What has been happening over the years?
   Developmental
   Physical
   Social and family

Psychological
Assessment/treatment

7. Adolescent's mental and physical state
8. Observations on health or behavior of others involved
9. Differential diagnoses, if any
10. Formulation of the situation
11. Specific short-term and long-term risks to adolescent/others
12. Management plan which includes timing, place (e.g., out-patient care, admission), people (e.g., nursing staff)
13. Explanation/information to patient, family, professionals

TWO EMERGENCIES

The following two emergencies involving adolescents illustrate several of the points made in this chapter. (The cases cannot be identified from the information given.)

Example 1

A 14-year-old girl is referred by her family doctor because of her misbehavior. He does not know her well, but he is aware that there is a history of family breakdown and recurrent misbehavior and school problems, with the repeated involvement of school authorities and social services.

Why has the family doctor become involved? The parents, mother and stepfather, think the girl is "crazy." It seems that she has been found by the police trying to solicit passing men in the city center's red-light area, and in the police station she has become aggressive and abusive. The family doctor and the police consider that she is a typically misbehaving youngster from a chronically disrupted background. They also feel that she should be placed in a young people's secure remand and assessment center for full assessment. The parents, however, think she should be admitted to a hospital. The doctor would like the psychiatrist's opinion in the near future; the parents think she should be hospitalized at once and keep calling the psychiatrist to tell him so. He has not seen the girl yet, as she was taken straight from the city center to the police station. Her aggressive behavior includes biting several officers and trying to break the place up.

The parents speak on the telephone to the psychiatrist, and it emerges that although the girl has been a school-avoider and absconder and generally difficult, her behavior has been characterized more by misery and anxiety than aggressive, extroverted behavior. Her poor social and school behavior has been characterized by isolation, withdrawal, and poor motivation, and therefore her present behavior is out of character. They are able to describe: (1) a typical story of family breakdown and recurring behavioral problems and (2) a period of quite severe depression followed by, for the past week, mounting excitability, elation, and sexually disinhibited behavior. The mother then describes her own past depressive illnesses and the serious depressive state which led to her own mother's death.

The family doctor agrees with the possibilities of the present disorder being mania or drug intoxication rather than rage and misbehavior. He hopes the psychiatrist will see the girl. The police accept the parents' word that although this sort of behavior is not unfamiliar to the police, it is quite out of character even for this disturbed girl.

The psychiatrist sees the girl within a few hours, confirms that she has the characteristic features of a manic state, and notes her hoarse voice and near-exhaustion. He confirms that the mother and father have authority to overrule the girl's refusal to accept hospital admission and treatment, there being no outstanding custody issue. He further notes that no social worker is actively involved and arranges urgent admission for full assessment. There is no evidence of drug misuse of physical disorder, and she is given sedation. A date is fixed for a few days hence when the parents can review the situation. The girl has a good relationship with her natural father, too, so it is agreed that he should be involved if this is useful and does not undermine the mother's and stepfather's position.

Decisions which are important but can wait include: (1) the possible need for continuing medication and perhaps the use of lithium; and (2) attention to the girl's many other problems, whatever the nature of their interaction with affective illness. Because manic adolescents can be extremely difficult to manage and their arousal resistant to high doses of medication, the situation is full of hazards; therefore, a detailed care plan is worked out with the nursing staff with this in mind.

Example 2

A psychiatrist requests the immediate admission to an adolescent unit of a 16-year-old girl with anorexia nervosa. She is losing weight rapidly, and her mother is now in a state of extreme anxiety because the outpatient work is having no useful effect. The girl's mother has been telephoning the child's psychiatrist daily demanding action, saying she will not be able to stand another weekend of anxiety over the girl's refusal to eat.

The following facts emerge. First, the child psychiatrist is the third the girl has seen because she has "not got on" with the previous psychiatrists. With the first, "she didn't understand what he was talking about." The second wanted to involve the girl's father, which was not possible because of his work as a busy executive who traveled widely nationally and internationally. The third was recommended as a remarkably good psychiatrist by a friend who worked in a child care charity and was slightly acquainted with him. In the initial meetings with this third psychiatrist, it was conveyed that "at last" the anorexic girl had found someone who understood her; the disappointment felt now at his "failure" is mutual.

The following conversation might have taken place when the hospital psychiatrist was contacted by the referring psychiatrist.

Hospital: Why treatment in hospital as an emergency?

Psychiatrist: Because a firmer line can be taken; it's now urgent.

Hospital: But the girl has three times evaded treatment, and in any case, she is 16 years old. Do you think that she should come in on a compulsory treatment basis?

Psychiatrist: Not necessary; she is actually a most compliant girl who does as her mother says. Of course, you could always detain her later if you thought it necessary.

Hospital: Does her father agree with her mother?

Psychiatrist: He is always happy to leave decisions like this to her.

Hospital: He does not undermine them, for example, by not attending the family appointments?

Psychiatrist: Not really. The point is the girl's behavior was better at that time because he was around more. In any case, it was a joint decision by both parents that he did not need to attend.

Hospital: It all sounds very confusing.

Psychiatrist: It's not at all confusing! This will be the fourth attempt at treatment. Minimum risk of a fourth failure is particularly important because the key issue is one of adult authority, and the girl is learning that adults cannot be relied upon to stop her starving herself to death.

Psychiatrist: That is rather a harsh way to put it.

Hospital: The girl is in no immediate physical danger. The greatest risk to her life and health does not lie in her being at home and not eating for a few more days, but rather in finding that a fourth attempt at treatment fails. The most urgent, necessary step is for the treatment team to meet the girl and both parents to explain that she is starving herself to death and to ask who is going to make her eat. Either the parents will do this, together, or the girl will agree to a treatment contract that includes bed rest and insistence on eating until she gains weight. Alternatively, the parents will have to consider, together, seeking legal authority for compulsory treatment. I do not see any other way of starting treatment on a firm basis.

Psychiatrist: That seems a rather rigid approach to me. Why can't you just get her in and sort out those details after the weekend?

Hospital: Without planning between the treatment team and family, we are likely to be as unsuccessful as the previous therapists, which should be avoided for the reasons I have explained. And there happens to be no reason for an urgent admission.

Psychiatrist: That's all very well, but her mother's beside herself with anxiety.

Hospital: What's the girl like?

Psychiatrist: She wants to go out with some friends.

Hospital: Please tell her and her mother that we will see the whole family, father too, on Tuesday to discuss a workable way of helping. Also that there seems no point in getting anxious about the girl's diet this particular weekend. Do you think those messages will contain the mother's anxiety?

Psychiatrist: I expect so. The problem is that I had promised to arrange the girl's admission today. That's what her mother is expecting now.

The family attended a few days later, and was not distressed at the delay, nor at the two week interval for family meetings that preceded a planned and wholly successful admission. The key to this "emergency," and which could have led to a fourth precipitate, unplanned and unsuccessful psychiatric encounter, lay in the transaction between an anxious woman, isolated with her daughter's problem within her family, and a psychiatrist who had been maneuvered onto a pedestal and whose effectiveness and pride were being severely challenged. Anyone dealing with disturbed children can be put into this position. This imaginary conversation therefore illustrates an occupational hazard of which clinicians should be aware.

SOME SPECIAL CIRCUMSTANCES

The Neglect and Abuse of Children

The neglect and physical and sexual abuse of young people is by no means confined to preadolescent children, although it has not received the same detailed attention (see review by Mrazek & Mrazek, 1985). The accusation or suspicion of physical or sexual abuse requires urgent attention because of the young person's distress and possible risk of further harm and because of the young person's distress and possible risk of further harm and because of the risk of harm to other and perhaps younger children in the family. The distress of the parent, too, should not be forgotten in the enquiry for the "culprit." The problem is rarely isolated, other family disturbance and dysfunction being common in cases of both sexual abuse (Mrazek & Bentovim, 1981) and physical abuse (Green, Liang, Gaines, & Suttan, 1980; Martin, 1980; Lieh-Mak, Chung, & Liu, 1983).

Unexplained or inadequately explained injury should lead to the suspicion of abuse, but remember that some physical injury and sexual abuse or exploitation can be the result of neglect and inadequate supervision by the parents of a disturbed child rather than direct abuse by them.

It is important to remember in such cases that there are three interrelated but separate aspects to dealing with such situations. First, there is the practical necessity of preventing further harm to the adolescent or anyone else. Second, there is therapeutic work to be done to relieve distress, aid normal development and by way of prophylaxis. Third, there are the legal requirements concerned with the care and protection of children and with the identification of offenders. The legal position and availability of helping and advisory services will vary from place to place, and the best advice that can be given here is that the clinician should be familiar with local provision and expectations.

The neglect and abuse of children is always difficult to deal with because of conflicting aspects of the previously mentioned requirements (e.g., apprehension and punishment of an offending adult and the reinstatement of positive family relationships), because of the general anxiety and uncertainty such problems arouse, and because of the fear of making an unjustified accusation. Indeed, it will feel like an accusation however the issue is raised. However difficult it is to handle, the suspicion of child abuse, like the suspicion of physical illness mentioned earlier, cannot be put aside while the clinician wonders whether to act. The difficult question must be faced: Do I believe that abuse has taken place?

The adults concerned must be asked about it. However difficult the situation and however distressed the parents, proper concern for the child means that the question must be raised. Should the "cause" (e.g., of unexplained relatively minor injuries) persist as a mystery, then parents and clinicians must agree to some form of supervision and "reporting" on an individual and family basis about what occurs, when, and how. If the child does indeed seem to be at serious risk, judged by the nature of the injury or the attitude or personality of the adults, separation is required. Such separation can be achieved either by admission to a hospital, if appropriate, or by removal to a children's home. In the United Kingdom, a Place of Safety Order can be obtained as an emergency, followed by an application for a Care Order. Real concern for the child is sufficient; the clinician does not have to have a watertight case. It is the court's work to ensure that proper evidence is obtained and the right action followed.

Large numbers of anxious workers can become involved with such cases. I recommend care being taken to clarify and separate the following roles: a therapeutic worker with the child; a therapeutic worker (or pair of workers) with the family; and a separate worker, preferably from outside the therapeutic team, to pursue legal matters. This is not to say that therapeutic workers should avoid matters of fact (on the contrary), but it is to say that evidence for a court must be distinguished clearly from the material used in therapy. It is essential to keep scrupulous records of who said what to whom, with times and dates noted, and to have at least drawings and preferably photographs of any injuries along with explanations for them. Go by the overall picture, not by so-called 'pathognomonic signs.'

Finally, do not be rushed by the excitement of other people into being inquisitorial or too laid back. Just get the facts of the case, with courtesy and respect for privacy, and where common sense or the law requires breach of confidentiality, say so. When in doubt, the clinician's priority should be what, in good faith, he or she considers to be in the child's interests.

Hospital Admission

Different adolescent inpatient units have varying admission policies. It is right that this should be so, because the range of demands that can be made on them, from psychotherapy through behavioral treatment to the containment of violent behavior, would be daunting for many general adult psychiatric hospitals, which characteristically parcel out such different functions into different units (Steinberg, 1982). Nonetheless, it has been pointed out that adolescent units can also become too specialized and exclusive.

My own view is that for *planned* admissions, any reasonable use of inpatient facilities should be open for discussion. However, the *immediate, unplanned admission* of a boy or girl to a psychiatric unit should be reserved for acute individual disorder. That is, the problem is perceived as being primarily in the adolescent, not in the family; it is seen as illness rather than misbehavior, for which care and control would be more appropriate (Steinberg, 1981, 1982); and day and night supervision by a medical and nursing team is really needed. In practice, I place in this category depressed young people threatening or contemplating suicide or injury to others; adolescents with acute psychotic illness; or adolescents experiencing extreme distress and who have not been helped by alternative care. Rapid physical deterioration in self-neglectful young people or adolescents with anorexia nervosa may require urgent admission, but careful consideration should first be given to whether a general hospital admission would be more appropriate.

In the following discussion of problems for the staff of inpatient units, it is suggested that requests for admission must sometimes be refused, and this may happen in the cases of adolescents who do need admission to a hospital. In such circumstances, I do not share the view that admission to an adult hospital while waiting for an adolescent unit place is an automatic disaster. Very often the adult unit will not have quite the same approach as an adolescent unit. For example, the adult unit may not provide for spending time with families, and it may not maintain an educational and therapeutic milieu for a wide range of very different patients, involving a great deal of parenting, nurturing, and limit-setting behavior. Accordingly, it is easier for a general unit to "hold" an acutely ill adolescent for a while, and at short notice.

Other inpatient teams have other views. The best thing for the clinician to do is to find out what they are and to become acquainted with the staff, their approach, and their reasons. Commonly, there will be gaps in residential provision for adolescents, and joint consultation and planning of services is preferable to occasional rows and mutual recrimination over a "hard to place" boy or girl.

Crises in Residential Units

Any residential unit for adolescents, psychiatric or otherwise, is vulnerable to pressures from within and without of the type to which much of this chapter has referred. There will be "straight" emergencies concerned with the threat of suicide or the development of acute psychosis, the absconding of a boy or girl at risk, or the sudden impact of parental anxiety, illness, or complaint on the residential staff.

The admission of a disturbed or demanding child when the nursing staff is already fully stretched (or even when one link in the day-and-night chain of nursing cover is fully stretched) can cause a crisis, too. Sometimes the excess demand comes not from the patient but from the admitting clinician, who prescribes what he or she wants in the way of supervision and management without first checking its feasibility. My own view is that it is bad practice, if not irresponsible, for a psychiatrist to insist on the admission of an adolescent patient on the grounds that "a bed is available," without discussing fully with the nursing staff what care will be expected for the adolescent and whether it can be done. Simply placing the adolescent on an available mattress would be a novel treatment of unproven efficacy. Those responsible for inpatient units must on the one hand help their teams provide as flexible and responsive a service as possible but on the other hand be sensitive to what the staff can manage. They must be prepared on occasion to say "no."

In addition to such practical problems, adolescent units tend to be vulnerable to emotional pressures which arise from the demands made on staff by disturbed young people and their families. Adolescents' problems cause anxiety, ambivalence, and uncertainty, and they require the help of people with very different training, aptitudes, and roles. Such people as psychiatrists, nursing staff, teachers, psychologists, psychotherapists, occupational therapists, social workers, and others are required. Maintenance of a reasonably consistent and therapeutic response from a staff group containing such diversity, without slipping into anarchic chaos on the one hand or an excessively autocratic, narrowly oriented regime on the other, is a challenge that, with colleagues, I have described elsewhere (Steinberg, 1986).

This chapter is not the place to attempt to describe the systems and strategies that may help keep a treatment organization therapeutic, creative, and human. Nor is it the place to explain how to respond to periods of turbulence and emergency and how to minimize less useful crises. When crises and emergencies do arise, however, the strategy to adopt should in essence be that which has formed the theme of this chapter. Identify someone who is senior and experienced to chair a meeting—which could be a meeting between two people in doubt, dispute, distress, or difficulties; a meeting of the whole community of staff and patients; or a meeting of any size group in between. Who gets together depends on the criteria given earlier: Who is concerned about what? Who has the necessary information? Who is in a position to help? The difference between the management of emergencies that arise "outside," and the crises within a treatment team, is that in the latter case, staff should be trained to know that such turns of events are as natural to a therapeutic unit as are changes in the weather to a ship at sea.

Much is expected from that elusive notion of "staff support." I believe that the best form of "support" is in training and supervision, and in systems of organization that take account of feelings and staff group dynamics as well as the more concrete aspects of management. All these are equally important and should result in a service that can anticipate problems and respond to them with competence.

SUMMARY

Both acute clinical disorder in the individual and situations of social and family crisis contribute to emergencies in adolescent psychiatry. In this chapter, we have seen how the former is sometimes present, and the latter is always present. Management strategies are described which take this fact into account. The point is made that the many characteristics of crises involving adolescents add to their complexity: the direct involvement of several other people; age-dependent issues of consent to treatment; diagnostic problems in this age group; issues concerning the adolescent's emotional maturity and physical status; and cultural attitudes toward adolescence. Assessment and treatment strategies are described in relation to each of these, and a general approach to management is described, in which particular attention is paid to the management of anxiety and the clarification of problems as perceived by the various people involved. The special situations of physical or sexual abuse, hospital admission, and crises occurring in treatment teams are briefly discussed in relation to the general strategies described.

REFERENCES

American Psychiatric Association (1987). *Diagnostic and statistical manual of mental disorders* (3rd ed., rev.). (DSM-III-R). Washington, DC: Author.

Bolton, D., Collins, S., & Steinberg, D. (1983). The treatment of obsessive-compulsive disorder in adolescence: A report of 15 cases. *British Journal of Psychiatry, 142,* 456–464.

Brandon, S. (1970). Crisis theory and the possibilities of therapeutic intervention. *British Journal of Psychiatry, 117,* 627–633.

Brook, E. M. (1974). *Suicide and attempted suicide* (Public Health Paper No. 58). Geneva: World Health Organization.

Brooksbank, D. J. (1985). Suicide and parasuicide in childhood and early adolescence. *British Journal of Psychiatry, 146,* 459–463.

Bruce, T. (1978). Group work with adolescents. *Journal of Adolescence, 1,* 47–54.

Bruggen, P. (1979). Authority in work with young adolescents: A personal review. *Journal of Adolescence, 2,* 345–354.

Bruggen, P., Byng-Hall, L. J., & Pitt-Aikens, T. (1973). The reason for admission as a focus of work in an adolescent unit. *British Journal of Psychiatry, 122,* 319–329.

Caplan, G. (1970). *The theory and practice of mental health consultation.* London: Tavistock.

Dare, C. (1985). Family therapy. In M. Rutter & L. Herson (Eds.), *Child and adolescent psychiatry: Modern approaches* (pp. 809-825). Oxford: Blackwell.

Eisenberg, L. (1975). The ethics of intervention: Acting amidst ambiguity. *Journal of Child Psychiatry and Psychology, 16,* 93–104.

Freud, A. (1966). *Normality and pathology in childhood.* London: Hogarth Press.

Garralda, M. E. (1985). Characteristics of the psychoses of late onset in children and adolescents: A comparative study of hallucinating children. *Journal of Adolescence, 8,* 195–207.

Golombek, H., & Garfinkel, B. D. (1983). *The adolescent and mood disturbance.* New York: International Universities Press.

Graham, P., & Rutter, M. (1985). Adolescent disorders. In M. Rutter & L. Hersov (Eds.), *Child and adolescent psychiatry: Modern approaches* (pp. 352–367). Oxford: Blackwell.

Green, A. H., Liang, V., Gaines, R., & Sultan, S. (1980). Psychopathological assessment of child-abusing, neglecting and normal mothers. *Journal of Nervous and Mental Disease, 168,* 356–360.

Hawton, K., Cole, D., O'Grady, J., & Osborn, M. (1982a). Motivational aspects of deliberate self-poisoning in adolescents. *British Journal of Psychiatry, 141,* 286–291.

Hawton, K., O'Grady, J., Osborn, M., & Cole, D. (1982b). Adolescents who take overdoses: Their characteristics, problems and contacts with helping agencies. *British Journal of Psychiatry, 140,* 118–123.

Hawton, K., Osborn, M., O'Grady, J., & Cole, D. (1982c). Classification of adolescents who take overdoses. *British Journal of Psychiatry, 140,* 124–131.

Heard, D. H. (1974). Crisis intervention guided by attachment concepts: A case study. *Journal of Child Psychiatry and Psychology, 15,* 111–122.

Holinger, P. C. (1978). Adolescent suicide: An epidemiological study of recent trends. *American Journal of Psychiatry, 135,* 754–756.

Holinger, P. C. (1979). Violent deaths among the young: Recent trends in suicide, homicide and accidents. *American Journal of Psychiatry, 136,* 1144–1147.

Holinger, P. C., & Offer, D. (1986). Suicide, homicide and accidents among adolescents: Trends and potential for prediction. In R. A. Feldman & A. R. Stiffman (Eds.), *Advances in adolescent mental health* (Vol. 1, B, pp. 119–145). Greenwich, CT: JAI.

Hughes, L., & Wilson, J. (1986). Social work on the bridge. In D. Steinberg (Ed.), *The adolescent unit: Work and teamwork in adolescent psychiatry* (pp. 1–18). New York: Wiley.

Lampen, J. (1978). Drest in a little brief authority: Controls in residential work with adolescents. *Journal of Adolescence, 1,* 163–175.

Leese, S. M. (1969). Suicide behaviour in 20 adolescents. *British Journal of Psychiatry, 115,* 479–480.

Lieh-Mak, F., Chung, S. Y., & Liu, Y. W. (1983). Characteristics of child-battering in Hong Kong: A controlled study. *British Journal of Psychiatry, 142,* 89–94.

Lumsden-Walker, W. (1980). Intentional self-injury in school-age children: A study of 50 cases. *Journal of Adolescence, 3,* 217–228.

Martin, H. P. (1980). Working with parents of abused and neglected children. In R. Abidin (Ed.), *Parent education and intervention handbook* (pp. 252–271). Springfield, IL: Thomas.

Mrazek, P., & Bentovim, A. (1981). Incest and the dysfunctional family system. In P. B. Mrazek & C. H. Kempe (Eds.), *Sexually abused children and their families* (pp. 167–178). Oxford: Pergamon.

Mrazek, D., & Mrazek, P. (1985). Child maltreatment. In M. Rutter & L. Hersov (Eds.), *Child and adolescent psychiatry: Modern approaches* (pp. 679–697). Oxford: Blackwell.

McClure, G. M. G. (1986). Recent changes in suicide among adolescents in England and Wales. *Journal of Adolescence, 9,* 135–143.

Prins, H. (1986). *Dangerous behaviour, the law, and mental disorder.* London: Tavistock.

Rutter, M., Graham, P., Chadwick, O., & Yule, W. (1976). Adolescent turmoil—fact or fiction? *Journal of Child Psychiatry and Psychology, 17,* 35–56.

Rutter, M., Shaffer, D., & Shepherd, M. (1975). *A multi-axial classification of child psychiatric disorders.* Geneva: World Health Organization.

Sainsbury, P., Jenkins, J., & Levey, A. (1980). The social correlates of suicide in Europe. In R. T. D. Farmer & S. R. Hirsch (Eds.), *The suicide syndrome* (pp. 38–53). London: Croom Helm.

Shaffer, D. (1974). Suicide in childhood and early adolescence. *Journal of Child Psychology and Psychiatry, 15,* 275–291.

Shaffer, D., & Fisher, P. (1981). The epidemiology of suicide in children and young adolescents. *Journal of the American Academy of Child Psychiatry, 20,* 545–565.

Steinberg, D. (1979). Some common psychiatric problems in adolescence. *Journal of the Irish Medical Association, 72,* 366–370.

Steinberg, D. (1981). *Using child psychiatry: The functions and operations of a specialty.* London: Hodder and Stoughton.

Steinberg, D. (1982). Treatment, training, care or control?: The functions of adolescent units. *British Journal of Psychiatry, 141,* 306–309.

Steinberg, D. (1983). *The clinical psychiatry of adolescence: Clinical work from a social and developmental perspective.* Chichester, UK: Wiley.

Steinberg, D. (1985). Psychotic and other severe disorders in adolescence. In M. Rutter & L. Hersov (Eds.), *Child and adolescent psychiatry: Modern approaches* (2nd ed.) (pp. 567–583). Oxford: Blackwell.

Steinberg, D. (Ed.). (1986). *The adolescent unit: Work and teamwork in adolescent psychiatry.* New York: Wiley.

Steinberg, D. (1987). *Basic adolescent psychiatry.* London: Blackwell.

Steinberg, D., Galhenage, D. P. C., & Robinson, S. C. (1981). Two years' referrals to a regional adolescent unit: Some implications for psychiatric services. *Social Science and Medicine, 15E,* 113–122.

Steinberg, D., & Hughes, L. (1987). The emergence of work-centered problems in consultative work. *Journal of Adolescence, 10,* 309–316.

Steinberg, D., & Yule, W. (1985). Consultative work. In M. Rutter & L. Hersov (Eds.), *Child and adolescent psychiatry: Modern approaches* (2nd ed.) (pp. 567–583). Oxford: Blackwell.

Tyrer, P., & Steinberg, D. (1987). *Models for mental disorder: Conceptual models in psychiatry.* New York: Wiley.

Winnicott, D. W. (1971). *Playing and reality.* London: Tavistock.

Zeitlin, H. (1986). *The natural history of psychiatric disorder in childhood.* University of London: Institute of Psychiatry Maudsley Monographs.

CHAPTER SEVEN

Suicide

Cynthia R. Pfeffer

"Apparent Pact Leads To Death of 18-Year-Old: Victim's Girlfriend, 16, Is Also Found Stabbed" (Purdum, 1986). This newspaper headline depicts the shocking phenomenon of teenage suicide which has provoked extensive sociopsychological morbidity in families, friends, and the community. Although the general public is alarmed and frightened by the high incidence of teenage suicide, relatively little research exists about this adolescent problem. In fact, most research on youth self-destructive behavior is centered on suicidal attempts, and these studies often assume that this kind of research will elucidate the characteristics of actual adolescent suicide. However, this assumption has not been tested adequately. Research studies comparing systematically teenagers who exhibit nonfatal and fatal suicidal behavior are just beginning to emerge, and they promise to elucidate distinctions between suicidal behavior and actual suicide.

This chapter will tackle the difficult task of synthesizing data about adolescent suicide. Much of it must be considered preliminary. When appropriate, information about suicidal behavior will be presented to supplement the newly emerging data about teenage suicide. Furthermore, this chapter, written primarily for clinicians, will attempt to prepare them for effective teenage suicide prevention and management.

ADOLESCENT SUICIDE AND THE CLINICIAN

Teenage suicide, like AIDS and drug abuse, has been a focus of intensive coverage by the media. For example, a June 6, 1986, *New York Times* article headlined the following:

> *Runner Badly Hurt in Leap Off Bridge: Attempted Suicide. Cathy Ormsby of North Carolina State, who broke the collegiate record for the women's 10,000 meter run seven weeks ago, was hospitalized with a serious spinal injury today after she bolted from another 10,000 meter race Wednesday night and apparently attempted to commit suicide by jumping off a bridge (Litsky, 1986).*

Another newspaper report on June 15, 1986, featured a discussion of the role of the media in suicide prevention: "Call-In Shows Are Tapping TV's Ability To Inform. What are the good things television can do? It can, evidence suggests, promote good health habits and inculcate what researchers call 'prosocial values'" (Corry, 1986). As a result of such reports, the general public has been extensively stimulated by the "facts" that have been presented. This heightened state of awareness impacts on the clinician in numerous ways.

Clinicians are pressed to provide answers to numerous queries about this problem. Certainly, it is a well-considered premise that educating the public about an illness or a disorder is an important prevention technique.

Thus clinicians must be able to serve as consultants to those educators who can teach the public about this problem. However, all too often clinicians find themselves discussing and answering questions about adolescent suicide without the benefit of information derived from systematic research. The media focuses on issues that take on qualities of fact well before they have been analyzed by systematic investigations. Thus the public may get information not grounded in adequate research.

The demands of the public for a remedy to decrease teen suicide further press on the clinician. In fact, clinicians may be forced to plan, consult to, and carry out prevention programs in a premature manner. Such approaches often lack adequate evaluation of their effectiveness. This has been especially evident in the development of school suicide prevention programs, which have been widely instituted and publicized. Clinicians also have been asked by avid zealots to consult for documentaries about teenage suicide. These media presentations, whose purpose is to prevent teen suicide, may actually have adverse effects (Corry, 1986). "Thus, there have been both drama and nonfiction programs about suicide among young people before, but no matter how well intended the programs, they can be disconcerting. They do not mean to do it, but they make suicide into a rather attractive possibility" (Corry, 1986). Indeed, there may have been a premature use of fictionalized media presentations as a vehicle for suicide prevention.

Paradoxically, when clinicians advise about measures for suicide prevention, their advice may go unheeded. This is dramatically illustrated by the resistance of some sections of the community to a plan to install protective barriers on bridges in the District of Columbia ("Suicide Problems," 1986).

After 34 suicides in 7 1/2 years at two bridges, the District of Columbia said it would install protective fences on the structures. The National Trust for Historic Preservation and some residents objected. . . . The Trust, fearing "an eyesore" and damage to the "architectural integrity and historic character" of the bridge, sued in Federal court to bar the work until public reaction could be sought. Residents concerned about esthetics asked the District Supreme Court to halt the work.

On a clinical level, resistance is often demonstrated by families through noncompliance with treatment plans. As a result, an adolescent may drop out of treatment and attempt to commit suicide. Clinicians, therefore, should educate families on the importance of maintaining the continuity of treatment (Taylor & Stansfeld, 1985), even allowing for the fact that further research is still necessary to determine whether adequate treatment in fact decreases the risk of suicide.

It is imperative that clinicians working with suicidal adolescents be aware of the most current systematically derived findings about adolescent suicide. Repeated educational courses should be mandatory for clinicians

(Editorial, *British Medical Journal,* 1981). The field of suicidology has rapidly advanced in the last few years. Some older notions are no longer valid and have been replaced by newer insights about trends in epidemiology, adolescent psychopathology, and its natural course. Patients and families, who are educated about this problem in a variety of ways, come to clinicians with a diverse set of beliefs, fantasies, requests, and expectations about the problems and the clinician's ability to be of assistance. Because of this, the clinician must be adequately armed with the latest systematically derived information in order to discuss with confidence the concerns and questions of the patients and families. Such knowledge also will enhance the clinician's skills in the appraisal of the patient's condition. However, the clinician must accept the fact that certain questions are not readily answerable. Under such circumstances, a clinician must be able to tolerate a patient's and his or her own anxiety.

The pressures on a clinician treating teenage suicidal behavior are often much greater than those encountered in treating other adolescent disorders. However, the management of adolescent suicidal behavior and consultation to community services on suicide prevention have an inherent challenge and excitement not evident in other clinical work. This makes the work of suicide management and prevention particularly worthwhile and rewarding.

SUICIDE AND SUICIDAL BEHAVIOR

One of the current controversies about suicidal behavior is whether individuals who commit suicide have different characteristics from those who make suicidal attempts. Because of the paucity of research data about suicide among adolescents, this issue cannot be settled definitively in this age group.

There are at least two schools of thought on this issue, both based primarily on evidence from adults who attempt and commit suicide. One is that suicidal behaviors show a continuity in characteristics and that the differences in characteristics between suicide and suicide attempts are mostly quantitative. Justification for this view lies in the finding that the diagnoses and symptoms for individuals who commit or attempt suicide appear to be similar. For example, both groups often show depressive symptoms and carry similar diagnoses such as major depressive disorder and alcohol abuse (Dorpat & Ripley, 1960; Guze & Robins, 1970; Barraclough, Bunch, Nelson, & Sainsbury, 1974).

Another view is that individuals who commit suicide are different from those who attempt suicide (Stengel, 1962). Although there is some overlap, the two groups are in fact discrete. Arguments for this view are based primarily on epidemiological data derived from prospective follow-up studies: Only a small proportion of individuals who previously attempted suicide later commit suicide. Also, retrospective studies indicate that among individuals who commit suicide only a small proportion have previously attempted suicide. Finally, there is a gender difference between the two groups (Weissman, 1974; Eisenberg, 1984): Men commit suicide more frequently, but women attempt suicide more often.

Shneidman (1985), who has vast clinical experience working with suicidal individuals, believes that suicide is different from suicidal behavior. He has suggested that the psychodynamic features in these two groups of individuals are distinct.

Whether these two points of view can apply to adolescents who attempt or commit suicide will require further study. Specifically, developmental issues, whether psychodynamic, genetic, environmental, or biological, need to be considered in this age group. In fact, systematic comparisons are needed between individuals who attempt or commit suicide at different phases of the life cycle before their relationship can be clarified.

THE EPIDEMIOLOGY OF ADOLESCENT SUICIDE

In 1984, suicide was the third leading cause of death for adolescents and young adults age 15 to 24 years, following only accidents and homicide (Monthly Vital Statistics Report of the National Center for Health Statistics, 1986). To illustrate the extent of the problem, in 1984, suicide was the eighth leading cause of death for all ages. In that year, there were 29,060 suicidal deaths in the United States. This amounted to a suicide rate of 12.3 per 100,000 population. In contrast, the age-specific suicide rate for 15- to 24-year-olds in 1984 was 12.2 per 100,000 population. There were over 5000 suicides for this group in 1984. Furthermore, it is estimated that for every suicide there are at least 100 adolescents who attempt suicide (Eisenberg, 1984). Thus suicidal behavior among adolescents and young adults is a major cause of concern.

However, despite these grim figures, suicide rates more recently have been decreasing or leveling off for adolescents and young adults. In 1977, the suicide rate for this age group reached a peak of 13.6. This rate declined to 12.4 in 1979, 12.3 in 1980 and 1981, 12.1 in 1982, and 12.2 in 1984 (Monthly Vital Statistics Report of the National Center for Health Statistics, 1979, 1984a, 1984b, 1986). Why this decrease has occurred is not entirely clear; several possible explanations will be discussed later in this section.

Differences in suicide rates occur among different gender and racial groups. White males have the highest suicide rate followed by nonwhite males, white females, and nonwhite females, respectively (Monthly Vital Statistics Report 1984b). For example, in 1982, the suicide rate per

100,000 population in the groups were: white male 20.7, nonwhite male 10.3, white female 6.1, nonwhite female 2.5.

Numerous questions remain about what may affect the national adolescent suicide rates. From a sociocultural perspective, it has been hypothesized that increased mobility, decreased family support, increased competition for jobs and educational opportunities, and increased coverage of the topic of suicide in the media may adversely affect suicide rates in adolescents. Determining just how specific they are requires further study.

In addition, recent research has offered two other explanations for changes in the national adolescent suicide rate during this century. The first is that the suicide rate of adolescents reflects the population changes among this age group (Holinger & Offer, 1982). Holinger and Offer found that between 1933 and 1975, the number of adolescents in the population at a given time is positively correlated with the adolescent suicide rate: When there are more adolescents in the population at a given time, the adolescent suicide rate increases. However, the authors found no similar relationship between the number of elderly in the population and the elderly suicide rate. They therefore proposed that this effect of population change on suicide rate among adolescents may be related to the increased competition for jobs and educational advancement that occurs when there are more adolescents. Their findings also suggest a method of predicting adolescent suicide rates.

A second explanation involves cohort effects and has been tested in three studies in different countries: United States, Canada, and Australia (Hellon & Solomon, 1980; Solomon & Hellon, 1980; Murphy & Wetzel, 1980; Goldney & Katsikitis, 1983). Each population was divided into groups or cohorts which were defined by their years of birth. All subjects born within a given 5-year period form one cohort. Thus all people born between 1930 and 1934 were in one cohort, while those born between 1935 and 1939 were in another cohort, and so forth. It was found in all three studies that with each successive birth cohort, the suicide rate for individuals who were 15 to 24 years old was higher than for the previous cohorts. In addition, it was noted that within a cohort, as individuals got older, their suicide rates increased. While the cause of this cohort effect remains unknown, it could be predicted that the youth suicide rate would continue to increase in future years. These findings also suggest that "whatever the cause of this effect, it is early and lasting" (Murphy & Wetzel, 1980).

FACTORS ASSOCIATED WITH ADOLESCENT SUICIDE

Suicide is a complexly determined event that occurs when combinations of factors are present simultaneously. Among the factors etiologically associated with suicide are disturbances in: (1) affects such as depression and aggression, (2) ego functioning that involve impulse control, judgment, and cognition, (3) interpersonal relations, (4) early developmental experiences (Pfeffer, 1986b). Although more research is needed to rank the significance of these factors, increasing evidence indicates that they are etiologically related to adolescent suicide.

Affective Disturbance

Although strong evidence exists for a relation between child and adolescent suicidal behavior and depressive symptoms (Carlson & Cantwell, 1982; Garfinkel, Froese, & Hood, 1982; Clarkin, Friedman, Hurt, Corn, & Aranoff, 1984; Meyers, Burke, & McCauley, 1985; Robbins, & Alessi, 1985; Pfeffer, 1986; Pfeffer, Plutchik, Mizruchi, & Lipkins, 1986), the relation between adolescent suicide and depression is surprisingly less obvious. In an early report of adolescent suicide, Shafii and associates (Shafii, Carrigan, Whittinghill, & Herrick, 1985) studied 20 adolescents, all 12 to 19 years of age, who committed suicide in Jefferson County, Kentucky, between January 1980 and June 1983. The authors obtained extensive retrospective information on these subjects by interviewing their relatives and acquaintances, using a psychological autopsy technique. Eighteen of the victims were male. Eighty-three percent of the families agreed to participate in this study. Of these participants, 95 % were white and 5% were black.

Shafii and associates noted that the teenagers who committed suicide, in contrast to a comparison group of nonsuicidal adolescents matched on sex, age, race, and social status, had significantly more of the following symptoms: previous suicidal ideas, threats, or attempts; frequent use of nonprescription drugs or alcohol; antisocial behaviors and inhibited personality. These adolescents, were very quiet, lacked close friends, did not openly talk about problems, and were lonely and extremely sensitive. In addition, they got into fights, had extensive school problems, sold drugs, and had other legal difficulties. There was little discussion about the association between depressive symptoms and suicide, but this finding must be considered tentative because the suicide victims were not directly evaluated before their death. It is commonly recognized that symptoms of depression are often not reliably reported by parents, but that externalizing behaviors such as assaultiveness, drug dealing, and school problems are reliably reported (Weissman, Orvaschel, & Padian, 1980; Kazdin, French, & Unis, 1983; Kazdin, Esveldt-Dawson, Unis, & Rancurello, 1983; Kashani, Orvaschel, Burk, & Reid, 1985; Moretti, Fine, Haley, & Marriage, 1985). Only by means of prospective studies of youngsters who commit suicide can this issue be more clearly understood.

Shaffer (1974), however, suggested that there is an association between child and adolescent suicide and depression. In a retrospective record review, he studied 31 youngsters, 14 years or younger, who committed suicide in England and Wales between 1962 and 1968. However, the study lacked a comparison group, and it was conducted on youngsters who had died more than 20 years ago. With regard to the affective and behavioral disturbances among these teenagers, Shaffer discerned that 4 (13%) had depressive symptoms, 17 (57%) had mixed affective and antisocial features, 5 (17%) had only antisocial symptoms, and 4 (13%) had neither affective nor antisocial features. While depressive symptoms were present, significant antisocial features also existed. Shaffer therefore proposed that not all teenagers who commit suicide are depressed and that conduct problems may also be an important risk factor. Shaffer and colleagues have recently undertaken a very large study of adolescent suicide in the New York area. They, too, are using the psychological autopsy method, and they are directly interviewing adolescent suicide attempters and their families as well as normal adolescents and their families. This study may therefore identify the characteristics of teenage suicide victims as well as clarify the continuity/discontinuity issue regarding adolescent suicide and suicide attempts.

Currently, there is almost no research regarding the types of psychiatric diagnoses that are associated with teenage suicide. Based on descriptions of symptoms by family and acquaintances, many of these teenage suicide subjects evidently had affective and conduct disturbances. However, because of the lack of systematic prospective assessments, more precise diagnoses usually cannot be assigned. Nevertheless, a few studies (Shaffer, 1974; Shafii et al., 1985;) do indicate that adolescents who commit suicide also frequently have a psychiatric disorder. It is, therefore, highly unlikely that suicide among teenagers can simply be attributed to a manifestation of adolescent turmoil. Rather, the evidence indicates that suicide occurs among those who are psychiatrically disturbed.

Another intriguing issue that may have some bearing on the increase in adolescent suicide in recent decades involves the changing epidemiology of depression during this time. Klerman and associates (1985) reported that there is a progressive increase in rates of depression as well as an earlier age of onset of depression in each successive birth cohort. This study, which was part of the National Institute of Mental Health-Clinical Research Branch Collaborative Program on the Psychobiology Depression Clinical Study, evaluated 2289 relatives of 523 subjects with an affective disorder. The findings of this study parallel trends suggestive of cohort effects for suicide and other violent deaths as well as for social phenomena involving economic and labor trends, marital profiles, and childbearing characteristics. Further evaluation of these parallel trends is required to clarify their potential relationships.

Ego-Functioning Disturbance

Ego functioning can be conceptualized as a person's intrapsychic functioning manifested by the degree of impulse control, judgment, and perceptions of current as well as past and future circumstances. Studies in adults suggest that ego-functioning disturbance may be an important risk factor for suicide. Strong evidence exists for a relationship between hopelessness and suicide. Beck and colleagues (Beck, Steer, Kovacs, & Garrison, 1985) studied 207 adult inpatients who had suicidal ideation but had made no attempt at the time of their index hospitalization. Fourteen patients committed suicide 5 to 10 years after discharge. Of all the variables studied, hopelessness and pessimism at the time of hospitalization predicted subsequent suicide. Shneidman (1980) offered a revealing description of disturbed ego functioning in suicidal adults. He proposed that at the time of suicide, the individual is in a heightened state of ego constriction. He described this constriction as a "narrowing of the range of perception, of opinions and of options that occur to the mind. The person is not only opinionated and prejudiced, but more importantly, suffers from a kind of 'tunnel vision'" (p. 12). Because of the failure to perceive and develop alternative plans for action, it appears that such individuals believe the only option is to commit suicide. In fact, Shneidman proposed that intervention should focus on decreasing the state of ego constriction and helping individuals perceive and develop alternative solutions to their dilemma.

The relationship between disturbed ego functioning and suicide in teenagers requires further study. Shaffer (1974) observed that teenage suicide seems to occur as a reaction to an immediate emotional crisis involving a family dispute or a disappointing or humiliating experience. However, the limitation of Shaffer's study lies in the fact that it was a retrospective study and lacked a control population.

Motto (1984), in a seven-year follow-up study of 122 male adolescents who were psychiatrically hospitalized for suicide attempts, found that 11 (9%) had committed suicide by the time of follow-up. "Fear of losing one's mind" and feelings of hopelessness at index hospitalization were the features that distinguished between those who committed suicide and those who did not. Both studies, therefore, lend some support to the view that ego functioning disturbance may be associated with adolescent suicide.

Interpersonal Relations

A great deal is yet to be learned about the interpersonal relations of adolescents who commit suicide. Anectodal statements of adolescents who later committed suicide suggest that they felt alone, abandoned, or had lost the support of an important friendship. One of the most revealing and detailed accounts of the depressing and painful experience of an isolated and suicidal adolescent girl was offered by Mack and Hickler (1981) in their book, *Vivienne: The Life and Suicide of an Adolescent Girl:* Among the immediate precipitants for the suicide of this girl, who died by hanging herself in her parent's home, was the loss of her favorite teacher who moved away. Signs of her intense depression and suicidal preoccupations, however, were evident before this teacher moved. Thus the factors contributing to her suicide were more than just the loss of her idealized teacher and apparently included problems such as identity diffusion, low self-esteem, and the nuances of a disturbed family relationship. Finally, Vivienne, like many teenagers who contemplate suicide, described herself as socially inept.

Motto (1984) in an important prospective follow-up study of 122 psychiatrically hospitalized teenagers who attempted suicide, found that many factors that strongly predicted subsequent suicide were those describing the individual's interpersonal relations. Suicide victims were more often interpersonally comprised. Further, although they had sought psychiatric help, they were very conflicted about entering into a therapeutic alliance with their therapist. They did not communicate openly, and it was therefore impossible to gain a clear insight into their fantasies, preoccupations, and feelings. As a result, these adolescents appeared to be quite unpredictable.

The aforementioned findings have major implications for adolescent suicide risk assessment. A clinician should always evaluate the quality of the patient's openness, his or her truthfulness and clarity of thinking. A systematic evaluation of such factors may allow the clinician to gauge the suicidal potential of the patient's self-destructive behavior.

Early Developmental Experiences

Vulnerability to suicide may be determined by an individual's adverse early life experiences. Numerous experiences have been identified for adults who committed suicide. These include death of parents, family loss, death or parental separation at an early age, affective disorders in family members, and suicide of relatives (Pfeffer, 1986a). These factors may operate either through a genetic and/or an experiential component. Unfortunately, little has been written about the early life experiences of adolescent suicide victims.

Being raised by a parent who has a severe affective disorder may influence the individual's behavior and development (Pfeffer, 1986a). Children whose parents have a major affective disorder have a threefold risk for developing a variety of psychiatric symptoms and disorders when compared with children of normal parents (Weissman et al., 1984). The most common psychiatric diagnoses of 6- to 18-year-old children of parents with severe depression are major depression, attention deficit disorder, and separation anxiety disorder.

A unique study that examines the adolescent suicide victim's early life experience was carried out by Salk, Lipsitt, Sturner, Reilly, and Levat (1985). Forty-six factors from the prenatal, birth, and neonatal records of 52 adolescents who committed suicide were compared to similar records of matched adolescents who did not commit suicide. The factors more commonly found in the suicide victims were respiratory distress for more than 1 hour after birth, no antenatal care before 20 weeks of pregnancy, and chronic disease of the mother. Although these results require further validation, they are intriguing because, like the cohort studies, they suggest a relationship between adolescent suicide and early life risk factors. This study clearly shows the importance of longitudinal prospective studies in the investigation of early risk factors in adolescent suicide.

Biological Factors

There are at present relatively few data on the role of biological factors in adolescent suicide. Those that exist are based on studies in adults, and they are not extensive. Recent research has focused on neuroendocrine and neurotransmitter physiology. Cortisol, a hormone, and serotonin, a neurotransmitter, have received the greatest attention.

Among the innovative approaches were studies that originated with the work of Asberg and colleagues (1976), who investigated the relation between suicide and low levels of 5-hydroxyindolacetic acid (5-HIAA) in the spinal fluid. These studies stimulated other studies that also have suggested a relation between violent suicide acts and low 5-HIAA, a metabolite of serotonin. Prospective research of adolescents at risk of suicide are necessary to determine which biological factors are important as predictors of suicide.

Special Issues

Adolescents may be highly susceptible to certain social and peer pressures. One type of such pressure is that of imitation, which may be particularly relevant to adolescent suicide. Imitation may lead to a contagion phenomenon, and evidence is accumulating that such a phenomenon for adolescent suicide does exist (Pfeffer, 1985). In the nineteenth century a cluster of adolescent suicides occurred after the publication of Goethe's book; *The Sorrows of Young Werther*. It appeared that vulnerable adolescents had identified themselves with Werther, the hero in the novel who died by shooting himself in the head. Recent research on the effects of media coverage of suicide also suggests elements of imitation and identification. Phillips (1974), investigating the effects of newspaper reports of the suicides of famous people, found that the national suicide rate increased significantly within approximately two weeks after such newspaper reports. He also noted that the more famous the person, the greater was the subsequent increase in suicide. This finding is also true for adolescents.

Some support for the phenomenon of adolescent suicide contagion is found in the study of the adolescents in Micronesia (Rubinstein, 1983), where since 1960 there had been an unusual increase in suicides among the 15- to 24-year-old males. On the one hand, this increase seemed to have resulted from a cohort effect that was related to the adolescents' dramatic shift away from the traditional communal village life. This shift increased the tension of their interpersonal relationships and the tension between them and their families. In particular, suicides among male adolescents seemed to result from their disturbed relationship with their parents. On the other hand, the increase may have been related to an imitative element among Micronesian youths which seemed to further increase their tendency to commit suicide.

There is little doubt that certain cultural factors can sometimes promote youth suicide. Specific populations of adolescents, such as certain Native Americans and homosexuals, are at high risk. These teenagers often encounter certain unique personal and social stresses: problems with identity, self-esteem, social denegration, and isolation. However, there is as yet insufficient research on their developmental, constitutional, sociocultural, and psychological aspects in regard to their increased suicide risk.

PREVENTION OF ADOLESCENT SUICIDE

This section will discuss the clinician's levels of involvement in adolescent suicide prevention. Foremost among these are the clinical tasks of recognition and intervention of adolescents at risk. In addition, a clinician often acts as a consultant to community groups involved in educating the public about teenage suicide.

Recognition of Adolescents at Risk

Early recognition of an adolescent at risk is a major factor in suicide prevention. Such a youngster may be successfully treated before suicide is actually attempted. The key to successful prevention is the early detection of the high risk signs. Among the most important of the early signs is a change in the individual's usual behavior, which is often associated with the development of depressive symptoms. For example, changes in eating and sleeping habits should always put the clinician on alert. Potentially suicidal adolescents frequently complain that they cannot sleep; they may have trouble falling asleep, may awaken frequently in the middle of the night, or may wake up early. Some may sleep more than usual; Motto (1984) has reported that they may withdraw into a state of hypersomnia. Loss of weight or excessive weight gain are also risk features. Social withdrawal is yet another important risk factor. Many distressed teenagers abandon their usual activities with friends and family. They prefer to be alone and brood. They often lack energy and no longer enjoy the once pleasurable activities. Some appear to be more tense and agitated. They have a heightened activity level but at the same time have difficulties concentrating. School performance deteriorates and grades fall.

Often, seriously distressed adolescents become more argumentative, angry, and belligerent. Such early warning signs frequently go unrecognized, however, because they are not perceived as signs of distress. Such behaviors provoke anger, bewilderment, and withdrawal in others, and the distressed adolescents are seen as a nuisance. Therefore, a clinician should always regard increased irritability and anger as serious signs of distress.

Somatic complaints of headaches, stomachaches, and other physical ailments may be manifestations of psychological distress, although they should always be thoroughly evaluated by a physician. School refusal may be another warning sign; the adolescent simply feels unable to cope with school.

Many teenagers who commit suicide have been excessively preoccupied with death for a significant time. Vivienne, the 14-year-old who hung herself in the basement of her parents' house, wrote extensive poetry involving themes of death (Mack & Hickler, 1981). Other adolescents dream about others getting killed or dying. Some dream of their own death. They also worry frequently about their relatives dying. Such excessive death preoccupation may be one of the earliest clues to youth suicide (Pfeffer, 1986b). A particularly high risk situation occurs in an adolescent who has experienced the recent death of a relative or friend. As part of the mourning reaction, the adolescent may dwell on scenes of death and harbor a wish or fantasy that the dead person would return. At times, however, this preoccupation takes the form of a more extensive rumination and propels the adolescent into a state of wishing to die. In sum, any evidence of repetitive death preoccupation merits careful exploration (Pfeffer, 1986b).

Of even greater significance than death preoccupation are specific statements about suicide. Motto (1984) found that the adolescent suicide attempters who subsequently committed suicide, in contrast to those who did not, more often clearly communicated their suicidal intent to someone before an attempt. Thus any talk of suicide should be taken seriously and evaluated carefully. In fact, during any clinical assessment of an adolescent, the clinician always should ask specifically about suicidal ideation and intent: Have you ever felt hopeless? Have you ever felt that life is not worth living? Have you ever wished to die? Have you ever thought about hurting yourself or committing suicide? Have you ever tried to hurt yourself or to attempt suicide? Furthermore, such questions should be asked at different times in the interview process rather than just once (Pfeffer,

1986b). Often the adolescent initially denies any such ideation or intent but when trust develops during the interview, speaks about these issues more openly.

Finally, in evaluating suicide risk, the clinician must always try to gather information from those around the patient, such as parents, teachers, siblings, and peers. While there may be discrepancies between the patient's and the observers' reports, information from multiple sources is nevertheless invaluable to the clinician in assessing suicidal risk.

Interventions for Suicidal Adolescents

A clinician should utilize a combination of interventions in working with suicidal adolescents. The most important approach is individual therapy with the teenager (Pfeffer, 1986b), whether inpatient or outpatient. The clinician must spend time with the adolescent to evaluate and explore the issues within the atmosphere of a secure and trusting therapeutic alliance. The importance of this empathic atmosphere cannot be overemphasized because the suicidal adolescent must feel free to discuss any issue relevant to his or her condition.

Suicidal adolescents often perceive themselves as devoid of certain essential emotional needs or as being unworthy of having such needs met. They may be deficient in skills that would allow them to achieve emotional satisfaction. Treatment, therefore, should focus on helping the adolescent identify needs and develop ways to satisfy such needs. The therapist should encourage the patient to describe personal expectations and fantasies, and each of them should be explored and discussed in detail. At times, the therapist becomes a "negotiator" who suggests options to counteract the adolescent's arbitrary and limited skills to develop alternative approaches for achieving emotional gratification. Repeated intensive discussions on these options are again indicated. Cognitive methods that include explicit suggestions on how to respond to situations, direct statements that enhance the self-esteem of the adolescent, and instructions on how to overcome helplessness and hopelessness are probably the most suitable for working with a suicidal adolescent.

At times of acute suicidal risk, the clinician must also work intensively with the parents (Pfeffer, 1986b). Therapy with the parents should focus initially on discovering parental attitudes, family communication patterns, and relationships. The strengths of the family should be mobilized to support the distressed teenager, while the more adverse family interactions should be decreased. It is essential to encourage the parents to maintain an honest, open, and determined attitude that the adolescent patient must remain alive and that no one in the family should die from suicide.

With regard to specific family dynamics in relation to suicide, Sabbath (1966) described the presence of several characteristics that often seemed to imply that the adolescent was "an expendable child." Moreover, the parents often considered the adolescent to be responsible for their problems. The adolescent thus perceived the parents' overt or covert rejection as a wish that he or she should die. A sense of mutual oppression, rejection, sadism, and lack of support were apparently common in such families. While these findings were preliminary, the clinician should be sensitive to such issues and work to resolve them. Sometimes families of youngsters who committed suicide overly focused on certain attributes of the adolescent (Corder & Haizlip, 1984). Unfortunately, these attributes may become overidealized and thus unrealistic, and when this family expectation fails to become realized, the adolescent may feel deeply humiliated and suicide may follow.

Medication is another significant treatment modality. The type of medication used will depend upon the symptoms and psychiatric diagnosis of the individual. An empirical approach to utilization of medications is recommended. Medication should be targeted at specific symptoms that are not ameliorated by other therapeutic techniques. For example, antidepressants may be essential for an unremitting depression. Currently, there is no specific medication that is unique to suicidal behavior.

Because suicidal adolescents attempt suicide by a variety of methods that are potentially highly lethal (Holinger, 1978), such as shooting, hanging, overdose or ingestion of poison, running into traffic, and self-stabbing, they are often treated initially in medical settings. If this is the case, the mental health professional should be involved immediately. It is essential that the assessment of the risk factors and psychotherapy begin as soon as possible (Lewis & Solnit, 1963).

Regardless of where the suicidal adolescent is first recognized and evaluated, a paramount objective in the intervention is to protect the teenager from self-harm (Pfeffer, 1986b). If social supports (particularly those from the family) are not adequate, the adolescent may need to be moved to a safe and supportive environment. Immediate psychiatric hospitalization may be necessary for an acutely suicidal youngster and is often the single most effective intervention, particularly for those at serious risk (Pfeffer et al., 1986).

In addition to enhancing familial support and protecting the youngster from harm, the clinician must also develop other environmental supports. Liaison with school professionals, for example, is essential since adolescents spend a major portion of their days in school. Ideally, the school should be able to work closely with the adolescent, parents, and therapists. The therapist may be able to achieve this working relationship by inviting the school counselor or a teacher who is closely involved to a case conference or even a meeting with the patient and the family. In such a setting, specific strategies can be developed. Of course, prior approval from the patient and/or parent is necessary for such a meeting.

Education and Consultation to the Community

One of the most important roles for the clinician in suicide prevention is to provide consultation to community resources as well as mental health professionals. Besides providing the most current and solid findings on suicide, the clinician must inform the lay community and professionals that the single most important prevention measure is appropriate and adequate treatment for the suicidal adolescent. It is apparent that adolescents who demonstrate repetitive suicidal behavior have often signed out of treatment against medical advice or have not followed through with treatment recommendation.

Clinicians, serving as educators, must capture the attention and enthusiasm of both the public and the professionals so that together they may form an effective community network for suicide prevention (Pfeffer, 1985). Many preventative measures can be instituted only with wide community support. Programs to limit access to guns and other lethal weapons and programs to put up barriers on high places are two such examples. In addition, clinicians should assist in the development of new curricula or review existing ones for educating the public regarding suicide. Consultation with media professionals about programs on adolescent suicide is another important area of prevention. It is essential that the topic is not glamorized; otherwise, such programs may inadvertently provoke the contagion phenomenon.

Finally, clinicians must work with the community and other professionals to ensure that suicide prevention efforts are maintained by legislation. Collaboration among government agencies, funding sources, professionals, and the general public must exist in order to develop effective and long-range suicide prevention strategies.

SUMMARY AND DIRECTIVES FOR THE FUTURE

The aim of this chapter is to bring together the current information about adolescent suicide; therefore, the chapter could be considered a "state of the art" description. Remarkably, although suicide is one of the most common causes of death for adolescents and young adults, significant gaps still exist in our knowledge on the topic. Fortunately, much enthusiasm exists among researchers on this topic, and in the next few years, there promises to be an explosion of research data about adolescent suicide.

One of the most pressing concerns is whether actual suicide has similar features to suicidal behavior. This is an especially critical concern because of the implications for suicide prevention. Unfortunately, research data are lacking in this area. However, data derived from empirical and epidemiological research must still be interpreted by the clinician. In a clinical setting, the clinician must focus on the unique risk factors of his or her particular patient. Pokorny (1983) noted that diagnosis of suicidal risk "consists of a sequence of small decisions. . . . the first decision might be based on some alerting note or sign, and the decision would be to investigate further" (p. 257).

There is no doubt that suicide is a complex phenomenon involving various biopsychosociocultural factors. Thus future adolescent suicide prevention must utilize information derived from different vantage points. Furthermore, it seems increasingly unlikely that a clinician in solo practice can offer effective intervention and prevention. Instead, a team of professionals should collaborate in the treatment of suicidal adolescents (Pfeffer, 1985). Each member of the team may offer a unique input and also provide support for the other team members in caring for suicidal adolescents. Meanwhile, although the social taboos surrounding adolescent suicide have lessened, more effort needs to be directed to reduce the stigmas attached to families bereaved by adolescent suicide. More effective help for such families through their bereavement needs to be developed. Finally, more efforts must be directed toward educating families and schools to enable them to identify the adolescent at risk.

REFERENCES

Asberg, M., Traskman, B., & Thoren, P. (1976). 5-HIAA in the cerebrospinal fluid: A biochemical suicide predictor? *Archives of General Psychiatry, 33,* 1193–1197.

Barraclough, B., Bunch, J., Nelson, N., & Sainsbury, P. (1974). A hundred cases of suicide: Clinical aspects. *British Journal of Psychiatry, 125,* 355–373.

Beck, A. T., Steer, R. A., Kovacs, M., & Garrison, B. (1985). Hopelessness and eventual suicide: A 10-year prospective study of patients hospitalized with suicidal ideation. *American Journal of Psychiatry, 142,* 559–563.

Carlson, G. A., & Cantwell, D. P. (1982). Suicidal behavior and depression in children and adolescents. *Journal of the American Academy of Child Psychiatry, 21,* 361–368.

Clarkin, J. F., Friedman, R. C., Hurt, S. W., Corn, R., & Aranoff, M. (1984). Affective and character pathology of suicidal adolescent and young adult inpatients. *Journal of Clinical Psychiatry, 45,* 19–22.

Corder, B. F., & Haizlip, T. M. (1984). Environmental and personality similarities in case histories of suicide and self-poisoning by children under ten. *Suicide and Life-Threatening Behavior, 14,* 59–66.

Corry, J. (1986, June 15). Call-in shows are tapping TV's ability to inform. *New York Times.*

Dorpat, T. L., & Ripley, H. S. (1960). A study of suicide in the Seattle area. *Comprehensive Psychiatry, 1,* 349–359.

Editorial (1981). Children and parasuicide. *British Medical Journal, 283,* 337–338.

Eisenberg, L. (1984). The epidemiology of suicide in adolescents. *Pediatric Annals, 13,* 47–54.

Garfinkel, B. D., Froese, A., & Hood, J. (1982). Suicide attempts in children and adolescents. *American Journal of Psychiatry, 139,* 1257–1261.

Goldney, R. D., & Katsikitis, M. (1983). Cohort analysis of suicide rates in Australia. *Archives of General Psychiatry 40,* 71–74.

Guze, S. B., & Robins, E. (1970). Suicide and primary affective disorders. *British Journal of Psychiatry, 117,* 437–438.

Hellon, C. P., & Solomon, M. I. (1980). Suicide and age in Alberta, Canada, 1951 to 1977: The changing profile. *Archives of General Psychiatry, 37,* 505–510.

Holinger, P. C. (1978). Adolescent suicide: An epidemiological study of recent trends. *American Journal of Psychiatry, 135,* 754–756.

Holinger, P. C., & Offer, D. (1982). Prediction of adolescent suicide: A population model. *American Journal of Psychiatry, 139,* 302–307.

Kashani, J. H., Orvaschel, H., Burk, J. P., & Reid, J. C. (1985). Informant variance: The issue of parent-child disagreement. *Journal of the American Academy of Child Psychiatry, 24,* 437–441.

Kazdin, A. E., Esveldt-Dawson, K., Unis, A. S., & Rancurello, M. D. (1983). Child and parent evaluations of depression and aggression in psychiatric inpatient children. *Journal of Abnormal Child Psychology, 11,* 401–413.

Kazdin, A. E., French, N. H., & Unis, A. S. (1983). Child, mother, and father evaluations of depression in psychiatric inpatient children. *Journal of Abnormal Child Psychology, 11,* 167–179.

Klerman, G. L., Lavori, P. W., Nice, J., Reich, T., Endicott, J., Andreasen, N. C., Keller, M. B., & Hirschfield, R. M. A. (1985). Birth-cohort trends in rates of major depressive disorder among relatives of patients with affective disorder. *Archives of General Psychiatry, 42,* 689–693.

Lewis, M., & Solnit, A. J. (1963). The adolescent in a suicidal crisis: Collaborative care in a pediatric ward. In A. Solnit & S. Provence (Eds.), *Modern Perspectives in child development.* New York: International Universities Press.

Litsky, F. (1986, June 6). Runner badly hurt in leap off bridge: Attempted suicide. *New York Times.*

Mack, J. E., & Hickler, H. (1981). *Vivienne: The life and suicide of an adolescent girl.* Boston, MA: Little Brown.

Monthly Vital Statistics Report of the National Ctr. for Health Statistics (1979). Final mortality statistics, 1977.

Monthly Vital Statistics Report of the National Ctr. for Health Statistics (1984a). Advance report of final statistics, 1981.

Monthly Vital Statistics Report of the National Ctr. for Health Statistics (1984b). Advance report of final mortality statistics, 1982.

Monthly Vital Statistics Report of the National Center for Health Statistics (1986). Preliminary 1984 suicide statistics.

Moretti, M. M., Fine, S., Haley, G., & Marriage, K. (1985). Childhood and adolescent depression: Child-report versus parent-report information. *Journal of the American Academy of Child Psychiatry, 24,* 298–302.

Motto, J. A. (1984). Suicide in male adolescents. In H. S. Sudak, A. B. Ford, & N. B. Rushforth (Eds.), *Suicide in the young.* Boston, MA: PSG.

Murphy, G. E., & Wetzel, R. D. (1980). Suicide risk by birth cohort in the United States, 1949 to 1974. *Archives of General Psychiatry, 37,* 519–523.

Myers, K. M., Burke, P., & McCauley, E. (1985). Suicidal behavior by hospitalized preadolescent children on a psychiatric unit. *Journal of the American Academy of Child Psychiatry, 24,* 474–480.

Pfeffer, G. R. (1985, September 18–20). Suicide prevention: Current efficacy and future promise. Presented at the Conference on Psychobiology of Suicidal Behavior, sponsored by The New York Academy of Sciences and National Institute of Mental Health, New York, NY.

Pfeffer, C. R. (1986a, May 8–9). Family factors in youth suicide. Presented at National Institute of Mental Health and Human Services Task Force on Risk Factors for Youth Suicide, Bethesda, MD.

Pfeffer, C. R. (1986b). *The suicidal child,* New York: Guilford.

Pfeffer, C. R., Plutchik, R., Mizruchi, M. S., & Lipkins, R. (1986). Suicidal behavior in child psychiatric inpatients and outpatients and in nonpatients. *American Journal of Psychiatry, 143,* 733–738.

Phillips, D. A. (1974). The influence of suggestion on suicide: Substantive and theoretical implications of the Werther effect. *American Sociological Review, 39,* 340–354.

Pokorny, A. D. (1983). Prediction of suicide in psychiatric patients. *Archives of General Psychiatry, 40,* 249–257.

Purdum, T. (1986, April 30). Apparent pact leads to death of 18-year-old. *New York Times.*

Robbins, D. R., & Alessi, N. E. (1985). Depressive symptoms and suicidal behavior in adolescents. *American Journal of Psychiatry, 142,* 588–592.

Rubinstein, D. H. (1983). Epidemic suicide among Micronesian adolescents. *Social Science Medicine, 17,* 657–665.

Sabbath, J. C. (1966). The suicidal adolescent—the expendable child. *Journal of the American Academy of Child Psychiatry, 5,* 272–289.

Salk, L., Lipsitt, L. P., Sturner, W. O., Reilly, B. M., & Levat, R. H. (1985). Relationship of maternal and perinatal conditions to eventual adolescent suicide. *The Lancet,* March 16, 624–627.

Shaffer, D. (1974). Suicide in childhood and early adolescence. *Journal of Child Psychology and Psychiatry, 15,* 275–291.

Shafii, M., Carrigan, S., Whittinghill, J. R., & Herrick, A. (1985). Psychological autopsy of completed suicide in children and adolescents. *American Journal of Psychiatry, 142,* 1061–1064.

Shneidman, E. (1985). *Definition of suicide,* New York: Wiley.

Shneidman, E. (1980). *Voices of death,* New York: Harper & Row.

Solomon, M. I., & Hellon, C. P. (1980). Suicide and age in Alberta, Canada, 1951 to 1977: A cohort analysis. *Archives of General Psychiatry, 37,* 511–513.

Stengel, E. (1962). Recent research into suicide and attempted suicide. *American Journal of Psychiatry, 118,* 725–727.

Suicide Problem at Twin Bridges. (1986, May 4). *New York Times.*

Taylor, E. A., & Stansfeld, S. A. (1985). Children who poison themselves: II. Prediction of attendance for treatment. *British Journal of Psychiatry, 146,* 132–135.

Weissman, M. M. (1974). The epidemiology of suicide attempts, 1960 to 1971. *Archives of General Psychiatry, 30,* 737–746.

Weissman, M. M., Orvaschel, H., & Padian, N. (1980). Children's symptom and social functioning self-report scales: comparison of mother's and children's reports. *Journal of Nervous and Mental Disease, 168,* 736–740.

Weissman, M. M., Prusoff, B. A., Gamnon, G. D., Merikangas, K. R., Leckman, J. F., & Kidd, K. K. (1984). Psychopathology in the children (ages 6–18) of depressed and normal patients. *Journal of the American Academy of Child Psychiatry, 23,* 78–84.

CHAPTER EIGHT

Legal Issues

Gary B. Melton
Linda K. Schmechel*

* Dr. Schmechel's work on this chapter was supported by a National Research Service Award from the National Institute of Mental Health to the University of Nebraska-Lincoln (Grant No. 5 T32 MH16156-06), where she was a postdoctoral fellow.

The fact that this volume includes a chapter on legal issues in adolescent mental health marks it as a product of the 1980s. Culminating in the Supreme Court's landmark decision in *Parham v. J. R.* (1979), questions about special legal problems in adolescent mental health generally did not reach the courts and the legislatures until the 1970s. Even today, the law is unsettled in regard to many practical problems of adolescent mental health law and policy (see generally Melton, 1987d; Melton & Spaulding, in press), and the law has yet to recognize adolescence as a special status (Melton, 1987d, in press; Zimring, 1982). The current state of the law is a conflict-laden and sometimes incoherent array of assumptions and doctrines that often leave considerable ambiguity about the correct answer to legal problems of adolescent mental health practice.

To understand these developments, a brief historical overview is helpful. Although "infants" always have been accorded solicitude in Anglo-American law, minority as a special legal status accompanied by special legal institutions is a more recent invention. At the last turn of the century, the first juvenile courts were organized, and the first child labor laws and compulsory education laws were enacted. At the same time, adolescence began to be recognized as a separate developmental stage (see, e.g., Hall, 1904). Most social historians have argued that the confluence of events was not accidental (see, e.g., Bakan, 1971; Kett, 1977; Platt, 1977). The invention of juvenile courts resulted in the invention of adolescence. By establishing special structures for the regulation of the lives of minors, the law increased scrutiny of young people in order to socialize immigrant youth and maintain control over youth in rural America. Whereas teen-agers had previously been counted upon to be productive members of the workforce, they were thrust into a conflict between actual competence and ascribed incompetence and between social expectations of productivity and legal requirements for dependency. The much ballyhooed identity crisis of youth apparently was largely nonexistent until the law reified such conflicts of role.

The invention of juvenile court was not the first time the law had established special rules for dealing with minors. However, until then, special institutions were not present, and the scope of special legal provisions was not nearly so broad in either the range of conduct to be regulated or the length of dependency. In Anglo-American common law, infancy was available as an irrebuttable defense in criminal and tort law for minors under the age of 7 and a rebuttable defense for minors age 7 to 14. Infants were regarded as incapable of moral reasoning and, therefore, deserving of protection but unentitled to the rights accorded moral and legal persons. In order to ensure that their estates were not squandered, the law as *parens patriae* (sovereign parent) assumed the role of benevolent overseer to ensure that minors, presumed totally dependent on competent adults to care for them, were always supervised by adult guardians who acted in their stead. The unity of interest between state and child* and, in most cases, parent and child was not challenged.

The major problem of this body of law is that it was uncritically applied when the jurisdiction of the juvenile court expanded in the first half of the twentieth century. Older adolescents were treated as infants, and the law assumed that it could oversee a wide range of youthful conduct effectively without undue harm to families or adolescents themselves. The actual complexity of relationships among child, parent, and state was overlooked.

Not until the late 1960s did serious questions arise about the status of children and the unity of their interests with those of their parents and the state. However, confusion has persisted even within the contemporary children's rights movement about the nature of the rights to which children are entitled and, therefore, the level of deference owed children's judgments (apart from those of their parents) about matters of personal significance, such as mental health. Although they commonly concede that children do have some independent rights, legal authorities and mental health professionals alike have been divided by their variant views of the proper moral and legal status of children in their assessment of what those rights are.

At least overtly, the several orientations to children's rights are based on divergent perceptions of the empirical realities of child development and family life. For the most part, these schools of thought can be categorized by their views of children's competency as decision makers and their vulnerability to psychological ill effects of bad decisions. One group, colloquially labeled "child savers," perceives children as incompetent and vulnerable and therefore dependent on adult protection. They argue that the state should enforce special entitlements for children (e.g., rights to education, health care, and even a loving family), but they regard recognition of rights to autonomy and privacy for children as unimportant and even ill-advised. To summarize, child savers would like recognition of rights for children to do or have what is good for them.

On the other hand, "kiddie libbers" perceive children, especially adolescents, as more like than unlike adults. They emphasize the significance of civil liberties in the lives of children as well as their parents, and thus they believe minors are entitled to protection of privacy and basic freedoms of self-expression, even when such rights bring them into conflict with their parents as well as the state. In sharp contrast to the child savers, the kiddie libbers emphasize that respect for persons includes the recognition of the right to be wrong, although they do not expect adolescents to be wrong more frequently than most adults whose right to self-determination is unquestioned.

Empirically, attitudes toward children's rights do load on two factors corresponding to these two broad perspectives: self-determination and

* Because the law has not discriminated between children and adolescents, we will lapse into use of the term "child" for convenience, except when we are distinguishing developmental findings. Obviously, the term should be read to include adolescents.

nurturance (see Melton, 1983a; Rogers & Wrightsman, 1978). However, within a given school of thought, other specific attitudes and beliefs may affect views on particular policies. For example, contemporary intellectual heirs to turn-of-the-century child savers believe that family privacy has been overvalued (see e.g., Feshbach & Feshbach, 1978; Garbarino, Gaboury, Long, Grandjean, & Asp, 1982). At least implicitly, they favor broad state involvement in the lives of families and their communities in order to protect the welfare of children. On the other hand, Goldstein, Freud, and Solnit (1973, 1979) and their followers start from the same assumptions about children's incompetence and vulnerability, but they favor almost unfettered parental action because of the significance they ascribe to parental authority in the psychological development of the child.

On some issues, child savers and kiddie libbers may advocate the same result, although for different reasons. For example, child savers may favor minors' independent access to mental health services because they want to ensure that children in need of services obtain them, while kiddie libbers may advocate the same policy because of respect for individual privacy in personal decisions. Similarly, both groups of child advocates may support entitlements to education. However, the liberationist group supports recognition of such entitlements, not because it believes that children need protection, but because education may be necessary to acquisition of the skills necessary to assert one's autonomy. (In both examples, the purists in the two groups would part company about whether children should have a right to refuse services.)

Obviously, most people's attitudes do not fit on the extremes of the two factors. Also, as previously noted, the two major schools of child advocates are not in constant conflict. However, the point still is important that discussion of "children's rights" is not helpful in forming policy unless the discussion includes detailed identification of the interests at stake, the level of claim attached to them, and the nature of assumptions on which various claims are based. As we shall see, such scholarly analyses commonly have eluded both judges and advocates. Moreover, because ambivalence about children's status and the nature of their interests persists, legal holdings often are ambiguous, particularly given the lack of forthright analysis of the degree of congruence and ultimate primacy of the various interests of child, family, and state.

THE DEVELOPMENT OF CASE LAW ON CHILDREN'S RIGHTS

Pre-Gault

The muddled approach to children's rights is not new. In the first half of this century, the Supreme Court decided three "children's rights" cases. In the first case in that series (*Meyer v. Nebraska,* 1923), the Court held that a state law barring instruction of any subject in a foreign language violated the due process clause of the Fourteenth Amendment. *Meyer* was followed by *Pierce v. Society of Sisters* (1925), in which the Court struck down a state law mandating that children attend *public* schools.

Neither case is very clear as to whose interests were vindicated, but what is certain is that independent interests of children were given little consideration. *Meyer* recognized the teacher's "right . . . to teach and the right of parents to engage him so to instruct their children," pursuant to the parental "right of control" (p. 400). Although the pleadings of the appellees in *Pierce* referred to "the right of the child to influence the parents' choice of a school," they also argued that the state law requiring attendance in public schools violated "the right of parents to choose schools where their children will receive appropriate mental and religious training," "the right of schools and teachers therein to engage in a useful business and profession," and the right of the Society of Sisters, as a private corporation, to make use of its property (p. 400). The Court itself concluded that the compulsory public education law "interfere[d] with the liberty of parents and guardians to direct the upbringing and education of children *under their control.* . . . The child is not the mere creature of the state; those who nurture him and direct his destiny have the right, coupled with the high duty, to recognize and prepare him for additional obligations" (pp. 534–535, emphasis added).

By contrast, in *Prince v. Massachusetts* (1944), the Court affirmed the conviction of a 9-year-old's guardian for violation of child labor laws by permitting the child to sell a magazine published by the Jehovah's Witnesses. The Court acknowledged "the rights of children to exercise their religion, and of parents to give them religious training" (p. 165). Citing *Meyer* and *Pierce,* the Court recognized that the state was invading a "private realm of family life"; it asserted a "cardinal [principle] . . . that the custody, care and nurturance of the child reside first in the parents, whose primary function and freedom include preparation for obligations the state can neither supply nor hinder" (p. 166).

Nonetheless, the *Prince* Court adopted a philosophy of protection by the state:

> . . . *It is the interest of youth itself, and of the whole community, that children be both safeguarded from abuses and given opportunities for growth into free and independent well-developed men [sic] and citizens.* . . . *Acting to guard the general interest in youth's well being, the state as parens patriae may restrict the* parent's control *by requiring school attendance, regulating or prohibiting the child's labor, and in many other ways.* . . .
>
> *The state's authority over children's activities is broader than over like actions of adults.* . . . *A democratic society rests, for its continuance, upon the healthy well-rounded growth of young people into full maturity as citizens, with all that*

*implies. It may secure this against impeding restraints and dangers, within a broad
range of selection [of matters for regulation]. . . .*

*. . . Parents may be free to become martyrs themselves. But it does not follow
they are free, in identical circumstances, to make martyrs of their children before
they have reached the age of full and legal discretion when they can make that
choice for themselves. (pp. 165–166, 168, and 170, emphasis added)*

The three "foundation cases" for children's rights are filled with
quotable dicta about the nature of childhood and family life, but the
principles for which they stand are not clear. They offer neither a bright
line that the state may not cross in matters of childrearing nor a clear
formulation of the degree that children's interests are coextensive with
either parents or the state. To the extent that the child's interests are
considered, the "liberty" that is recognized is a mere right to obey—to
follow the direction of the parents or state authority. *Meyer, Pierce,* and
Prince may have laid the foundation for recognition of a constitutional
right to privacy (see *Roe v. Wade,* 1973), but they have been mislabeled as
children's rights cases.

In re Gault

The Supreme Court did not directly deal with the question of *children's*
rights until 1966. The turning point came in the case of *In re Gault.*
Accused of having made an obscene telephone call including comments of
"the irritatingly offensive, adolescent variety" (p. 4), 15-year-old Gerald
Gault was taken into custody without parental notification. He was de-
tained on the basis of a hearing in which no record was made, witnesses
were not confronted, and the privilege against self-incrimination was not
recognized. Without specific judicial findings, he was committed to a
juvenile correctional facility for an indefinite period that might have extended to age 21. Overturning the juvenile court's finding that Gault was
a delinquent and its order of commitment, the Supreme Court held that
respondents in delinquency proceedings have a right to most of the procedural protections owed adult defendants: timely written notice of the
charges, the right to counsel, the right to confront and cross-examine
witnesses, and the privilege against self-incrimination.

Gault had two major effects. First, the Court made clear that it no longer
would uphold the verdicts of a lawless "kangaroo court" (p. 28) for juveniles
accused of delinquent offenses. Even if grounded in a protectionist philosophy, juvenile proceedings not only were not benign but indeed were "the
worst of both worlds" (p. 18, note 23). They lacked the procedural protections of criminal courts while providing services that not only were not
effective but indeed were harsh and iatrogenic. In short, the Court sent a

message that a therapeutic rationale cannot be used as an all-purpose justification for practices that really are indefensible.

Second, the Court announced for the first time that minors are "persons" within the meaning of the Bill of Rights and the Fourteenth Amendment, which makes the Bill of Rights applicable to the states. The Court thus made clear that, as individuals, minors do possess fundamental rights recognized in law. However, because no one seriously argues that *all* age-graded distinctions are without compelling justification, *Gault* opened the door to questions about the limits of minors' autonomy. Indeed, *Gault* itself raised one such issue. The Court forthrightly held that the Fifth Amendment protects juvenile respondents from self-incrimination despite the "civil" nature of juvenile proceedings. However, noting concerns that juveniles might be overwhelmed by skillful police interrogation (cf. *Haley v. Ohio*, 1948), the Court indicated that special care should be taken to ensure that juveniles' waivers of their rights are not "the product of ignorance of rights or adolescent fantasy, fright or despair" (*In re Gault*, 1966, p. 55). Thus at the same time that the Court recognized the application of constitutional rights to juveniles, it raised questions about whether limits might be legitimately placed on minors' self-determination in order to protect them from harm.

Gault also failed to offer much clarification of the separability of the interests of child, family, and state. For example, *Gault* requires notice to "the child and his parents" (p. 41) of the child's right to counsel, thus raising questions of who really is being represented.

Post-Gault

Gault did indeed open the gate to a flood of cases about the limits of minors' autonomy and privacy. The topics are diverse: access to contraception and abortion; access to pinball parlors; school prayer and school-based religious organizations; the right to a jury trial in delinquency proceedings; censorship of school campaign addresses and newspapers; waiver of Fifth and Sixth Amendment rights; application of compulsory school attendance laws to Amish teenagers; admission to mental hospitals; preventive detention of juveniles accused of delinquent offenses; access to pornography.

Most of the children's rights cases actually have involved adolescents. In some instances, patterns of both biological and social development guarantee that questions of autonomy and privacy will be raised only by older minors. For example, most of the cases in which a minor seeks to have an abortion without parental knowledge or consent involve 16- and 17-year-olds (see for reviews, Melton, 1987b; Melton & Pliner, 1986). Delinquent behavior is largely an adolescent phenomenon (Rutter & Giller, 1984); therefore, it is unsurprising that cases about exercise of rights in investigations of delinquent behavior (e.g., *Fare v. Michael C.*, 1979; *New Jersey v.*

T.L.O., 1985), juvenile detention (*Schall v. Martin,* 1984), and juvenile adjudicatory proceedings (e.g., *Breed v. Jones,* 1975; *McKeiver v. Pennsylvania,* 1971) have involved adolescents. Similarly, the population of residential treatment centers consists largely of adolescents (see, for reviews, Melton, 1987a; Melton & Spaulding, in press), so it is unsurprising that *Parham v. J.R.* (1979) involved adolescents as representatives of the class of institutionalized minors.

In general, the Court has treated minors as "half-persons," entitled to some but not all of the rights accorded persons, with state intrusions on minors' rights subject to less scrutiny than attempts to limit the rights of people without respect to age (see for review, Melton, 1984; for illustrative cases, see Wadlington, Whitebread, & Davis, 1983). For example, the Court has recognized the right to privacy as applying to minors, but it has required only "significant" (rather than "compelling") state interests to justify legal requirements that pregnant adolescents convince a judge of their maturity or the desirability of an abortion before their decision in that regard will be honored. The pattern in the post-*Gault* cases is for the Court to recognize minors' rights in the abstract but then to place much greater attention on reasons to limit those rights.

Except perhaps in the Court's establishment of "mature minor" provisions in abortion cases, the law still does not recognize adolescents as a class. As will be discussed in the following section, a substantial body of research has confirmed adolescents' ability to make medical and educational decisions in the same manner as adults, but the law generally still fails to distinguish between adolescence and "infancy." There seems to be an implicit recognition that civil rights for adolescents would conflict with the state's paternalist heritage. The assumption of children's dependency and incompetency has passed from presumption to myth—a legal fiction (Melton, 1987d).

ADOLESCENTS' RIGHTS IN OUTPATIENT MENTAL HEALTH SERVICES

So far, we have attended primarily to developments in constitutional law; such cases most vividly illustrate the conflicts related to children's rights. Because mental health services occur in consensually recognized zones of privacy, consent to mental health treatment also touches on constitutionally protected interests (see e.g., *Merriken v. Cressman,* 1973; *Milonas v. Williams,* 1982; *Mills v. Rogers,* 1982; *Parham v. J.R.,* 1979). However, most of the law related to mental health treatment of minors is found in the statute books and the common law of torts. Indeed, the mature minor rule, which has been elevated to a principle of constitutional law in adolescent abortion cases, developed as a pragmatic response in tort cases in which physicians were sued for "technical" batteries (acts of nonconsensual touch-ing) for having treated older minors without the consent of their parents but with the informed consent of the minors themselves (Wadlington, 1973, 1983).

As in the constitutional cases, the relevant law is largely derived from and applicable to cases involving adolescents. As a practical matter, statu-tory revisions to increase minors' opportunities for self-determination in such matters as treatment decisions have affected only adolescents (Melton, 1981), perhaps because younger minors have been uninterested or simply did not know how to make use of the opportunities.

The Nature of Informed Consent

Legal problems of outpatient mental health services for adolescents gener-ally are related to issues of consent.* Like professional ethics codes (see e.g., American Psychological Association [APA], 1981, Principle 6), the law requires that a client give informed consent before health services can be provided (for excellent reviews of the state of the law, see Katz, 1984, and Lidz, Meisel, Zerubavel, Carter, Sestak, & Roth, 1984). As applied to adults, the purposes of this requirement are clear: (1) to protect autonomy and privacy by barring intrusion into one's body or mind without consent, and (2) to promote shared decision making between doctor and patient by "humanizing" their relationship.

Disclosure.   For consent to be informed, adequate information about treatment alternatives must be disclosed, the individual must be competent to give consent, and the consent must be given voluntarily. Historically, the standard in tort law for adequate disclosure has been essentially the same as for professional negligence (malpractice). That is, health professionals have not been found liable for failing to obtain informed consent if they disclosed the same information as would any reasonable health professional in his or her community. Although it is still the law in some jurisdictions, such a standard is inconsistent with the purposes of informed consent.

The majority rule at this point is *materiality.* Under such a rule, the health professional must inform patients about any information that might be material to their decision (i.e., information that might affect the deci-sion). In general, patients must be informed about the nature, risks, and

---

* Although confidentiality usually is analyzed as a separate problem from consent to services, ethical and legal issues related to confidentiality can be understood as a subset of consent issues. First, insofar as the limits of confidentiality are material to a prospective client's deci-sion whether to seek treatment, consent is not truly informed if such limits are not fully and accurately disclosed. Second, where confidentiality is breached without the prior consent of the client, the major ethical insult is the client's loss of control over information that may be related to preservation of personal dignity.

benefits of the proposed treatment and any alternatives, presumably including no treatment.

In determining the specific information that must be disclosed, most states require only that the clinician describe the aspects, risks, and benefits that would be material to a reasonable person. Such a rule is called an objective standard, which has the advantages of consistency and efficiency. Objective standards permit clinicians to develop standard protocols for disclosure of information to patients making decisions about treatment. However, objective standards are less protective of individual autonomy and, therefore, less rigorous ethically than subjective standards of materiality. Under the latter type of rule, the clinician must disclose whatever information would be material to a particular individual, given his or her own values. Although a subjective standard sacrifices efficiency, it effectively requires clinicians to develop a relationship with their patients sufficient to learn and honor their idiosyncratic preferences.

Competence. Standards for competence to consent are even more complex, largely because courts and legislatures rarely have enunciated the elements of competence (see Weithorn, 1982, for discussion). As a practical matter in the treatment of noninstitutionalized adults (who are presumed competent), the standard is *expression of a preference.* Under such a standard, which is very protective of individual autonomy, patients' decisions are honored unless they are unable to indicate their preference. Assessment of a patient's competence under such a standard usually is easy. It is problematic only when patients are so ambivalent that they are unable to provide an unambiguous answer whether they will accept a given treatment.

A somewhat more complex standard is *understanding.* Under such a standard, patients are competent if they comprehend material information that has been disclosed to them. Obviously, the standard of understanding leaves the question of how much one must know to be competent and how well one must appreciate the significance of the information for oneself.

A still higher standard is a *reasonable process* of decision making. Under that standard, patients must be able not only to comprehend material information but also to weigh the risks and benefits of the various alternatives in a rational manner.

The standard that is least respectful of individual autonomy in a *reasonable outcome* of decision making. Under such a standard, it makes no difference how well one comprehends and weighs the information that has been disclosed. As long as the choice made is one that a reasonable person would have made, the patient is viewed as competent. Such a standard implies rejection of the individual's own values and effectively abrogates the underlying theory of informed consent.

Voluntariness.   Determinations of voluntariness necessarily must be made on a case-by-case basis. Assessment of voluntariness is a commonsense moral inquiry about the level of threat of punishment for failure to accept a recommended treatment and, conversely, the level of inducement for conformity to the professional's recommendations. Voluntariness diminishes as perceived freedom to decline recommendations diminishes.

In that regard, institutional pressures in the health care system must be considered. Given the power and prestige of health professionals, patients may perceive that they will be denied any care or privileges or that they will simply be shamed if they do not comply with clinicians' recommendations.

Exceptions.   The general rule that informed consent is necessary for the legal administration of treatment is not absolute. The least controversial exception, the *emergency exception,* is one that permits treatment without informed consent when the patient is unable to consent but in need of treatment to avoid death or serious harm. The emergency exception rarely arises in mental health.

On the other hand, *therapeutic privilege* may be especially commonly invoked in mental health. Such a doctrine permits withholding of material information when the clinician reasonably believes that its disclosure would harm the patient. Thus mental health professionals may decline to inform patients about their diagnoses although such information may be helpful in making treatment decisions. Because it is inconsistent with the goal of protecting patient autonomy, therapeutic privilege has lost acceptance as a justification for failure to obtain fully informed consent. As a matter of both ethics and defensive practice, clinicians probably should not rely on it.

Somewhat less controversial is the practice of patients' waiving the right to make treatment decisions. If we fully respect patients' decisions, then we should honor their decision, when competently made, to delegate specific decisions to a proxy, whether it is the patient's therapist or another individual. Two problems arise, however, in determining whether to accept such waivers. First, unforeseen situations may arise that the patients did not take into account at the time of the waiver but that are especially germane to them given their values. Such an objection has led some commentators (Dresser, 1982; Ennis, 1982) to doubt the legal enforceability of psychiatric wills (Szasz, 1982) designed to carry out the wishes of competent people about what should be done if they should become incompetent. Second, if the proxy has a stake in the decision (e.g., if the proxy is a treating health professional), the conflict of interests may influence decisions ostensibly on behalf of the patient.

Finally and most germane to our discussion, patients may be treated without informed consent if they are incompetent and a proxy decision maker has given permission for their treatment. Because they are presumed incompetent to consent, this exception is especially relevant to treatment of adolescents.

Adolescents and Consent

The State of the Law. In general, the law does not recognize adolescents' competence to consent, whatever their de facto competence. Decisions about treatment of minors usually are reserved for their parents or guardians, who act as proxies for their children or wards. In such a circumstance, the purposes of informed consent are obfuscated. Because a third party has made the decision, the consent process cannot be said to have promoted either the patient's autonomy or a contractual relationship between health professional and patient. Consent procedures in minors' cases more directly serve parental autonomy and family privacy. They also protect parents from financial obligations entered into by their children, and they may provide scrutiny necessary to increase the likelihood that clinicians offer good care to their children. In short, proxy consent may protect both parents and children, but it fails to support the autonomy of de facto competent youth and to make them partners in their treatment.

Although per se incompetence to consent is the general rule, circumstances do exist in which the law recognizes informed consent by de facto competent minors. The most common exception arises when the public health is at stake and minors might not seek treatment if parental permission were required. For example, all states permit minors to consent to evaluation and treatment for venereal disease. Statutes permitting minors to consent to treatment for substance abuse (when analogous provisions are not available for other reasons for mental health services) also may reflect a concern with the welfare of the public more than the adolescents themselves.

Minors also are able to consent independently to health services in instances in which individual privacy interests are recognized. Most notably, contraception and abortion generally are available without parental consent. A plausible argument could be made that privacy interests of equal significance are implicated in mental health treatment. However, constitutional claims of privacy are not as likely to prevail in such a context as they are in matters involving procreation (compare *Parham v. J.R.*, 1979, with *Carey v. Population Services International*, 1977, and *Planned Parenthood of Central Missouri v. Danforth*, 1976). The lesser protection of privacy in matters related to minors' mental health probably reflects two facts: The law of privacy happens to have developed in cases about reproductive decisions, and decisions about procreation are essentially irreversible and cannot be delayed until the minor reaches the age of majority. Nonetheless, even if states are not constitutionally required to recognize minors' privacy in decisions whether to seek the assistance of a mental health professional, they are free to adopt the same logic in enacting statutory exceptions to the usual requirement for parental permission for treatment of minors.

Parental permission also is not required if the state considers the minor to be emancipated and, therefore, legally independent of parents' control. Although the requirements for emancipation vary across jurisdictions, they generally relate more to financial independence than psychological maturity. Among the bases for emancipation in various states are marriage, parenthood, enlistment in the military, and independent domicile (in effect, running away). Emancipation statutes typically are a pragmatic response to problems of financial responsibility more than a recognition of independent interests in autonomy and privacy.

Mature minor rules commonly are based on a combination of the factors involved in privacy and emancipation exceptions. In tort law, the mature minor rule arose as a pragmatic doctrine to protect health professionals from liability when they treated obviously competent minors without the consent of their parents (Wadlington, 1973, 1983). When the age of majority was 21, courts reasonably concluded that it would be unjust to hold physicians civilly liable for failing to obtain informed consent when, for example, the patient was a junior in college and full disclosure had been made of material information. Thus in common law, a rule has developed validating consent by de facto competent older minors who, having been fully informed, consent to medical procedures for their own benefit.

However, black-letter law remains that minors are per se incompetent to consent. Therefore, some states have adopted a statutory mature minor rule, in which de facto competent minors can consent to treatment. Whether such rules are intended primarily to protect health professionals from liability or to respect the privacy of "mature" adolescents, their effect is to emancipate mature minors for the limited purpose of consenting to treatment. (Under such statutes, unlike most general emancipation statutes, the minor would remain de jure incompetent to contract for goods and services other than health services.)

Mental Health Exceptions.   Recognition of a special exception to permit minors to consent independently to mental health treatment has been advocated on the basis of two somewhat conflicting rationales. Child savers make the paternalist argument that children who need such treatment (e.g., victims of abuse) may not receive it if parental permission is required. In keeping with the state's interest in promoting the health and welfare of minors, child savers argue that access to treatment should be promoted even if family privacy is invaded. Child libertarians, on the other hand, advocate independent access to treatment in order to protect the fundamental interests in individual privacy that they believe are involved in mental health treatment of children and adolescents.

Child libertarians' arguments are bolstered by the research showing adolescents to be as competent as adults according to all four standards of competence to consent to treatment (see e.g., Adelman, Kaser-Boyd, & Taylor, 1984; Adelman, Lusk, Alvarez, & Acousta, 1985; Belter & Grisso, 1984; Kaser-Boyd, Adelman, & Taylor, 1985; Koocher, 1983; Melton, 1983d, 1984; Taylor, Adelman, & Kaser-Boyd, 1985; Weithorn, 1982; Weithorn & Campbell, 1982). Such research suggests that adolescents are at no more risk than adults for "bad" decisions and resulting harm. They are able to weigh risks and benefits rationally and thus to satisfy the most rigorous ethical standards for recognition of personhood.

Child libertarians also note the research indicating that, independent of levels of competence, decision making itself has positive effects (Melton, 1983b) as does recognition of zones of privacy (Melton, 1983c). Therefore, the risk of harm is small, and the benefit may be substantial when a marginally competent minor is permitted to make independent treatment decisions.* Among the positive effects are increased sense of personal control, increased self-esteem, increased competence of legal reasoning, diminished anxiety, and increased treatment compliance and efficacy.

Whatever their reasons for doing so, most child mental health professionals sometimes treat adolescents without parental consent even without a legal imprimatur for doing so. However, they do not publicize the availability of treatment to adolescents even when the state statutes expressly permit treatment without parental consent (Melton, 1981). Statutory exceptions permitting minors to consent to treatment thus may serve merely to protect mental health professionals from liability for what they would do even in the absence of express statutory authority.

The lack of impact of special consent laws may result in part from the fact that such laws often raise more questions than they answer (see for review, Ehrenreich & Melton, 1983). Does a right to consent imply a right to consent *confidentially?* If so, does it apply even to those minors who are brought for treatment by their parents? Does a right to consent independently of parents imply a right to refuse treatment arranged by parents? In either instance, who bears financial responsibility? Can parents be held liable for treatment that they did not authorize? Can billings be sent to third-party insurers without breaching confidentiality, given that private coverage of minors typically is pursuant to their parents' policies? In view of other statutes governing special educational services and school

* The risk of harm is minimized further by the fact that even elementary-school-age children tend to make the same treatment decisions as adults, even though they generally are less competent than adolescents and adults in comprehending and weighing treatment information (Lewis, 1983; Weithorn & Campbell, 1982). Therefore, for routine treatment decisions, the concern with competence may be misplaced even for younger minors.

records, do statutes permitting minors to consent to mental health treatment apply to school-based services? If so, do they apply differentially to school health professionals (e.g., nurses and possibly psychologists) and nonmedical guidance counselors?

In the face of such ambiguities, mental health professionals may avoid dealing with minors seeking treatment independently. The problems that remain when legislatures act to ensure minors' access to treatment highlight the need for mental health professionals to give careful thought to ethical issues involved in treating adolescents. Although clinicians generally should defer to the community's moral judgments as embedded in law (APA, 1981, Principles 3c and 3d), such a rule does not dissolve their ethical responsibility. The law serves as a guidepost to moral conduct, but it does not end ethical inquiry. As we shall discuss in more detail later, mental health professionals who work with adolescents have a duty to weigh carefully the application of general principles of ethics to the special situations encountered in services to adolescents.

CIVIL COMMITMENT OF MINORS

Parham v. J.R.

No issue in adolescent mental health has engendered more vitriolic commentary about the state of the law than the standards and procedures to be applied to the admission of minors to inpatient programs. In brief, the issue is whether minors are due the same process as adults when they are potentially subject to deprivation of liberty and intrusions on privacy for the purpose of treatment. Specifically, can parents or guardians (including state social workers) "volunteer" minors for residential treatment?

The Supreme Court's answer to the latter question in *Parham v. J.R.* (1979) was a qualified "yes." Although the Court recognized that minors did have an independent liberty interest at stake, it asserted that parents, through their "natural bonds of affection" (p. 602), generally guard the interests of their children. In any event, the admitting mental health professional acting as "neutral factfinder" (p. 606) offered sufficient scrutiny to the parents' decision to protect the child's independent interests. To justify this holding, Chief Justice Burger wrote a lengthy opinion mythologizing the family and the mental health system and generally conflicting with social science knowledge (Melton & Spaulding, in press; Perry & Melton, 1984).

Although the Court largely ignored the facts presented by the appellants at trial in *Parham* (Melton & Spaulding, in press), it did attend to certain evidence that suggests some limits to the *Parham* holding. The majority emphasized that thorough evaluations had been conducted and community-based treatment had been attempted. It also assumed that admitting professionals would obtain information from parents, schools, and social service agencies and that they would be free to decline admissions. Therefore, more procedural protections may be required when such evidence is unavailable.

The Court also indicated that it was limiting its holding to preadmission procedures. The majority declined to reach the question of the postadmission procedures necessary to meet the requirements of due process, although they indicated that postadmission review need not be in the form of an adversary hearing.

Responses to Parham

The mental health professions have been divided in their response to *Parham* and related cases (for review and analysis of the various commentary, see Melton & Spaulding, in press, Chapter 7). The American Psychiatric Association (1982) generally has minimized the need for procedural protection. It has argued that formal nonmedical reviews interfere with treatment by fractionating families, undermining parental authority, and supporting resistance to treatment. Like the *Parham* Court, the American Psychiatric Association has emphasized the benevolent intentions of parents (even when the "parent" is a state social worker) and mental health professionals and the incompetence and vulnerability of minors.

By contrast, the American Psychological Association and the American Orthopsychiatric Association have emphasized the liberty and privacy interests intruded upon by psychiatric hospitalization. They have noted the frequency of hospitalization for administrative convenience, the fractionation already present in families in which placement of a child is sought, and the competence of adolescents to participate in treatment decisions. Although the advocates of increased procedural protection rarely have done so on purely utilitarian grounds, they have rebutted the proponents of a paternalist approach by arguing that due process and treatment efficacy are compatible. The logic is similar to that of the Supreme Court in *Gault:* "the appearance as well as the actuality of fairness, impartiality and orderliness—in short, the essentials of due process—may be a more impressive and more therapeutic attitude so far as the juvenile is concerned" (*In re Gault,* 1966, p. 26).

We have argued previously that *Parham* and the commentary surrounding it have served largely symbolic purposes (Melton, 1984, 1987d; Melton & Spaulding, in press; Perry & Melton, 1984). Commentary has focused on the historic issue of the degree of identity of interests among child, family, and state and the related problem of the allocation of decision-making authority. As a practical matter, however, that issue has little significance in determining the disposition in cases involving troubled and troubling adolescents. The more critical problem is constructing a policy that will minimize the restrictiveness and intrusiveness of placement when troubled and troublesome youth have no place to go.

The Nature of the Residential Treatment System

Discussions of policy on admissions to psychiatric facilities often have been divorced from the realities of who is served and why patients are institutionalized. Despite the prevailing rhetoric about deinstitutionalization, rates of psychiatric hospitalization and other forms of residential treatment have risen steadily (Kiesler, 1982), especially among adolescents (see e.g., Lerman, 1980). The de facto policy in children's services is to rely on restrictive forms of care.

The choice of the term *children's services* instead of *child mental health services* was intentional. Child mental health policy is so difficult to formulate because all of the major systems for services to minors with behavior disorders—mental health, juvenile justice, special education, child welfare—have a primary goal of treatment. Each system serves essentially the same clients: conduct disordered adolescent males from families under stress, many of whom are already wards of the state (see for review, Melton & Spaulding, in press, Chapter 5). With the increase in private programs, the services themselves often are the same. That is, a single facility may be a mental health facility, a therapeutic school, a group care facility, and a program for juvenile offenders. At the same time, none of the systems in most states has developed a continuum of services in which alternatives to residential treatment other than traditional outpatient psychotherapy are available.

In such a context, the likelihood is that tightening procedures for admission to the mental hospitals without similar constraints on the other child treatment systems will result simply in a movement across systems to other residential treatment programs. Such a possibility was demonstrated dramatically by the "transinstitutionalization" that occurred after status offenders were barred from juvenile correctional facilities (Costello & Worthington, 1981; General Accounting Office, 1985; Hinckley & Ellis, 1985; Krisberg & Schwartz, 1983; Van Dusen, 1981; Warren, 1981). Reform is needed throughout the children's service system, not just in the mental health system.

Recent innovations in intensive home-based services and day treatment have demonstrated that residential placement usually is unnecessary (see e.g., AuClaire & Schwartz, 1986; Behar, 1985, 1986; Heying, 1985; Hinckley & Ellis, 1985; Kettlewell, Jones, & Jones, 1985; Kinney, Madsen, Fleming, & Haapala, 1977; Leeds, 1984; Pecora, Delewski, Booth, Haapala, & Kinney, 1985; Tolmach, 1985). Indeed, not a single study has demonstrated inpatient treatment to be superior to alternatives (see for reviews, Kiesler, 1982; Melton & Spaulding, in press; Miller & Hester, 1986).

In that regard, the much touted conflict between parents and children at admission to psychiatric facilities is likely to be illusory. Development of alternatives that protect the child's autonomy and privacy also promote family integrity. Exploration of alternatives and development of individualized alternatives commonly is welcomed by parents even in states in which adversary procedures are used for commitment of minors (Perlin, 1981). The child's attorney often will be working in concert with the parents to find less restrictive alternatives to hospitalization.

SUMMARY

Perhaps the strongest message from our review is the complexity of the law and ethics of adolescent mental health services. As the discussion of civil commitment indicates, the dilemmas that are present in adolescent mental health services often are not "simply" a matter of balancing the interests of child, family, and state. In the diffusion of responsibilities that commonly occurs in the child treatment system, such considerations often only begin the inquiry.

The law rarely presents a command: "You must treat," or "you must not treat." Although some behavior is so violative of individual rights that it presents clear "do's" or "don'ts," more commonly clinicians are left with choices. Even where "do's" and "don'ts" may be present in law, they may be arguable. For example, it can be argued that a right to consent to treatment independently, when granted by statute, implies a right to control over the records arising from that treatment. Insofar as the purpose underlying such a statute is promotion of personal autonomy and privacy, such a result is sensible. On the other hand, it could be argued that, even if it is a wise policy to permit adolescents to seek treatment on their own, parents need information about what is happening in treatment in order to fulfill their duty of protecting their child. Moreover, as a practical matter, other agencies may not honor the adolescent's waivers of confidentiality that are necessary to secure releases of information.

To deal with such legally and ethically ambiguous situations, clinicians must consider carefully the implications of legal doctrines and fundamental ethical principles. Consistent with the basic principle of respect for the dignity of persons (APA, 1981, Preamble), we believe that the first attention must be given to protection of the autonomy of competent adolescents, but we also support promotion of family privacy whenever feasible.

This general rule can be applied even when the law apparently is to permit parents sole power of consent. In that instance, nothing prohibits the clinician from adopting a model of shared decision making in which adolescents themselves are informed of information relevant to treatment decisions and are permitted to share in the decision making. In fact, the clinician can even recognize a power of assent and treat only those adolescents who are willing to accept treatment. (The converse, of course, also may be true. For sophisticated discussions of the ethical alternatives in allocation of decision-making authority and the psychology of preparing children and youth to exercise varying levels of autonomy, see Taylor & Adelman, 1986; Weithorn, 1983.) Koocher (1983) has offered still other "realistic alternatives," including mediation between parents and the adolescent.

In conclusion, a commitment to due process may have substantial long-term effects for adolescents and the society as a whole:

> . . . *[P]sychologists [and other mental health professionals] can preserve those myths that express respect for human dignity and, in so doing, embody the highest principles of Western thought. The social contract that creates a duty of respect for autonomous persons in a state of equality (Rawls, 1971) is mythical, but its meaning is true. The most basic ethical obligation of psychologists is to "respect the dignity and worth of the individual and strive for the preservation of fundamental human rights" (APA, 1981, Preamble). . . . When we respect the autonomy and privacy of child clients . . . , we reify the symbols of personhood and the myths of equality in the moral community. We owe children no less. (Melton, 1987d, p. 352)*

REFERENCES

Adelman, H. S., Kaser-Boyd, N., & Taylor, L. (1984). Children's participation in consent for psychotherapy and their subsequent response to treatment. *Journal of Clinical Child Psychology, 13,* 170–178.

Adelman, H. S., Lusk, R., Alvarez, V., & Acousta, N. (1985). Competence of minors to understand, evaluate, and communicate about their psychoeducational problems. *Professional Psychology: Research and Practice, 16,* 426–434.

American Psychiatric Association. (1982). Guidelines for the psychiatric hospitalization of minors. *American Journal of Psychiatry, 139,* 971–974.

American Psychological Association. (1981). Ethical principles of psychologists. *American Psychologist, 36,* 633–638.

AuClaire, P., & Schwartz, I. M. (1986, December). *An evaluation of the effectiveness of intensive home-based services as an alternative to placement for adolescents and their families.* University of Minnesota, Hubert M. Humphrey Institute of Public Affairs, Center for Youth Policy.

Bakan, D. (1971). Adolescence in America: From idea to social fact. In J. Kagan & R. Coles (Eds.), *Twelve to sixteen: Early adolescence* (pp. 73–89). New York: Norton.

Behar, L. (1985). Changing patterns of state responsibility: A case study of North Carolina. *Journal of Clinical Child Psychology, 14,* 188–195.

Behar, L. (1986, May–June). A state model for child mental health services: The North Carolina experience. *Children Today,* pp. 16–21.

Belter, R. W., & Grisso, T. (1984). Children's recognition of rights violations in counseling. *Professional Psychology: Research and Practice, 15,* 899–910.

Breed v. Jones, 421 U.S. 519 (1975).

Costello, J. C., & Worthington, N. L. (1981). Incarcerating status offenders: Attempts to circumvent the Juvenile Justice and Delinquency Prevention Act. *Harvard Civil Rights-Civil Liberties Law Review, 16,* 41–81.

Carey v. Population Services International, 431 U.S. 678 (1977).

Dresser, R. S. (1982). Ulysses and the psychiatrists: A legal and policy analysis of the voluntary commitment contract. *Harvard Civil Rights-Civil Liberties Law Review, 16,* 777–854.

Ennis, B. J. (1982). The psychiatric will: Odysseus at the mast [Comment]. *American Psychologist, 37,* 854.

Ehrenreich, N. S., & Melton, G. B. (1983). Ethical and legal issues in the treatment of children. In C. E. Walker & M. C. Roberts (Eds.), *Handbook of clinical child psychology* (pp. 1285–1317). New York: Wiley.

Fare v. Michael C., 442 U.S. 707 (1979).

Feshbach, S., Feshbach, N. D. (1978). Child advocacy and family privacy. *Journal of Social Issues, 34*(2), 114–121.

Garbarino, J., Gaboury, M. T., Long, R., Grandjean, P., & Asp, E. (1982). Who owns the children? An ecological perspective on public policy affecting children. In G. B. Melton (Ed.), *Legal reforms affecting child and youth services* (pp. 43–63). New York: Haworth.

General Accounting Office. (1985). *Residential care: Patterns of child placement in three states* (Report No. GAO/PEMD–85–2). Washington, DC: Author.

Goldstein, J., Freud, A., & Solnit, A. J. (1973). *Before the best interests of the child.* New York: Free Press.

Goldstein, J., Freud, A., & Solnit, A. J. (1979). *Beyond the best interests of the child.* New York: Free Press.

Haley v. Ohio, 332 U.S. 596 (1948).

Hall, G. S. (1904). *Adolescence: Its psychology and its relations to physiology, anthropology, sex, crime, religion, and education.* New York: Appleton.

Heying, K. R. (1985). Family-based in-home services for the severely emotionally disturbed child. *Child Welfare, 64,* 519–527.

Hinckley, E. C., & Ellis, W. F. (1985). An effective alternative to residential placement: Home-based services. *Journal of Clinical Child Psychology, 14,* 209–213.

In re Gault, 387 U.S. 1 (1966).

Kaser-Boyd, N., Adelman, H. S., & Taylor, L. (1985). Minors' ability to identify risks and benefits of therapy. *Professional Psychology: Research and Practice, 16,* 411–417.

Katz, J. (1984). *The silent world of doctor and patient.* New York: Free Press.

Kett, J. F. (1977). *Rites of passage.* New York: Basic Books.

Kettlewell, P. W., Jones, J. K., & Jones, R. H. (1985). Adolescent partial hospitalization: Some preliminary outcome data. *Journal of Clinical Child Psychology, 14,* 139–144.

Kiesler, C. A. (1982). Mental hospitals and alternative care: Noninstitutionalization as potential public policy for mental patients. *American Psychologist, 37,* 349–360.

Kinney, J., Madsen, B., Fleming, T., & Haapala, D. (1977). Homebuilders: Keeping families together. *Journal of Consulting and Clinical Psychology, 45,* 667–673.

Koocher, G. P. (1983). Competence to consent: Psychotherapy. In G. B. Melton, G. P. Koocher, & M. J. Saks (Eds.), *Children's competence to consent* (pp. 111–128). New York: Plenum.

Krisberg, B. A., & Schwartz, I. M. (1983). Rethinking juvenile justice. *Crime and Delinquency, 29,* 333–364.

Leeds, S. J. (1984, March). *Evaluation of Nebraska's intensive services project.* Iowa City: University of Iowa School of Social Work, National Resource Center on Family Based Services.

Lerman, P. (1980). Trends and issues in the deinstitutionalization of youths in trouble. *Crime and Delinquency, 26,* 281–298.

Lewis, C. E. (1983). Decision making related to health: When could/should children act responsibly? In G. B. Melton, G. P. Koocher, & M. J. Saks (Eds.), *Children's competence to consent* (pp. 75–91). New York: Plenum.

Lidz, C. W., Meisel, A., Zerubavel, E., Carter, M., Sestak, R. M., & Roth, L. M. (1984). *Informed consent: A study of decisionmaking in psychiatry.* New York: Guilford.

McKeiver v. Pennsylvania, 403 U.S. 528 (1971).

Melton, G. B. (1981). Effects of a state law permitting minors to consent to psychotherapy. *Professional Psychology, 12,* 647–654.

Melton, G. B. (1983a). *Child advocacy: Psychological issues and interventions.* New York: Plenum.

Melton, G. B. (1983b). Decision making by children: Psychological risks and benefits. In G. B. Melton, G. P. Koocher, & M. J. Saks (Eds.), *Children's competence to consent* (pp. 21–40). New York: Plenum.

Melton, G. B. (1983c). Minors and privacy: Are legal and psychological concepts compatible? *Nebraska Law Review, 62,* 455–493.

Melton, G. B. (1983d). Toward "personhood" for adolescents: Autonomy and privacy as values in public policy. *American Psychologist, 38,* 99–103.

Melton, G. B. (1984). Development psychology and the law: The state of the art. *Journal of Family Law, 22,* 445–482.

Melton, G. B. (1987a). *Epidemiology of mental health problems in childhood and adolescence.* Lincoln: State of Nebraska, Department of Public Institutions.

Melton, G. B. (1987b). Legal regulation of adolescent abortion: Unintended effects. *American Psychologist, 42,* 79–83.

Melton, G. B. (1987c). *Service models in child and adolescent mental health: What works for whom?* Lincoln: State of Nebraska, Department of Public Institutions.

Melton, G. B. (1987d). The clashing of symbols: Prelude to child and family policy. *American Psychologist, 42,* 345–354.

Melton, G. B. (in press). Are adolescents people? Problems of liberty, responsibility, and entitlement. In J. Worell & F. Danner, *Adolescent development: Issues for education*. New York: Academic.

Melton, G. B., & Pliner, A. J. (1986). Adolescent abortion: A psycholegal analysis. In G. B. Melton (Ed.), *Adolescent abortion: Psychological and legal issues* (pp. 1–39). Lincoln: University of Nebraska Press.

Melton, G. B., & Spaulding, W. J. (in press). *No place to go: Civil commitment of minors*. Lincoln: University of Nebraska Press.

Merriken v. Cressman, 364 F. Supp. 913 (E.D. Pa. 1973).

Meyer v. Nebraska, 262 U.S. 390 (1923).

Miller, W. R., & Hester, R. W. (1986). Inpatient alcoholism treatment: Who benefits? *American Psychologist, 41,* 794–805.

Mills v. Rogers, 457 U.S. 291 (1982).

Milonas v. Williams, 691 F.2d 931 (10th Cir. 1982), *cert. denied,* 460 U.S. 1069 (1982).

New Jersey v. T. L. O., 469 U.S. 325 (1985).

Parham v. J. R., 442 U.S. 584 (1979).

Pecora, P. J., Delewski, C. H., Booth, C., Haapala, D., & Kinney, J. (1985). Home-based, family-centered services: The impact on worker attitudes. *Child Welfare, 64,* 529–540.

Perlin, M. (1981). An invitation to the dance: An empirical response to Chief Justice Warren Burger's "time-consuming procedural minuets" theory in *Parham v. J. R. Bulletin of the American Academy of Psychiatry and the Law, 9,* 149–164.

Perry, G. S., & Melton, G. B. (1984). Precedential value of judicial notice of social facts: *Parham* as an example. *Journal of Family Law, 22,* 633–676.

Pierce v. Society of Sisters, 268 U.S. 510 (1925).

Planned Parenthood of Central Missouri v. Danforth, 438 U.S. 52 (1976).

Platt, A. M. (1977). *The child savers: The invention of delinquency* (2nd ed.). Chicago: University of Chicago Press.

Prince v. Massachusetts, 321 U.S. 158 (1944).

Rawls, J. (1971). *A theory of justice*. Cambridge, MA: Harvard University Press.

Roe v. Wade, 410 U.S. 113 (1973).

Rogers, C. M., & Wrightsman, L. S. (1978). Attitudes toward children's rights: Nurturance or self-determination. *Journal of Social Issues, 34*(2), 59–68.

Rutter, M., & Giller, H. (1984). *Juvenile delinquency: Trends and perspectives*. New York: Guilford.

Schall v. Martin, 467 U.S. 253 (1984).

Szasz, T. (1982). The psychiatric will: A new mechanism for protecting persons against "psychosis" and psychiatry. *American Psychologist, 37,* 762–770.

Taylor, L., & Adelman, J. S. (1986). Facilitating children's participation in decisions that affect them: From concept to practice. *Journal of Clinical Child Psychology, 15,* 346–351.

Taylor, L., Adelman, J. S., & Kaser-Boyd, N. (1985). Exploring minors' reluctance and dissatisfaction with psychotherapy. *Professional Psychology: Research and Practice, 16,* 418–425.

Tolmach, J. (1985). "There ain't nobody on my side": A new day treatment program for black urban youth. *Journal of Clinical Child Psychology, 14,* 214–219.

Van Dusen, K. T. (1981). Net widening and relabeling: Some consequences of deinstitutionalization. *American Behavioral Scientist, 24,* 801–810.

Wadlington, W. J. (1973). Minors and health care: The age of consent. *Osgoode Hall Law Journal, 11,* 115–125.

Wadlington, W. J. (1983). Consent to medical care for minors: The legal framework. In G. B. Melton, G. P. Koocher, & M. J. Saks (Eds.), *Children's competence to consent* (pp. 235–260). New York: Plenum.

Wadlington, W. J., Whitebread, C. H., & Davis, S. M. (1983). *Cases and materials on children in the legal system.* Mineola, NY: Foundation Press.

Warren, C. A. B. (1981). New forms of social control: The myth of deinstitutionalization. *American Behavioral Scientist, 24,* 724–740.

Weithorn, L. A. (1982). Developmental factors and competence to make informed treatment decisions. In G. B. Melton (Ed.), *Legal reforms affecting child and youth services* (pp. 85–100). New York: Haworth.

Weithorn, L. A. (1983). Involving children in decisions affecting their own welfare: Guidelines for professionals. In G. B. Melton, G. P. Koocher, & M. J. Saks (Eds.), *Children's competence to consent* (pp. 235–260). New York: Plenum.

Weithorn, L. A., & Campbell, S. B. (1982). The competency of children and adolescents to make informed treatment decisions. *Child Development, 53,* 1589–1598.

Zimring, F. E. (1982). *The changing world of legal adolescence.* New York: Free Press.

Part III

Specific Disorders

CHAPTER NINE

Anxiety Disorders

Dennis P. Cantwell
Lorian Baker

INTRODUCTION

This chapter on anxiety disorders in adolescents will begin with the general concept and definition of anxiety and a review of some etiological theories. A discussion of the epidemiology of anxiety disorders and developmental issues will follow. Of interest here is the relationship of anxiety disorders in childhood, adolescence, and adult life. The differential diagnosis of anxiety symptoms will be reviewed, and there will be a detailed description of the various clinical problems subsumed under the anxiety disorders. The discussion of interventions will include pharmacological as well as psychodynamic and behavioral approaches. Directions for future research will be indicated in the summary.

As pointed out by Gittelman (1986), the concept of anxiety is crucial to all theories of psychopathology, whether one is considering psychopathology in children, adolescents, or in adults. There are different theories of the origins of anxiety, but all theoretical models of mental functioning integrate anxiety into their structure.

The definition of anxiety remains somewhat problematic; different definitions are discussed by Goodwin (1986), Beck and Emery (1985), and Werry (1986). Some distinguish between fear and anxiety (Beck & Emery, 1985), while others do not (Werry, 1986).

The DSM-III-R (APA, 1987) defines anxiety as "apprehension, tension, or uneasiness that stems from the anticipation of danger which may be internal or external." It also points out that other investigators distinguish anxiety from fear by limiting it to the anticipation of danger, the source of which is largely unknown. In contrast, fear is a response to an external threat or danger that is consciously recognized by the individual. However, because the manifestations of fear and the manifestations of anxiety are essentially the same and both include autonomic hyperactivity, apprehensive expectation, vigilance, scanning, and motor tension, DSM-III-R drops the distinction between the two.

Werry (1986) makes a useful distinction between anxiety symptoms, anxiety disorders, state anxiety, and trait anxiety. Werry defines a symptom as a behavior, an emotion, or a physiological response that is either unwanted or undesirable on the part of the individual. Anxiety may be experienced as subjective symptoms or associated with observable physiological, cognitive, and behavioral manifestations. Anxiety may be free-floating, or it may be provoked by specific situations or experiences. Anxiety symptoms include: shortness of breath, rapid heart beat, chest pain, dizzy spells, tingling in the hands and feet, sweating, fainting, trembling, or shaking. They also include: motor tension, autonomic hyperactivity, apprehensive expectation, obsessions and compulsions, and vigilance and scanning as manifested by difficulty in concentrating, insomnia, and irritability. However, these symptoms are not specific to an anxiety disorder. Obsessions and compulsions, for example, may occur in disorders other than anxiety disorders.

Werry distinguishes between anxiety symptoms and anxiety disorders. He defines a disorder as a unit consisting of symptoms which regularly occur together. Each unit is presumed to have a consistent clinical picture, a common outcome, a particular pattern of response to treatment, and specific etiologic factors. Werry's concept of a disorder is essentially similar to that of the DSM-III-R.

Werry points out that trait anxiety differs from an anxiety disorder in that trait anxiety is a universal characteristic present to some degree in all individuals and is assumed to be stable over time. In contrast, state anxiety (i.e., anxiety disorder) is assumed to be transitory and not characteristic of any individual at all times. State and trait anxiety are considered to be similar in one aspect: They are both assumed to be dimensional and measurable along a scale.

As Werry points out, clinicians sometimes conceptualize traits as disorders by the use of clinical judgment or by the use of severity cutoff scores. However, clinical judgment is often arbitrary, and a cutoff score may result in the creation of heterogeneous groups of individuals because a high severity score can be produced by different combinations of symptoms. Such an approach would fail, for example, to differentiate between children with a single extreme anxiety disorder and children with, for instance, conduct symptomatology mixed with anxiety and depressive symptomatology.

Etiologic theories of anxiety are multiple and have recently been reviewed by Goodwin (1986), Klein (1981), Shaffer (1986), and Trautman (1986). Goodwin reviews concepts of anxiety as espoused by philosophers such as Soren Kierkegaard and other existentialists, by physiologists such as Walter Cannon, Carney Landis, and William A. Hunt, and psychologists such as Konrad Lorenz and Donald Hebb.

Of particular interest to clinicians are the two major theories of anxiety proposed respectively by psychoanalysts and behaviorists. Trautman (1986) and Klein (1981) have both outlined the psychoanalytic theory of the origins of anxiety. Trautman describes how Sigmund Freud's theories of anxiety simultaneously evolved over a period of more than 30 years. Freud's earliest theory (1894/1962) defined anxiety as the discharge of a "quota of affect" or "sum of excitation," and described pathological anxiety as a failure of repression. Whenever psychic energy attached to unacceptable libidinal impulses became too strong to be repressed, it would break through in a distorted and disguised form to cause pathological anxiety. This theory of anxiety as caused by undischarged, repressed libido was revised in 1926 (Freud, 1926/1959) along with the development of the structural theory of the mind. While the first theory postulated that repressed, undischarged libido energy was transformed to anxiety, the second theory suggested that neutralized libidinal energy supplied the ego so that it would signal anxiety.

Anxiety was thus postulated as a response of the ego to a threat, a signal that the ego was in a dangerous situation. Anxiety led to repression in the second theory; repression led to anxiety in the first theory. In the first formulation, Freud (1894/1962) postulated that realistic anxiety arose when there was a real external danger that threatened the individual and neurotic anxiety arose when internal danger threatened the pleasure principle. In the 1926 reformulation, Freud (1926/1959), dropped the distinction between realistic and neurotic anxiety.

Klein (1981) and Trautman (1986) also discussed the role of separation anxiety and ethological findings in the formulation of the psychoanalytic theories of anxiety. Freud first mentioned the primary importance of separation from the mother and the origin of anxiety in his introductory lecture of 1917 (Freud, 1917/1963). Bowlby (1969, 1973), many years later, while studying infant-mother attachment, developed an ethological theory of anxiety which takes into account many of the phenomena of normal anxiety responses.

Learning theory (Shaffer, 1986) suggests that anxiety serves as a secondary drive and can be understood as the conditioned part of fear. The model, simply described, suggests that an unconditioned stimulus (UCS) causes unconditioned responses such as fear. Fear serves as a primary drive and leads to escape and avoidance behavior, which in turn leads to a decrease in fear, reinforcing the escape and avoidant behavior. A stimulus which often precedes an unconditioned stimulus will become a conditioned stimulus by simple classical contiguity conditioning. A conditioned stimulus then will serve as a signal of a yet to come UCS and will produce a conditioned response—anxiety. This anxiety serves as a secondary drive leading to avoidant behavior. The resultant escape from the UCS reduces the secondary drive of anxiety and reinforces the escape-avoidance behavior. However, as Klein (1981) points out, classical learning theory cannot generate a comprehensive theory of anxiety. For instance, it does not explain why phobias do not develop in response to multiple stimuli, although a later adaptive evolutionary preparedness theory (Garcia & Koelling, 1966) has been proposed to explain this.

Klein (1981) also points out that while classical learning theory may explain the therapeutic effect of certain behavior therapy procedures such as deconditioning, it does not explain the effectiveness of other procedures. In addition, neither learning theory nor psychoanalytic theory, both of which he considers to be similar in the end, distinguish between anticipatory anxiety, which is chronic, and panic attack, which is acute. While both psychoanalytic and learning theory have contributed to the understanding of the origin of anxiety disorders, both are lacking as comprehensive theories. They have led to treatment models, but neither has been subjected to rigorous scientific study, particularly in an adolescent population.

In a recent work, Beck and Emery (1985) assert that the traditional emphasis on the affective or feeling component of anxiety has drawn the attention of researchers and clinicians away from what they consider to be the central feature of anxiety disorders, that is, a person's preoccupation with danger and his or her response to that preoccupation. They suggest that more emphasis should be put into the cognitive or thinking component of anxiety. Interested readers are referred to their recent publication for a detailed exposition of their view and how their theory leads to a cognitive treatment approach for anxiety disorders.

There is a number of newer biological theories of anxiety based on studies of adults with various anxiety disorders. None has been specifically studied in adolescent patients. These theories are reviewed in detail by Gorman, Liebowitz, and Klein (1984). Brief mention will be made of each.

Recent interest in biological theories of anxiety has been driven by the increasing evidence of a genetic basis for the anxiety disorders. Anxiety disorders tend to run in families, as both family and family history studies have shown. However, this evidence is much stronger for panic disorder than it is for generalized anxiety disorder: Twin studies suggest greater concordance for monozygotic than dizygotic twins for anxiety disorders with panic attack, but not for generalized anxiety disorder. The evidence for agoraphobia is lacking since there are few family studies of this disorder. However, phobic disorders in general show higher concordance in monozygotic than dizygotic twins.

Recent studies of the children of adult patients with anxiety and depressive disorders also show increased rates of anxiety disorders in the children with some degree of concordance between parent disorder and child disorder (Weissman, Leckman, Merikangas, Gammon, & Prusoff, 1984).

The James-Lange theory is another biological theory which states that anxiety is a response to peripheral physical stimuli, such as increased heart rate and increased respiration. Studies to date are inconclusive as to whether these are the causes of panic attacks, or whether they are merely the consequences of a high level of anticipatory anxiety. However, there is an increased body of evidence to suggest that anxiety disorders are associated with increased levels of circulating catecholamines, especially epinephrine and norepinephrine. Platelet monoamine oxidase (MAO) and the beta adrenergic receptors also have been studied. Level of neurotransmitters has been studied as well as response of anxious patients to various provocative tests. The data from these studies suggest that beta-receptors are down-regulated in anxious patients, possibly a result of elevated plasma and urine catecholamine levels (Nesse, Cameron, Curtis, McCann, & Huber-Smith, 1984).

Cannon's argument (1929) is that anxiety disorders originate in the central nervous system and that peripheral events such as increased heart rate and increased respiration are secondary to the central nervous system arousal. Certain drugs known to curtail activity in the locus ceruleus can block panic attacks in anxious subjects. This area is currently the focus of intense research. The locus ceruleus may be considered the primary generator of panic attacks, or alternatively, panic may result from the locus ceruleus being overstimulated from other systems.

The neurotransmitter gamma amino butyric acid (GABA) increases binding of tritiated benzodiazepine to its receptor. This finding has led to a theory of how benzodiazepines alleviate anxiety in conjunction with GABA. Furthermore, a theory has been postulated that a compound present in the brain which binds to benzodiazepine receptors may cause anxiety.

Pitts and McClure (1967) were the first to demonstrate that sodium lactate infusion provoked panic attacks in patients with spontaneous panic attacks and not in normal controls. This has been replicated by several other investigators. There are several mechanisms whereby sodium lactate may cause panic attacks; for instance, lowering of ionized calcium (Pitts & McClure, 1967) or metabolic alkalosis may be responsible. Further research, using subjects of different age groups and different types of anxiety disorders as well as controls with other psychiatric disorders, is needed to clarify the exact mechanism.

Klein (1981) has postulated that the mechanism underlying normal human separation anxiety is defective in patients with panic disorder. He based this observation on the fact that a substantial number of adult patients (up to 50% in some studies) with a panic disorder also had a separation anxiety disorder in childhood.

Finally, there is a statistical correlation between mitral valve prolapse (MVP) and panic disorder in adult patients. MVP may be associated with panic disorder in patients who are prone to develop panic attacks following autonomic stress, of which MVP would be one. Also, panic disorder and MVP may both be manifestations of a basic generalized disturbance of autonomic function. Thus the existing evidence indicates that MVP does not cause panic disorder. Panic disorders with and without MVP seem to be similar in clinical features.

In summary, numerous biological theories of anxiety have arisen over the years. Most of these have been driven by the finding that anxiety disorders tend to run in families. However, all the studies have essentially been done in patients who are over the age of 18. The validity of these theories in adults remains to be verified, and the extent to which they overlap is still to be determined. Whether they apply to adolescent patients with various types of anxiety disorder remains a subject for future research. For a more detailed discussion of biological issues in anxiety disorders, the interested reader is referred to Rainey and Nesse (1985) and Wolkowitz and Paul (1985).

DIAGNOSTIC AND DEVELOPMENTAL CONSIDERATIONS

The epidemiology of anxiety disorders has been reasonably well studied in adults (for review, see Weissman, 1985). The recent studies have benefited from the use of specific diagnostic criteria that allow the prevalence of more precisely defined anxiety disorders to be determined.

The 1975 New Haven Community Survey (Weissman, Myers, & Harding, 1978) produced current prevalence rates of disorders according to Research Diagnostic Criteria (RDC) (Spitzer, Endicott, & Robins, 1978) diagnoses. From a population survey of over 1000 households, 511 adults with psychiatric disorder were found: 2.5% had generalized anxiety disorder; 1.4% had phobic disorder; and 0.4% had panic disorder. In the 1979 national survey of psychotherapeutic drug use, prevalence rates annually were 1.2% for agoraphobia and panic attack, 2.3% for other phobia, and 6.5% for generalized anxiety. Previous surveys of the population of several community mental health catchment areas (Myers, Lindenthal, & Pepper, 1975) showed the 6-month prevalence rates for panic disorder ranged from 0.6% in New Haven to 1.0% in Baltimore. These surveys were all done with adult populations.

Orvaschel and Weissman (1986) recently reviewed available epidemiological data for childhood anxiety disorders. Generally the subjects surveyed were under the age of 12, but many were as young as 3. Their conclusion was that the only data available were those on anxiety *symptoms.* They found that anxiety symptoms were more prevalent in girls than in boys, but that the prevalence varied considerably, depending on the age of the child and the type of anxiety symptom. Fears and worries were present in 43% of 6- to 12-year-olds in Lapouse and Monk's studies (1958, 1959) but in only 4% in the Kastrup (1976) study of 5- to 6-year-old children. On the other hand, worries and fears ranged 2% to 43% and 4% to 33%, respectively in the Japanese study (Abe & Masue, 1981) of subjects 11 to 12 years of age.

Some more specific data on DSM-III (APA, 1980) diagnoses are provided by several other studies. Silva's study (Silva, Justin, McGee, & Williams, 1984) in New Zealand generated DSM-III diagnoses in 792 11-year-olds (416 boys and 376 girls). Anxiety disorders totaled 9.7% of the sample. Some of the children had multiple anxiety disorder diagnoses. Separation anxiety disorder affected 3.5% of the sample (mostly females); generalized anxiety disorder, 2.9% (mostly males); simple phobia, 2.4% (mostly females); and social phobia, 1% (mostly females).

Offord's (1985) epidemiological studies in the Province of Ontario in Canada have an overall category of neurosis, which includes both anxiety disorders and depression. In a random sample, 7.9% of males and 11.9% of females in the 4- to 16-year age range had a neurosis diagnosis.

Epidemiological studies of specific anxiety disorders, especially those using more recent diagnostic criteria, are very limited in children or adolescents. The developmental significance of anxiety symptoms and/or disorders in childhood and their natural development through adolescence and adult life is not well known. Much of the early work on developmental psychopathology in the anxiety area was done on heterogeneous groups of disorders classified as "emotional disturbances" (Rutter & Garmezy, 1983). It is clear that overall the group of disorders labeled "emotional disorders" is different from the disruptive behavior disorders (such as attention deficit disorder and conduct disorder) in a number of ways such as: sex ratio, association with family discord, association with learning disorders, prognosis, and long-term outcome. There is less agreement as to whether the finer differentiations among anxiety disorders (to be described in the next section) are supported by external validity studies in children and adolescents.

The link between anxiety disorders in childhood and adolescence and those in adulthood appears tenuous. Robins' (1966) data suggest that most emotional disorders of childhood do not persist into adult life. Other data (Zeitlen, 1983; Marks, 1969; Lader & Marks, 1971) suggest that most anxiety disorders in adults did not begin in childhood. Orvaschel and Weissman (1986) have reviewed issues of stability and continuity of anxiety symptomatology across all age groups. They concluded that childhood anxiety disorders are related to adult anxiety disorders in general but with little diagnostic specificity. For instance, school refusal and/or separation anxiety disorder may be related to adult anxiety disorders in *general* but not *specifically* to agoraphobia with or without panic attacks. However, they cautioned that the findings must be considered preliminary since there are no prospective, longitudinal data to support them. Indeed, more recent data do suggest that there may be some temporal continuity among various types of anxiety disorders in childhood, adolescence, and adulthood and that they remain diagnostically distinct over time (Rutter, 1986).

Phobias are more common in younger children than in older children or adolescents. Most phobic symptoms diminish with age. Obsessive-compulsive symptoms, when they occur, may show strong temporal continuity from childhood through adolescence and adult life. The usual age of onset is in adolescence, but data are conflicting as to whether they are associated with other anxiety disorders or whether they constitute a unique syndrome. Zeitlen's data (1983) suggested that the temporal continuity in obsessive-compulsive symptomatology was greater than for any other emotional or anxiety symptom.

Separation anxiety disorder in childhood may be associated with agoraphobia and panic disorder in adult life. Klein's retrospective data (1981) indicate that adults with panic disorder and/or agoraphobia report a high rate of childhood separation anxiety disorder. However, it is less clear in prospective studies whether separation anxiety disorder occurring for the first time in adolescence becomes panic disorder or agoraphobia in adulthood (Rutter, 1985).

Generalized anxiety disorders or, as Rutter and Garmezy (1983) call them, nonspecific emotional disturbances, show no great variation during the childhood years in prevalence, but they increase in adolescence. In addition, the similar sex ratio in childhood changes to a female preponderance in adolescence.

Diagnostic Issues

The diagnosis of any type of psychiatric disorder involves the use of a diagnostic *process*, which essentially includes: a series of questions to be answered about a particular patient, a set of diagnostic *tools* for collecting the data to answer the questions, a diagnostic *classification system* that specifies different types of disorders, and a *process of assimilation* through which one makes an interpretation of the data collected to arrive at a diagnostic statement.

The questions to be answered in evaluating an adolescent presenting with any type of psychiatric symptomatology include the following:

1. Does this adolescent have any type of psychiatric disorder? We define a psychiatric disorder as a significant problem in development, which may be manifested as an abnormality in behavior, an abnormality in emotional state, an abnormality in interpersonal relations, or an abnormality in cognition. Moreover, these abnormalities must be of sufficient severity and duration to cause significant functional impairment, which is defined as distress, disability, or disadvantage.

2. Does the clinical picture of this adolescent's disorder fit a known and recognized clinical syndrome? This implies that a particular classification system is being used that contains specific criteria to delineate and define the different disorders.

3. What are the differential diagnoses? According to the classification system being used, does the clinical picture also at least partially fit other clinical syndromes? (A more detailed description of the process of formulating differential diagnoses will follow.)

4. What are the possible etiological factors for this disorder? In adolescence, the etiology of any disorder is likely to be multifactorial: intrapsychic, familial, social, biologic, or some combination thereof. Therefore, the clinician also should ask: What are the relative strengths of the various etiological factors for this particular patient's disorder?

5. What forces are currently maintaining the disorder in this adolescent?

6. What forces are facilitating this adolescent's normal development?

7. What are this adolescent's strengths and competencies? What are the strengths and competencies of the family? And what are the strengths and competencies of the adolescent's overall psychosocial environment?

8. If untreated, what is the likely outcome of this disorder? The outcome of any disorder depends partly on its natural history and partly on factors such as those outlined in questions 4 to 7. In the case of anxiety disorders, each disorder has its own natural history, and it is the natural history that determines the type and urgency of intervention. A disorder that resolves rapidly without residual effect will require much less urgent and complex intervention than a disorder that leads to chronic and severe disability. The natural history of a disorder also serves as a standard by which the effectiveness of any intervention can be judged. An effective intervention ought to produce a better outcome than that which results from its natural history.

As already mentioned, the issue of differential diagnosis is crucial in the diagnostic process. This subject of the differential diagnosis of anxiety disorders has been reviewed by Shuckit (1981) and by Cameron (1985). Shuckit distinguishes between situational anxiety disturbance, primary anxiety disorders, and secondary anxiety disorders. Among the secondary anxiety disorders, he distinguishes those due to organic physical causes and those associated with other types of (nonanxiety) psychiatric disorders.

Cameron notes that among the factors relevant to the differential diagnosis are: the age of onset; associated findings, such as medical and neurological symptoms and signs and other psychiatric symptoms; presenting features; duration of illness; family history; predisposing factors; prevalence of the disorder; presence of phobic behavior; presence of psychic anxiety; and increased arousal, including increased metabolic state and adrenergic activity.

In DSM-III-R, the differential diagnostic process for adult anxiety disorders is set out in a decision tree (APA, 1987, pp. 384–385). The major difference between DSM-III and DSM-III-R is that the latter has largely abandoned the hierarchical approach used by the former, except when organic factors are involved. The DSM-III, for instance, would not make a diagnosis of an anxiety disorder when the anxiety symptoms occur concurrently with, say, schizophrenia; but the DSM-III-R now allows both diagnoses to be made independently if the anxiety symptoms extend beyond the schizophrenic episode. Cameron (1985) points out that many DSM-III psychiatric disorders may be associated with anxiety *symptoms* and may lead to diagnostic confusion. These disorders include: schizophrenia; depression; somatoform disorders; dissociative disorders; avoidant, dependent, and compulsive personality disorder; and some childhood disorders, such as attention deficit, schizoid, tic disorders, stuttering, enuresis, and sleep disorders. In addition, there may be overlaps among disorders, and some disorders, such as anxiety and depression, may occur together. The changes in the DSM-III-R are therefore welcome.

The DSM-III-R differential diagnostic process for symptoms of irrational and excessive anxiety or worry, avoidance behavior, or increased arousal not attributable to a psychotic disorder involves successive considerations of the presence of the following: (1) organicity; (2) recurrent panic attacks; (3) fear and avoidance of being in certain places, separation from attachment figures, or being in certain social situations; (4) obsessions and compulsions; (5) 6-month duration of symptoms in the absence of a stressor; (6) a specific stressor; and (7) reexperiencing of a traumatic event. Age of onset, which was one of the main differential factors in the DSM-III, is now important only for item 3, separation anxiety disorder, and item 5, overanxious disorder (versus generalized anxiety disorder). As already mentioned, presence of other mood or psychotic symptoms would exclude a diagnosis of an anxiety disorder only if the anxiety symptoms occur exclusively during the course of a mood or psychotic disorder.

All clinicians and researchers use some diagnostic system to classify the anxiety disorders so they can be differentiated from each other and from other nonanxiety psychiatric disorders. The DSM-III-R classification, although popular and described in some detail here, is not the only one in use. The International Classification of Disease, Ninth Edition (ICD-9) differs from DSM-III and DSM-III-R in that it does not give operational criteria and it does not describe the disorders in as much detail. The ICD-9 classification is currently under revision. Cameron (1985) has proposed an even simpler classification of endogenous versus exogenous anxiety. Endogenous anxiety is presumed to be due to an abnormal psychophysiological state and is not caused predictably by identifiable environmental stressors. In contrast, exogenous anxiety is presumed to be that which is provoked regularly by specific environmental stimuli.

Werry (1986) describes a dimensional classification system that has been used particularly in children and adolescents. A dimensional or trait approach employs a quantitative cutoff score on a particular rating scale to define the presence of a disorder. The scores on the rating scales are then subjected to certain factor and cluster analyses. The great bulk of these analyses has produced two broad factors: (1) a factor of "externalizing disorders" that is somewhat equivalent to the DSM-III-R grouping of disruptive behavior disorder, and (2) a second "internalizing disorder" factor that encompasses mainly anxiety and depressive features. Some investigators, such as Achenbach (1980), have taken this approach one step further and moved from the rather broad band, internalizing group to the narrower band, more discrete internalizing disorders described as anxious-obsessive, uncommunicative, and somatic complaints. Whether the categorical or dimensional approach to diagnosis is superior is a subject for future research.

Diagnostic tools available to both the clinician and the researcher in evaluating adolescents include the following: interview with the parents about the adolescent; interview with the entire family; interview with the adolescent; behavior rating scales which may be completed by parents, teachers, significant others, and the adolescents themselves; physical and neurological examination; and various laboratory studies including psychological testing. A complete discussion of all these tools is beyond the scope of this chapter, but we will comment briefly on some of them.

Orvaschel (1985) has recently reviewed psychiatric interviews that are suitable for the evaluation of children and adolescents with psychiatric disorders, including anxiety disorders. The ones that seem to have the most to offer are the Children's Assessment Schedule (CAS) (Hodges, McKnew, Cytryn, Stern, & Kline, 1982), the Diagnostic Interview for Children and Adolescents (DICA) (Herjanic & Reich, 1983), the Diagnostic Interview Schedule for Children (DISC) (Costello, Edelbrock, Dulcan, Kalas, & Klaric, 1984), the Interview Schedule for Children (ISC) (Kovacs, 1978), and the Kiddie Schedule for Affective Disorders and Schizophrenia (K-SADS) (Spitzer & Endicott, 1978). Generally, these interviews contain a form to be used for the parents and a form for the adolescent. All of them are validated for adolescents up to age 17 but also may be used for older patients. They differ from each other in the time period that is covered in the interview, the time it takes to administer the interview, and the symptomatology that is examined. All have significant reliability data.

With regard to the anxiety disorders, these interview schedules all provide reasonable coverage. The CAS encompasses avoidant disorder, generalized anxiety, obsessive-compulsive disorder, overanxious, panic, phobic, and separation anxiety disorders. The DICA, DISC, and ISC do not cover generalized anxiety disorder, and the K-SADS does not cover avoidant disorder. The ISC is the only one giving any significant coverage of Axis II personality disorders. None covers agoraphobia per se. The interview schedules also vary in their coverage of other DSM-III-R disorders.

Behavior rating scales useful in the diagnosis of anxiety disorders in adolescents have been reviewed by Gittelman (1985) and by Werry (1986). Several scales that are designed to cover a wide range of psychopathology include the Behavior Problem Checklist for parents and teachers (Quay & Peterson, 1983), the Conners parent and teacher questionnaires (Conners & Barkley, 1985), and the parent and teacher questionnaires of Achenbach (Achenbach, 1986). They all have anxiety items, and they can be used to derive factors involving anxiety symptoms. Gittelman (1985a, 1985b) has revised the Conners parent and teacher rating scales by adding to them multiple anxiety and depressive items, thus increasing their coverage of anxiety symptoms.

The various self-report inventories and scales have been reviewed by Werry (1986) and Gittelman (1986). These include such scales as the

California Personality Inventories, the Minnesota Multiphasic Personality Inventory (MMPI), the Junior Eysenck Personality Inventory, and the Cattel 16 PF Tests. Clinicians and researchers have also used the Children's Manifest Anxiety Scale, the State-Trait Anxiety Scale, the Test Anxiety Scale for Children, and the Fear Survey Schedule.

While the physical and neurological examination rarely contributes to the diagnosis of a *specific* disorder in adolescence, Werry has discussed some physiological measures that may be related to anxiety symptoms. These include cardiovascular measures (such as pulse rate, blood pressure, vasoconstriction in the fingers), pupillary dilatation, respiratory rate, finger tremor, muscle tension, and other physiological measures such as the electroencephalogram (EEG), the contingent negative variation (CNV), various endocrine measures, and palm or sweat measures of conductance and habituation to novel stimuli. Other aspects of psychobiological measures of anxiety are discussed by Rainey and Nesse (1985). However, research in adolescent anxiety disorders has not made much use of psychobiological and physical measures. Claims that anxiety disorder adolescents have specific findings on projective psychological tests have been discredited (Gittelman, 1980; Werry, 1986).

In summary, the researcher and clinician use as diagnostic tools: interviews with parents, interviews with the adolescent, and various types of behavior rating scales completed by the adolescent, the parents, teachers, and possibly by significant others (such as peers).

Last, the diagnostic process involves the assimilation of the data collected and the making of a diagnostic statement. To make a diagnosis according to a particular classification system reliably and validly depends strongly on the correct use of the system. This aspect has been little studied in child and adolescent psychiatry. However, Elizabeth Costello's data (1982) on this issue are sobering. She found that in a division of child and adolescent psychiatry known for its emphasis on research, clinicians in diagnostic conferences seldom used the rules of DSM-III in arriving at a final diagnosis. DSM-III criteria were explicitly used only rarely. In the great majority of cases, either a "pattern matching" approach was used in which a diagnosis was made if the patient's clinical picture somewhat resembled the DSM-III criteria, or the clinician simply drew upon his or her own experience of what a particular disorder should look like and pronounced a diagnosis. Furthermore, the DSM-III diagnostic decision tree approach was almost never used: Disorders higher up in the hierarchy were not discussed in the diagnostic process and, consequently, were usually ruled out.

Thus the reliability or validity of any diagnostic system, such as the DSM-III or DSM-III-R, depends very heavily on whether the system is used in the way it is supposed to be used. At present, research studies usually specify the entry criteria, which are almost always based on a particular diagnostic system. However, this does not necessarily guarantee that the criteria are always used correctly. This may explain the discrepancies in the findings of some studies of similar design that claim to have used the same diagnostic criteria.

CLINICAL PROBLEMS

The specific anxiety disorders will now be discussed using the DSM-III-R framework. The DSM-III and DSM-III-R classifications for the anxiety disorders of childhood and adolescence are presented in Table 9.1. The DSM-III (1980) is now superseded by the revised version, DSM-III-R (1987). The major changes in the DSM-III-R involving anxiety disorders will now be discussed.

DSM-III, as previously stated, is based on a hierarchical system. This conceptualization has been removed from DSM-III-R except when organicity is involved. There are some changes in the wordings of the criteria for the diagnosis of separation anxiety disorder, avoidant disorder, and overanxious disorder. By and large, however, the criteria for these disorders remain relatively unchanged.

Agoraphobia with panic attacks in DSM-III is changed to Panic Disorder with Agoraphobia in DSM-III-R because clinical observation suggests that panic disorder almost always precedes agoraphobia, (i.e., the panic disorder is primary and the phobic avoidance secondary). DSM-III-R has defined attacks involving four or more symptoms as panic attacks and attacks involving fewer than four symptoms as "limited symptom attacks." The clinician can specify when diagnosing panic disorder whether limited symptom attacks are present. Agoraphobia without panic attacks is now called agoraphobia without history of panic disorder, because it is recognized that sometimes the anxiety attack in these individuals may not meet the full criteria for a panic disorder.

For social phobia, DSM-III-R elaborates upon the criteria for distress and avoidance, and it clarifies the relation of social phobia with other Axis I or Axis III diagnoses. It stipulates that anxiety upon exposure to the phobic stimulus is necessary and that the person must recognize that the fear is excessive or unreasonable. It also allows the clinician to specify whether the social phobia is generalized (i.e., the phobic response extends to most social situations), in which case an associated diagnosis of avoidant personality disorder should be considered.

In DSM-III-R, the duration for generalized anxiety disorder is 6 months instead of 1 month so that transient anxiety reactions are excluded. The revised symptom list provides a richer description of the disorder than it has in DSM-III. The DSM-III-R clarifies the relationship of the disorder with another Axis I disorder; in particular, it stipulates

Table 9.1. The DSM-III and DSM-III-R Classification of Disorders Involving Anxiety

DSM-III*	DSM-III-R**
Anxiety Disorders of Childhood	*Anxiety Disorders of Childhood or Adolescence*
Separation anxiety disorder	Separation anxiety disorder
Avoidant disorder	Avoidant disorder of childhood or adolescence
Overanxious disorder	Overanxious disorder
Anxiety Disorders	*Anxiety Disorders*
Phobic disorders	Panic disorder
Agoraphobia with panic attacks	with agoraphobia
Agoraphobia without panic attacks	without agoraphobia
Social phobia	Agoraphobia without history
Simple phobia	of panic disorder
Anxiety states	Social phobia
Panic disorder	Simple phobia
Generalized anxiety disorder	Obsessive-compulsive disorder
Obsessive-compulsive disorder	Post-traumatic stress disorder
Post-traumatic stress disorder	Generalized anxiety disorder
Acute	Anxiety disorder not otherwise
Chronic or delayed	specified
Atypical anxiety disorder	
Adjustment Disorders	*Adjustment Disorders*
With anxious mood	With anxious mood
With mixed emotional features	With mixed emotional features
With withdrawal	With withdrawal
Personality Disorders	*Personality Disorders*
Avoidant	Avoidant
Compulsive	Obsessive-compulsive

*Adapted from DSM-III, pp. 15, 18, & 19
**Adapted from DSM-III-R, pp. 4, 7, & 9

that the disturbance should not occur only during the course of a mood or psychotic disorder.

For post-traumatic stress disorder, DSM-III-R clarifies the nature of the stressor. Numbing symptoms have been expanded to include avoidance and amnesia, and physiological arousal symptoms have replaced miscellaneous symptoms. In the text, specific symptoms are listed for the disorder in childhood. A more detailed description of the clinical picture of these major disorders will follow. For further details, the interested reader is referred to DSM-III, DSM-III-R, Beck and Emery (1985), Goodwin (1986), Cameron (1985), and Gorman et al. (1984).

Separation Anxiety Disorder

Werry (1986) points out that the DSM-III classification of anxiety disorders of childhood and adolescence is consistent with age-specific types of anxiety. He thus conceptualizes overanxious disorder as an exaggeration of the normal elemental anxiety present at birth; avoidant disorder as persistent stranger anxiety; and separation anxiety as persistent separation fear, which normally occurs after the age of 6 months. Finally, phobic anxiety is conceptualized as specific conditioned anxiety. As already mentioned, DSM-III-R essentially uses the same conceptualizations.

Werry suggests that panic disorder probably does not occur in children and agrees with Klein (1981) that it may be a biogenic anxiety related to separation anxiety. While it is true that panic episodes do not occur independently in prepubertal children, they probably do occur in association with separation anxiety disorders in this age group.

Among the anxiety disorders of childhood and adolescence, separation anxiety disorder probably is the one that has been most systematically studied. Since separation anxiety is a normal developmental phenomenon, one of the key issues is to determine when such anxiety becomes deviant or pathological.

Gittelman (1984) has delineated the characteristics of pathologic separation anxiety. First, there must be very obvious distress on separation. In its most severe form, this distress becomes panic. Second, there must be morbid worries about the potential dangers that threaten the family. Finally, there must be an intense desire to be reunited with home and family to a degree that goes beyond the usual homesickness. These three characteristics may occur together or independently of one another. When they are considered to be symptomatic, they must be severe enough to interfere with the child's adaptive functioning, such as markedly restricting activities or impairing emotional well-being.

The cardinal feature of separation anxiety disorder in adolescence is the anxiety that occurs whenever the adolescent has to be away from home or familiar areas such as school, camp, or friends' houses. Even within his or her own house, instead of being able to stay alone in a room, the anxiety may compel the adolescent to follow other individuals around from room to room.

Somatic complaints are common. They may occur at the time of separation or when it is anticipated, for example, on Monday mornings when the adolescent is going back to school. Cardiovascular symptoms (such as palpitations, chest pain, choking, or smothering sensations) that are common complaints in adults are also common in adolescents. They are less frequent in younger children, who instead develop stomachaches, headaches, nausea, and vomiting. With separation, there is often a preoccupation with morbid fears such as those of being kidnapped, of never being able to see their parents again, or of other disasters that may happen to them. Often the fears also center around the well-being of their parents.

Compared to younger children, adolescents more often demonstrate anticipatory anxiety of separation and fears toward potential identifiable dangers such as that of the father dying while taking an airplane trip for business. Adolescent patients may deny fear of separation or fear that their parents will come to harm, yet their behavior will betray their morbid anxiety and fear. They may therefore show a reluctance to leave home, to sleep over in a friend's house, or to go to camp. They may also demonstrate certain specific fears (such as fears of the dark or fear of ghosts) and may show demanding, intrusive, and attention-seeking behavior.

The separation anxiety may begin in the preschool years. However, the most extreme forms of the disorder, especially those that involve school refusal, usually begin around the age of 12. The disorder may appear suddenly in an adolescent who has previously not demonstrated any significant type of psychopathology, or it may occur as an acute episode in one who has previously had subclinical chronic separation anxiety. This disorder may remit completely spontaneously, in contrast to more chronic childhood disorders such as Attention Deficit Disorder.

While school refusal is a common presenting symptom of separation anxiety disorder and often is what leads the adolescent to referral, separation anxiety disorder is not always manifested by school refusal. There are very few studies comparing separation anxiety disorder and school phobia, a term which should be used for an actual phobic disorder of school. One recent study by Last and her colleagues (Last, Hersen, Kazdin, Finkelstein, & Strauss, 1987) indicated that when children and adolescents with pure separation anxiety disorder were compared to those with a true phobic disorder of school, they differed on a number of dimensions, including age, sex, social class, presence of other psychiatric disorder, and psychopathological aggression of depression in mothers. Subjects with separation anxiety disorder were mostly female, prepubertal, and came from a lower social class. Those with true school phobia were mostly male and from a higher social class. Furthermore, those with separation anxiety disorder were more likely to have an additional DSM-III diagnosis and to have mothers with affective disturbances.

The natural history of separation anxiety disorder generally consists of periods of remission and exacerbation which may last over several years, although it may also remit spontaneously after just one episode. Some cases persist into young adult life, with an exacerbation of anxiety when the individual is confronted with situations such as leaving home to go to college or to take a job in another city. Some authors have suggested that childhood and adolescent separation anxiety disorder may predispose the individual to develop agoraphobia in adult life. Follow-up studies of adolescents with school phobia, most of whom probably had separation anxiety disorder, suggest that they are more likely to develop work phobia later in life (Coolidge, Brodie, & Feeney, 1964).

Avoidant Disorder of Childhood and Adolescence

Avoidant disorder was described for the first time in DSM-III, but the description was based on clinical observations rather than on scientific studies. The DSM-III-R retains this diagnostic entity. The cardinal feature of the disorder is a persistent and excessive shrinking from contact with strangers that is severe enough to interfere with normal social functioning and the development of peer relationships. However, the adolescent with an avoidant disorder must also desire acceptance and affection, in contrast to a schizoid individual who does not. Moreover, relationship with familiar figures, such as family members and close family friends, must be warm and satisfying, demonstrating that the adolescent does have the capacity for close relationships.

Younger children with this disorder generally are clinging and become anxious and tearful when confronted with the need for contact with strangers. They are easily embarrassed and timid although they seem interested in developing social relationships. In adolescence, lack of assertiveness, poor self-concept, and sexual inhibition may also be present.

The disorder may develop as early as 2 1/2 years of age, when normal stranger anxiety usually disappears. It is unclear if the disorder can develop for the first time in adolescence, but it seems unlikely. The natural history of this disorder seems variable; some may improve spontaneously while others may develop a chronic illness persisting into adolescence and later life.

If the social discomfort, fear of negative evaluation, and timidity is pervasive, a diagnosis of avoidant personality disorder is given. Such individuals have a lifelong pattern of avoidant behavior which is not episodic or related to other illness. They also show social withdrawal, unwillingness to enter into relationships unless uncritical acceptance is guaranteed, hypersensitivity to rejection, and low self-esteem. In order for the disorder to be diagnosed, it must be of sufficient severity to cause subjective distress, and this must be accompanied by a desire for affection and acceptance. Cantwell and Baker (1987) found avoidant disorder to be a common diagnosis in children and adolescents with communication disorders as did Beitchman and his colleagues (Beitchman, Nair, Clegg, Ferguson, & Patel, 1986) in their epidemiological study of younger children with communication disorders. However, there is an extensive behavioral literature on the treatment of severely shy children, and while there may be many reasons for extreme shyness, some of these subjects may have qualified for a diagnosis of avoidant disorder in childhood or avoidant personality disorder in adolescence.

Overanxious Disorder of Childhood and Adolescence — Generalized Anxiety Disorder

When DSM-III was formulated, one of the conceptualizations (retained by DSM-III-R) was if a disorder that began regularly in infancy, childhood, or adolescence resembled another disorder occurring in later life, it was listed and described as a separate disorder with a different name. Thus overanxious disorder is, in essence, generalized anxiety disorder occurring in childhood with a slightly different clinical picture.

The cardinal feature of overanxious disorder of childhood and adolescence is generalized persistent anxiety, generalized in the sense that the anxiety is not related to a specific situation or a specific object. The symptoms, according to DSM-III, must persist for 6 months. According to DSM-III-R, the diagnosis may be made in the presence of another Axis I disorder, provided the anxiety and worry extend beyond the focus of that disorder. For instance, overanxious disorder and obsessive-compulsive disorder may both be diagnosed if generalized anxiety symptoms are present and are not limited to those of the obsessive-compulsive disorder.

In childhood, overanxious patients may have unrealistic worries about the future or about past behaviors that they consider embarrassing or inappropriate. They may have very unrealistic concerns about their competence. Adolescents with this disorder may worry greatly about their appearance, their abilities, or their performance, particularly in comparison with their peers. Many of these concerns occur even in normal adolescents, but they become pathological when they are excessive and persistent and interfere with functioning. Marked self-consciousness, tension, and the need for constant reassurance are characteristic. Multiple physical complaints such as headaches and stomachaches not due to organic causes are common, but these also can occur in somatization disorder or hypochondriasis. Anxiety about the future may include excessive worries about everyday activities such as going to the doctor, taking an examination, being invited to a party, or being able to keep a particular deadline for a paper in class.

Adolescents with an overanxious disorder may perceive various adult figures such as teachers and coaches as being hypercritical. Again, these concerns are typical adolescent ones, and they become pathological only when they are severe and persistent and interfere with functioning. These adolescents are often described as "good kids" because they are conforming, perfectionistic, and hypermature when talking to adults.

The onset of the disorder may be gradual or acute. Remissions and exacerbations may be related to a change in life events. The disorder may persist into adult life to become generalized anxiety disorder and perhaps social phobia; however, systematic prospective follow-up studies are lacking.

Last and her colleagues (Last et al., 1987), in a comparative study of children and adolescents with separation anxiety disorder and overanxious disorder, found that the two disorders differed in a number of ways. These included age, sex, social class, and the presence of another, coexisting, anxiety disorder. The mean age of children with separation anxiety disorder was approximately 9, whereas for overanxious disorder it was nearly 13 1/2. More of those with separation anxiety were female, while half of those with overanxious disorder were male. More of the children with separation anxiety disorder were from lower socioeconomic-class families. Those with overanxious disorder were highly likely to have another anxiety disorder—11.5% had avoidant disorder, more than a quarter had simple phobia, nearly 8% had social phobia, 8% had agoraphobia, 15% had panic disorder, and nearly 8% had obsessive-compulsive disorder. With separation anxiety disorder, the only other coexistent disorder was avoidant disorder in one child, slightly less than 5% of the sample. Affective disorders were relatively common in both groups but did not differ between the groups. Interestingly, attention deficit disorder was relatively common in both groups as was oppositional disorder.

Generalized anxiety disorder, the corresponding disorder to overanxious disorder if the patient was age 18 or older, has a set of more elaborate criteria: at least 6 months of persistent, unrealistic, or excessive worry, and the presence of 6 symptoms among 18 grouped according to motor tension, autonomic hyperactivity, and vigilance and scanning. An organic causative factor such as hyperthyroidism or amphetamine intoxication must not be present, although other Axis I disorders may be diagnosed. However, the focus of the symptoms cannot be related soley to that disorder if a concomitant diagnosis of generalized anxiety disorder is to be made.

The main symptomatic difference between generalized anxiety disorder and panic disorder is the presence or absence of discrete panic attacks. However, the two disorders may coexist.

Panic Disorder

Panic disorder in DSM-III is listed as one of the anxiety states under the overall heading of anxiety disorder. In DSM-III-R, panic disorder takes a more central role among the anxiety disorders. The subtypes are distinguished as panic disorder with agoraphobia and panic disorder without agoraphobia.

The characteristic features of a panic attack are the sudden and, at least initially, unpredictable onset of discrete periods of intense fear or discomfort accompanied by physical and other psychological symptoms. Somatic symptoms listed by DSM-III-R include dyspnea, dizziness, palpitations, trembling, sweating, choking, nausea, numbness, flushes or chills, and chest pains. Psychological symptoms include feelings of depersonalization or derealization, fear of dying, and fear of going crazy or doing something uncontrolled during the attack. DSM-III-R requires at least four of the symptoms during at least one of the attacks, and uses the term "limited symptom attack" for those involving less than four symptoms. In terms of frequency of attacks, it requires four attacks within a 4-week period or one or more attacks followed by at least 1 month of persistent fear of having another attack. DSM-III-R specifies that at some time during the illness, one or more panic attacks must be unexpected and not triggered by situations in which the individual was the focus of others' attention. A fourth criterion is that during at least some of the attacks, at least four of the symptoms should develop suddenly and increase in intensity within 10 minutes of the beginning of the first symptom. Finally, organic factors such as amphetamine intoxication or hyperthyroidism must be excluded.

Individuals who develop panic attacks also have varying degrees of between-attack anticipatory nervousness, apprehension, and fear of developing another attack. The onset is usually in early adult life, but it may begin in late adolescence. There is no evidence that the symptom pattern is different if the illness occurs in adolescence. Some evidence exists that separation anxiety disorder in childhood may predispose to panic disorder in adolescence or adult life, but this is not clearly established. Depression and alcohol abuse may occur to a greater degree in individuals with panic disorder. Cameron (1985) suggests that 3% of the general population have clinically significant panic disorder plus generalized anxiety disorder.

Agoraphobia

DSM-III-R (p. 403) defines a phobia as a persistent and irrational fear of a specific object, activity, or situation that leads to an overwhelming desire to avoid the phobic stimulus. Furthermore, the patient must recognize that this particular fear is unreasonable and excessive when compared to the actual dangerousness of the phobic stimulus.

Agoraphobia is characterized by an intense fear of being in particular places or in particular situations that would lead to unbearable embarrassment from which escape might be difficult or for which help might not be available should a panic attack occur. Moreover, this particular fear must result in functional impairment. The functional impairment may take the form of intense anxiety associated with the specific fear such as that of being alone, being in a strange place, being in closed places or elevators, or flying on airplanes; or it may be increasing constriction of normal activity so that, for instance, the individual cannot travel, cannot leave home alone, cannot ride in a car, or cannot fly in an airplane.

As already mentioned, agoraphobia in DSM-III is described as being with and without panic attacks, and panic disorder is considered separately. In DSM-III-R, panic disorder with agoraphobia and panic disorder without agoraphobia are considered to be subtypes of panic disorder. The reason for this change is that systematic studies have found that in most patients agoraphobia develops after panic attacks have occurred. The avoidant behavior in agoraphobia is conceptualized as being secondary to a fear of having a panic attack in a place (such as an elevator, a plane, or a train) where help would not be available and/or the attack would be embarrassing to the individual. Those cases of agoraphobia without panic attacks are given a separate classification in DSM-III-R, agoraphobia without history of panic disorder, and it should be specified if limited symptom attacks of panic have occurred. Depressive symptoms, generalized anxiety, minor obsessive rituals and checking behavior, or ruminations are also common accompaniments in agoraphobic individuals. The onset is generally in the late 20s, but it can occur later or earlier. Apparently, however, panic episodes do not occur in the absence of separation anxiety disorder. It is suggested that separation anxiety and sudden object loss or other sudden traumatic events may be predisposing factors to the development of agoraphobia. Prevalence in the general population is about 0.6% (Cameron, 1985).

The prognosis of agoraphobia is variable. In some cases, the disorder is quite disabling. In other cases, the severity may wax and wane over time with periods of remission. In addition, the actual phobic stimulus (such as leaving home, flying, falling, and being in open spaces) may change over time in the same individual.

Social Phobia

Individuals with social phobia avoid situations in which they expect to be scrutinized by others. They have an excessive fear of being the focus of others' attention and of behaving in a way which will be embarrassing or humiliating. Common examples of social phobias are fear of having to speak in public (i.e., a situation in which there is an audience, small or large), fear of using public lavatories, and fear of writing or eating in public. It is important to remember that the patient does not actually fear people or crowds, but fears scrutiny and the possibility that he will act in an embarrassing or humiliating way.

The anticipatory anxiety about facing these phobic situations may be marked. If the individual has to endure the situation, it is done so with intense distress. Panic attacks may occur but are not common. The disorder usually begins in late childhood or early adolescence. However, it may begin at any age from childhood to adulthood. No definitive predisposing factors have been delineated, but the disorder has not been studied extensively in childhood or adolescence. Theoretically, social phobia may lead to general avoidant behavior, and therefore the individual may be given a concomitant diagnosis of avoidant disorder of childhood or adolescence, or avoidant personality disorder.

While this disorder tends to run a chronic course, it rarely leads to severe incapacitation, but it may cause significant inconvenience if the individuals hold jobs that require performing or speaking in public or frequent traveling. These individuals may then be at risk for abuse of medication or alcohol with which they self-medicate to relieve anxiety.

Simple Phobia

Simple phobia in both DSM-III and DSM-III-R is a residual category. It is essentially a phobic reaction to a situation other than fear of having a panic attack, of being humiliated, of embarrassment in social situations, or of separation from familiar figures, since in these cases, the diagnosis of panic attack, social phobia, and separation anxiety disorder would be made respectively. DSM-III-R further stipulates that the phobic stimulus in simple phobia cannot be related to the content of obsessions or compulsions or the trauma of post-traumatic stress disorder. Beyond these restrictions, theoretically, almost any situation or object could be a phobic stimulus, although in actual practice, some are much more common than others. Animal phobias are probably the most common in the general population, but they are not necessarily the most common among those who come for treatment.

Cameron (1985) suggested that the rather nonspecific residual aspect of simple phobia as defined in DSM-III was probably incorrect. He pointed out that there were several specific situational phobias that were associated with panic disorder and/or agoraphobia. However, animal phobias did not belong in this grouping. He also suggested that fear of physical injury and fear of blood should be considered a separate class of simple phobias based on their distinctive psychophysiological reactions. Cameron therefore proposed that simple phobias be divided into: (1) animal phobias; (2) other single discrete phobias, such as fear of blood, illness, and injury, and (3) specific situational phobias which are variants of panic disorder and agoraphobia.

When all simple phobias are considered together, the mean age of onset is probably middle adolescence. However, different types of simple phobias have different ages of onset. Animal phobias almost always start in childhood, whereas the others usually occur in adolescence or later life.

The course of simple phobias that begin in childhood generally is one of remission without specific treatment. Those that persist into adulthood or begin later in life may require therapeutic intervention. Obviously, the impairment of a simple phobia is related to the prevalence in the general population of the feared object. Elephant phobia is unlikely to cause problems for urban city dwellers, but fear of heights in someone who works in a skyscraper and is unable to avoid that job may be incapacitating. No good evidence exists that there are any particular predisposing factors for simple phobias.

Obsessive-Compulsive Disorder

Obsessive-compulsive disorder is characterized by the presence of either obsessions or compulsions. Obsessions may be ideas, thoughts, or images. The defining characteristic is that they are recurrent and persistent and are unwanted by the individual, who clearly sees them as intrusive, senseless, and repugnant. The individual must recognize that these obsessions are products of his or her own mind rather than being imposed from some external source and that attempts are made to ignore, suppress, and neutralize them with some other thought or action.

Compulsions are acts that are intentional, purposeful, and repetitive. The individual performs these acts using certain rules or in a stereotyped fashion. To qualify for a compulsion, the behavior must be recognized by the individual as excessive and unreasonable, and it must be performed to prevent anxiety, discomfort, or some dreaded situation or event. The individual must recognize that the compulsive activity is not connected in any realistic way with the event that it is designed to prevent. The compulsion must cause marked distress and interfere with normal functioning.

Obsessions and compulsions are often associated with other disorders such as organic disorders, depression, schizophrenia, and Tourette's disorder. According to DSM-III-R, for an obsessive-compulsive disorder to be diagnosed, the obsessions and compulsions must not be related to the content of any other Axis I or Axis II psychiatric disorder. Cameron (1985) suggests that compulsions occur in about 75% of obsessive-compulsive patients and that multiple compulsions are uncommon, while obsessions occur in almost all the patients with many having more than one obsession. Cameron also suggests that true delusional beliefs may occur in obsessive-compulsive individuals, but even in these patients the obsessive-compulsive behavior remains egodystonic, in contrast to those in psychotic disorders.

Recent studies by Rapoport and her colleagues (Rapoport et al., 1981) suggest that depressive disorder is quite common in adolescents with obsessive-compulsive disorder. Phobic avoidance also may develop as the patient attempts to avoid situations that trigger obsessions. For instance, a patient who is fearful of contamination and infestation may avoid public lavatories.

The disorder may begin in childhood, but generally it begins in late adolescence or early adult life. Approximately 40% of obsessive-compulsive patients on follow-up remain unchanged, while 40% will show improvement and 20% will show complete remission (Cameron, 1985).

Despite its relative rarity, the disorder has been quite intensively investigated recently. Results from a National Institute of Mental Health (NIMH) study by Rapoport (Rapoport et al., 1981) of 27 children and adolescents with an obsessive-compulsive disorder have called into question whether the disorder should be classified as an anxiety disorder since it seems phenomenologically unrelated to the other anxiety disorders. In the sample studied, the age of onset was 2 to 4 years of age in 11%, 7 to 9 years in 26%, 10 to 14 in 56%, and 15 to 16 in 7%. The onset was generally gradual but was acute in some subjects. There was no solid evidence for any precipitating event or a distinct premorbid personality pattern. Particularly, the investigators did not find that these individuals were introverted or had obsessional personalities prior to the onset of their disorder. The symptom pattern and the extent of functional impairment in the adolescents and children were very similar to those seen in adults. Formal thought disorder was noticeably absent, but depression was common: only a few subjects met criteria for major depressive disorder at the time of the study, but most of them had the disorder at some point in the past.

The family history in Rapoport's group was interesting. The majority of parents were free of any psychiatric illness, and there was no particular pattern to the psychiatric disorders of the 39% of parents who had such a history. The investigators could find no peculiar parental attitude or distinctive child-rearing pattern in the families. Of the siblings younger than 18 years of age, 62% had no psychiatric diagnosis, and of those who had, conduct disorder and attention deficit disorder were the most common diagnoses. However, although more than half the siblings over the age of 18 also had no psychiatric disorder, 6% had an obsessive-compulsive disorder, 9% generalized anxiety disorder, 6% panic disorder, and 3% phobic reaction.

Of particular interest are the findings which suggest that there may be some type of neuropsychological deficit and altered neurological functioning in this sample of adolescents and children. On the neuropsychological test battery, the patient sample did as well as the controls on psychometric measures of attention, memory, and decision times. However, they made more errors on a road map test and on a stylus learning test, and took significantly longer to copy figures on a complex figure design test. Taken together, these findings suggested that the obsessive subjects had difficulty making spatial and directional judgments using their body as a reference, had difficulty discerning unstated patterns, took longer times to copy figures, and used less refined strategies on the complex figure copying task. These data are suggestive of frontal lobe dysfunction since similar patterns have been found in subjects with known frontal lobe damage. The deficits are relatively specific because there was an absence of evidence of general cognitive impairment and memory or attention difficulties.

Psycholinguistic testing revealed that the patients were similar to the controls on language expression and language comprehension. However, results from several tests such as the Dichotic Listing and the degree of left-handedness in the patients suggested that hemisphere dominance in this group was not as strong as it was in the control group of normal children.

EEGs were generally normal. Fifteen percent were mildly abnormal; another six EEGs did have intermittent slow wave activity, but this was not considered to be definitely abnormal. In computerized axial tomography

(CT scans), the obsessive group had higher mean ventricular to brain ratio (VBR) than the control group, and a quarter of the subjects had VBRs greater than two standard deviations above the mean.

In summary, there may be some type of central nervous system dysfunction in children and adolescents with an obsessive-compulsive disorder. However, while the different measures suggest cortical dysfunction, there was little correlation between the individual measures, indicating that the dysfunction is likely to be complex and subtle.

Post-Traumatic Stress Disorder

Post-traumatic stress disorder has been studied extensively in adults, particularly in military or veteran hospital populations. More recently, a growing body of literature has delineated the symptomatology of this disorder in children and adolescents. Much of the data has come from children who have experienced traumatic events such as the death of a parent and physical and/or sexual abuse. Some researchers in the area of sexual abuse feel that chronic sexual abuse may result in a rather particular syndrome that is a possible variant of post-traumatic stress disorder (Corwin, personal communication).

DSM-III-R stipulates that the traumatic event must be outside the range of usual human experience, an event that would be markedly distressing to almost anyone. The listed examples include a serious threat to one's life or physical integrity and sudden destruction of one's home or community.

A second requirement in DSM-III-R is persistent reexperiencing of the traumatic event as evidenced by at least one of four sets of symptoms: (1) recurrent and intrusive distressing recollections of the event, (2) recurrent distressing dreams of the event, (3) sudden acting or feelings as if the event is reoccurring, and (4) intense psychological distress at exposure to events that symbolize or resemble the event. For young children, the DSM-III-R specifically states that the reexperiencing of the event might be expressed in repetitive play involving themes or aspects of the trauma.

The third criterion in DSM-III-R stipulates persistent avoidance of stimuli associated with the trauma or numbing of general responsiveness as manifested by at least three of seven symptoms: (1) avoidance of rights and feelings associated with the trauma, (2) avoidance of activities or situations that arouse recollection of the event, (3) psychogenic amnesia, (4) loss of interest, and in young children, loss of recently acquired developmental skills (such as language skills or toilet training), (5) feeling of detachment, (6) restricted range of affect, and (7) sense of a foreshortened future (e.g., an adolescent does not expect to have a career, marriage, children, or long life). DSM-III-R includes as the fourth criterion persistent symptoms of increased arousal, as manifested by two out of six symptoms: (1) sleep

disturbance, (2) irritability, (3) difficulty concentrating, (4) hypervigi-
lance, (5) exaggerated startled response, and (6) physiological reactivity
occurring on exposure to events that symbolize or resemble an aspect of the
traumatic event. Finally, DSM-III-R stipulates that the duration of symptoms in criteria 2, 3, and 4 should be at least 1 month, and it further stipu-
lated that a delayed onset should be specified if symptoms began more than
6 months after the trauma.

In individuals with post-traumatic stress disorder, depression and other
anxiety symptoms may be present, and some adolescents may therefore
qualify for another diagnosis in addition to post-traumatic stress disorder.
The onset may be at any age from childhood to adult life. Symptoms may
begin immediately or soon after the trauma, or they may be delayed
following a latency period of months or years. The impairment produced
by the disorder can range from mild to severe. Good information is not
available on prevalence, sex ratio, and family aggregation of psychopathology of this disorder.

INTERVENTION

General Principles of Intervention

This section will discuss the general principles of intervention, various
therapeutic options, and the specific treatment of individual anxiety disorders. We may state at the onset that effective intervention rests upon the
following: (1) accurate diagnosis and differential diagnosis, (2) knowledge
of the available therapeutic options and their efficacy and safety, and (3)
careful implementation of the treatment plan with systematic monitoring
and periodic reevaluation. Furthermore, several general principles of intervention must be followed.

The first general principle is that no single treatment has been found to
be always effective for any one of the anxiety disorders, much less for all of
them. It is highly unlikely that a disorder with multifactorial etiology and
variable course and outcome will always respond to one type of treatment.
Multiple modes of treatment are therefore needed even for a single disorder. Furthermore, individual patients differ in their strengths and weaknesses, as do their environments. Thus a set of treatments effective in one
adolescent may prove to be ineffective in another, even for the same disorder. Finally, since the symptoms and the needs of a patient may change
over the course of the illness, different types of treatment for the same
disorder may be required at different times in the patient's life.

The second principle is that the final treatment goal is to return the
adolescent to normal functioning as rapidly as possible. Since adolescence
is a period of rapid development in many areas (psychosocial, cognitive,

etc.), it is important that the impact of the disorder on the individual's development be minimized. This can be done best by returning the adolescent to as many areas of normal functioning (school, home, leisure time, social activities, etc.) as possible without unnecessary delay.

The third principle is that simpler interventions should be tried first, and the use of more complex and difficult interventions with possibly more frequent or serious side effects should be considered only when the simpler ones have failed. The natural history of the disorder and the degree of functional impairment should determine the urgency and complexity of intervention.

A final general principle is that every treatment plan represents at best an educated guess. Since there are very few well-controlled treatment studies in adolescent anxiety disorders, it is hard to plan treatment based solely on proven findings. It is still a truism that interventions delivered to adolescents with anxiety, or for that matter, with any kind of psychiatric disorder, tend to reflect more the ideological bias of the clinician than the result of carefully conducted treatment studies.

Types of Intervention

Several general discussions of the treatments in anxiety disorders are available (Davis, Nasr, Spira, & Vogel, 1981; Schuckit, 1981; Ulenhuth, 1981; Carlson, Figueroa, & Lahey, 1986). These interventions fall under the following headings: (1) family and child counseling or supportive therapy, (2) behavior and cognitive behavioral interventions, (3) psychodynamically based individual and family intervention, and (4) psychopharmacological intervention.

Supportive Treatment

Family and child counseling include such supportive techniques as reassurance, advice, education, and environmental manipulation. Families and adolescents may benefit from a better understanding of the nature of the disorder, its natural history, and its likely etiological roots. Reassurance that the obsessive-compulsive symptoms are not signs of a severe psychiatric disorder may decrease the anxiety level in the patient and the family.

Schaefer and Millman (1981) have detailed how reassurance and advice may be given to parents to help their adolescents who demonstrate anxious and worrisome behavior. First, they outline how fearful and anxious behavior may develop, listing their causes, such as feelings of insecurity and guilt, defective parental modeling, and excessive frustration. They then describe ways for the parents to prevent fearful and anxious behavior in their children, outlining methods such as those that promote fostering, understanding, problem solving, security and self-confidence. They also urge the parents to accept the adolescents' sometimes unrealistic fantasies. Further, they suggest that the parents should accept the adolescents' anxious and fearful behavior, teach the adolescents relaxation and other antianxiety techniques, teach the adolescents to develop positive self-talk, and foster open expression of feelings in the family. They also recommend several books on anxiety and worrying for the family to read.

Schaefer and Millman use this approach for several types of symptomatic behavior, including anxious worrisome behavior, fearfulness, shyness, compulsive and perfectionistic behavior, and hypersensitivity to criticism. Since these behaviors may be present in all the anxiety disorders, we recommend their approach to all clinicians treating anxiety disorders in adolescents. These simple procedures may be very effective, but unfortunately, they tend to be overlooked in favor of more complex professional intervention.

If it is decided that professional intervention is necessary, the clinician has the choice of a variety of treatments which we will presently discuss. However, few of these interventions have been studied systematically in adolescents with anxiety disorders.

Behavior Modification

Carlson and her colleagues (Carlson et al., 1986) have described the use of behavior modification for children and adolescents. Among the specific behavioral and cognitive behavioral interventions for anxiety disorders are: relaxation training, systematic desensitization, implosion, flooding, aversion relief, thought stopping, modeling, and social skills training.

Relaxation training is an attempt to decrease anxiety through the use of specific techniques such as muscle relaxation, biofeedback, or transcendental meditation. For adolescents, this would seem to be most effective for overanxious disorder, panic disorder, and situational anxiety disorder such as adjustment disorders (Schuckit, 1981).

Systematic desensitization has been used for phobic disorders. This usually consists of the patient making successive approaches to the phobic object along with self-monitoring of anxiety level and the use of appropriate rewards (Schuckit, 1981). Flooding and implosion require confrontation with the anxiety-provoking stimuli. In contrast to desensitization where anxiety is kept to a minimum during confrontation, these approaches encourage the development of high levels of anxiety. In implosion, overwhelming anxiety is achieved through the patient's imagination of the phobic situation, but in flooding, actual confrontation with the phobic stimulus is used. These approaches are thought to be effective for phobic disorders including agoraphobia and separation anxiety and panic attacks (Schuckit, 1981). Phobic disorders also may be treated with aversion relief, which usually is done by delivering a mild shock to the patient's finger and then stopping the shock when the phobic stimulus is presented.

Thought stopping and response prevention have been used to treat obsessive-compulsive disorder. In the former, the therapist asks the patient to produce an obsessive thought or rumination and then to terminate it by loudly yelling "stop," banging on a table, or snapping a rubber band on his or her wrist. In response prevention, the patient is exposed to the stimuli that cause obsessive-compulsive symptoms but is then prevented from engaging in the ritualistic behavior. Initially the technique causes an increase in anxiety and obsessions, but after repeated sessions they may decrease. A hierarchy of stimuli exposure (from less to more anxiety provoking) and relaxation training may be used in conjunction with response prevention.

Modeling (exposure of the patient to a live demonstration of how a model approaches the phobic stimulus) may also be useful in phobic disorders, obsessive-compulsive disorders, and avoidant disorders. Social skills training would seem to be most useful for patients with an avoidant disorder or avoidant personality disorder.

Psychotherapy

Lewis (1986) has outlined the principles of intensive individual psychoanalytic therapy for anxiety disorder, and several authors have written on the use of family therapy for these disorders (Goldenberg & Goldenberg, 1985; Barker, 1981). With adults, there is some evidence (Schuckit, 1981) that psychotherapy alone is rarely effective for the primary anxiety disorders. However, intensive individual therapy and family therapy have not been studied systematically in adolescents with anxiety disorders. Most of the literature consists of individual case reports.

Pharmacotherapy

Medication treatment may be given to decrease anxiety symptoms, to increase adaptive functioning, and to treat any concomitant disorders. Despite the fact that pharmacotherapy for anxiety disorders in adults has been intensively studied, the literature dealing with such treatment for children or adolescents is very limited. Unfortunately, one cannot simply extend the adult pharmacotherapy data to adolescents or to children who have apparently similar disorders. Medications for the treatment of anxiety disorders in adolescents must be independently demonstrated to be effective and safe in this population in double-blind placebo-controlled studies.

Schuckit (1981) has reviewed the literature on pharmacotherapy of anxiety disorders in adults. Effective medications include the beta blockers, the monoamine oxidase inhibitors (MAOI), the tricyclic antidepressants (TCA), and various antianxiety agents such as the benzodiazepines, alprazolam, and buspirone.

Beta blockers such as propranolol (Inderal) are probably best used for panic episodes and for situational anxiety states with prominent somatic symptoms such as those that occur prior to taking an examination or performing in public. They are less useful for generalized anxiety disorders and phobic disorders including agoraphobia that are not accompanied or preceded by panic attacks.

The MAOIs are marketed primarily as antidepressants. However, they have been used with positive results in adults for agoraphobia, social phobia, panic attacks, and "atypical depression" in which anxiety and somatic symptoms predominate. However, the MAOIs may not completely abolish the anxiety symptoms, and they may take up to 6 to 8 weeks to work. Thus the MAOIs may not be as useful for situational anxiety or phobic disorders.

Tricyclic antidepressants likewise are marketed primarily as antidepressants. However, they also have been effective in adolescents with attention deficit disorder and enuresis. In adults, they are effective for agoraphobia and social phobia, but in adolescents their effects seem to be mixed (Gittelman & Koplewicz, 1986). Their antianxiety effect is probably not mediated secondarily through their antidepressant action, as there is no strong correlation between response and initial level of depression. They are probably best used in panic episodes, but because they may take several weeks to become effective, they are not useful for acute situational anxiety.

Gittelman and Koplewicz (1986) have discussed the pharmacotherapy of anxiety disorders in adolescents as have Simeon and Ferguson (1985). Gittelman and Koplewicz observe that over the past years numerous medications (including neuroleptics, psychostimulants, and antihistamines) have been tried on children with anxiety disorders. However, there is no scientific evidence that these are effective. Most of the literature on medication treatment of anxiety disorders in children consists of only limited case reports. In their literature review, Gittelman and Koplewicz found only three controlled studies of drug treatments for anxiety disorders in children, and these all involved TCAs.

One of the controlled studies was an early study by Gittelman-Klein and Klein (1971), examining the use of a TCA, imipramine, in children with school phobia. The drug was found to be effective both in helping children and adolescents to return to school and in decreasing anxiety and somatic symptoms. The second study (Berney et al., 1981) used clomipramine in a similar group of children, but the results were not striking, possibly due to the low dosage used. The third study by Rapoport and her colleagues (Rapoport, Elkins, & Mikkelsen, 1980) found higher doses of chlorimipramine were effective in reducing symptoms of obsessive-compulsive disorder in adolescents. Gittelman and Koplewicz conclude that the TCAs may be useful in the management of certain early anxiety disorders.

Simeon and Ferguson's literature review (1985) reaches similar conclusions, although these authors express concern that tricyclics may not be as safe as benzodiazepines. Among the antianxiety agents benzodiazepines have had the longest usage. They seem to decrease subjective feelings of anxiety and may be useful in acute situation anxiety and adjustment disorders. However, Schuckit (1981) feels that their effectiveness may wear off after several weeks of treatment. The benzodiazepines may cause impairment in motor and cognitive function and in some patients may increase feelings of hostility and frustration. They can produce psychological dependence and sometimes physical dependence with withdrawal symptoms. The benzodiazepines should therefore be used as adjuncts to behavior or cognitive behavior therapy for short periods of time (for instance, 3 weeks) for situational anxiety disorder. They are not useful for phobic or panic disorders.

Alprazolam, a triazolobenzodiazepine, has antianxiety and perhaps antidepressant properties. Its antianxiety properties are about equal to that of diazepam but with somewhat less sedation. Gittelman and Koplewicz suggest that alprazolam may be effective for adolescents with separation anxiety and panic disorder who are not responsive to psychotherapy.

Buspirone is a nonbenzodiazepine with antianxiety effects similar to alprazolam. A recent symposium (Rickels, 1981) discussed the use of buspirone in adults. As already mentioned, these data cannot be readily applied to adolescents without further study.

Simeon and Ferguson have treated adolescents with generalized anxiety and avoidant disorder with alprazolam. They report improvement with treatment and relapses after the drug is withdrawn. In the treatment of 12 patients, 7 showed marked or moderate improvement, and 5 showed minimal or no improvement. During the postdrug placebo period, 4 of the 12 relapsed, 4 maintained improvement, 3 continued to improve, and 1 improved for the first time. At follow-up after a drug-free period, 3 of the 12 patients relapsed further, 3 showed new relapse, and 1 had continued to improve. When alprazolam was reinstituted in 5 of the relapsed patients, 4 improved again, but 1 did not.

Further analysis of the data suggested that those individuals whose predominant symptomatology was inhibition, shyness, and nervousness, and who had good premorbid adjustment, responded well to benzodiazepines and showed further improvement after the medication was discontinued. However, those adolescents with poor premorbid personality development seemed to respond poorly, and the benzodiazepine may have had a disinhibiting effect. Even with initial improvement, they tended to relapse after the medication was discontinued.

In summary, the literature suggests that certain medications may be effective for childhood anxiety disorders. Unfortunately, treatments for childhood and adolescent anxiety disorders have not been systematically studied. Clinically, it is important to obtain good baseline measures of target behaviors and monitor them during treatment in order to determine if the treatment goals are met. Constant reevaluation of treatment is necessary. Currently, psychopharmacological interventions are most

Table 9.2. Treatments for Various Anxiety Disorders

TREATMENTS

Disorders	Nonspecific Counseling — Advice, Reassurance	Behavioral & Cognitive Behavioral — Relaxation Training	Social Skills Training	Desensitization Flooding, Implosion	Immersion Aversion	Modeling	Thought Stopping	Antidepressants — Clomipramine, Trazodone	Others
Separation anxiety disorder	X			X					X
Agoraphobia without panic	X			X					X
Panic disorder with and without agoraphobia	X	X							X
Generalized anxiety disorder	X	X							
Avoidant disorder	X		X			X			
Simple phobias	X			X	X	X			
Social phobias	X	X		X	X	X			
Obsessive-compulsive disorder	X	X		X		X	X	X	
Post-traumatic stress	X			?		?			

Table 9.2. **Treatments for Various Anxiety Disorders** *(continued)*

		TREATMENTS			
Disorders	MAO Inhibitors	Antianxiety Agents Alprazolam	Benzo-diazepines	Beta Blockers	Reenact-ment
Separation anxiety disorder	X	X			
Agoraphobia without panic	X	X			
Panic disorder with and without agoraphobia	X	X			
Generalized anxiety disorder			X	X	
Avoidant disorder					
Simple phobias			X		
Social phobias	X		X	X	
Obsessive-compulsive disorder					
Post-traumatic stress					X

commonly used in conjunction with psychosocial interventions. Table 9.2 presents a summary of the treatment approaches that may be useful for the specific types of childhood anxiety disorders.

FUTURE DIRECTIONS

Although much is known about anxiety disorders in adults, this review shows that much less is known about anxiety disorders in children and adolescents. More research is needed with regard to the essential and associated clinical features of anxiety disorders in children, the natural course and outcome of these disorders, and their responses to various treatment modalities.

Currently, there are numbers of tools available for quantifying anxiety symptomatology, including observational and self-rating scales, interviews, and physiological measurement techniques. These, along with rigorous diagnostic criteria such as DSM-III and DSM-III-R, will permit the identification of more homogeneous groups of children suffering from various subtypes of anxiety disorders. Systematic collection of data on these groups will be necessary, particularly with regard to family and demographic features, and concomitant psychiatric symptomatology (such as depression, obsessions, and compulsions).

The observation of such groups over time will provide valuable information on the natural outcome of these disorders and their association with the adult anxiety disorders. As already mentioned, controlled treatment studies of the various childhood and adolescent anxiety disorders are urgently needed.

SUMMARY

This chapter begins with a discussion of the general concept and the various definitions of anxiety. Various etiologic theories are then discussed. The epidemiology of anxiety disorders in children and adolescents is reviewed, along with the developmental issues and the relationship between the disorders of childhood, adolescence, and adult life. The chapter then discusses the diagnosis and differential diagnosis of anxiety disorders and outlines the presenting clinical problems using the DSM-III-R framework. Finally, interventions, both pharmacological and nonpharmacological, are discussed for the various anxiety disorders in children and adolescents.

REFERENCES

Abe, K., & Masui, T. (1981). Age-sex trends of phobic and anxiety symptoms. *British Journal of Psychiatry, 138,* 297–302.

Achenbach, T. (1980). DSM-III in light of empirical research on the classification of child psychopathology. *Journal of the American Academy of Child Psychiatry, 19,* 395–412.

Achenbach, T. (1986). *Assessment and taxonomy of child and adolescent psychopathology.* New York: Sage Publications.

American Psychiatric Association (1952). *Diagnostic and statistical manual of mental disorders* (1st ed.). Washington, DC: Author.

American Psychiatric Association (1980). *Diagnostic and statistical manual of mental disorders* (3rd ed.). (DSM-III). Washington, DC: Author.

American Psychiatric Association (1987). *Diagnostic and statistical manual of mental disorders* (3rd ed., rev.). (DSM-III-R). Washington, DC: Author.

Barker, P. A. (1981). *Basic family therapy.* Baltimore: University Park Press.

Beck, A. T., & Emery, G. (1985). *Anxiety disorders and phobias: A cognitive perspective.* New York: Basic Books.

Beitchman, J. H., Nair, R., Clegg, M., Ferguson, B., & Patel, P. G. (1986). Prevalence of psychiatric disorders in children with speech and language disorders. *Journal of the American Academy of Child Psychiatry, 25,* 528–533.

Berney, T., Kolvin, I., Bhate, S. R., Garside, R. F., Jeans, J., Kay, B., & Scarth, L. (1981). School phobia: A therapeutic trial with clomipramine and short-term outcome. *British Journal of Psychiatry, 138,* 110–118.

Bowlby, J. (1969). *Attachment and loss (Vol. I: Attachment).* New York: Basic Books.

Bowlby, J. (1973). *Attachment and loss (Vol. II: Separation anxiety and anger).* New York: Basic Books.

Cameron, O. G. (1985). The differential diagnosis of anxiety. *Psychiatric Clinics of North America, 8,* 3–24.

Cannon, W. (1929). *Bodily changes in pain, hunger, fear and rage.* New York: Appleton-Century-Croft.

Cantwell, D. P., & Baker, L. (1985). Psychiatric and learning disorders in children with speech and language disorders: A descriptive analysis. *Advances in Learning and Behavioral Disabilities, 4,* 29–47.

Cantwell, D. P., & Baker, L. (1987). The prevalence of anxiety disorders in children with communication disorders. *Journal of Anxiety Disorders, 1,* 239–248.

Carlson, C. L., Figueroa, R. G., & Lahey, B. B. (1986). Behavior therapy for childhood anxiety disorders. In R. Gittelman (Ed.), *Anxiety disorders of childhood* (pp. 204–232). New York: Guilford.

Conners, C. K., & Barkley, R. A. (1985). Rating scales and checklists for child psychopharmacology. *Psychopharmacology Bulletin, 21,* 809–815.

Coolidge, J. C., Brodie, R. D., & Feeney, B. (1964). A ten-year follow-up study of sixty-six school-phobic children. *American Journal of Orthopsychiatry, 34,* 675–684.

Corwin, D. (1985, October 26). Personal communication.

Costello, E. J. (1982, October). Clinical decision making in child psychiatry. Paper presented at the 29th Meeting of the American Academy of Child Psychiatry, Washington, DC.

Costello, A., Edelbrock, C., Dulcan, H., Kalas, R., & Klaric, S. (1984). Diagnostic Interview Schedule for Children (DISC). Western Psychiatric Institute, Pittsburgh, PA. Unpublished.

Davis, J. M., Nasr, S., Spira, N., & Vogel, C. (1981). Anxiety: Differential diagnosis and treatment from a biologic perspective. *Journal of Clinical Psychiatry, 42,* 4–14.

Freud, S. (1959). Inhibitions, symptoms and anxiety. In J. Strachey (Ed. & Trans.), *Standard edition* (Vol. 20, pp. 75–175). London: Hogarth. (Original work published in 1926.)

Freud, S. (1962). The neuro-psychoses of defence. In J. Strachey (Ed. & Trans.), *Standard edition* (Vol. 3, pp. 43–61). London: Hogarth Press. (Original work published in 1894.)

Freud, S. (1963). Introductory lectures on psychoanalysis. Lecture 25: Anxiety. In J. Strachey (Ed. & Trans.), *Standard edition* (Vol. 16, pp. 392–411). London: Hogarth. (Original work published in 1917.)

Garcia, I., & Koelling, R. A. (1966). Relation of cue to consequence in avoidance learning. *Psychonomic Science, 4,* 123–124.

Gittelman, R. (1980). The role of psychological tests for differential diagnosis in child psychiatry. *Journal of the American Academy of Child Psychiatry, 19,* 413–438.

Gittelman, R. (1984). *Anxiety disorders in children. Psychiatric update* (Vol. 3). Washington, DC: American Psychiatric Press.

Gittelman, R. (1985). Ratings for anxiety disorders. *Psychopharmacology Bulletin, 21,* 933–950.

Gittelman, R. (1985a). Parent's questionnaire (modified Conners); Anxiety and mood items added. *Psychopharmacology Bulletin, 21,* 939–944.

Gittelman, R. (1985b). Teacher rating scale (modified Conners); Anxiety and mood items added. *Psychopharmacology Bulletin, 21,* 945–950.

Gittelman, R. (Ed.) (1986). *Anxiety disorders of childhood.* New York: Guilford.

Gittelman, R., & Koplewicz, H. S. (1986). Pharmacotherapy of childhood anxiety disorders. In R. Gittelman (Ed.), *Anxiety disorders of childhood* (pp. 188–203). New York: Guilford.

Gittelman-Klein, R., & Klein, D. F. (1971). Controlled imipramine treatment of school phobia. *Archives of General Psychiatry, 25,* 204–207.

Goldenberg, I., & Goldenberg, H. (1985). *Family therapy: An overview.* Monterey, CA: Brooks/Cole.

Goodwin, D. W. (1986). *Anxiety.* New York: Oxford.

Gorman, J. M., Liebowitz, M. R., & Klein, D. F. (1984). Panic disorder and agoraphobia (Monograph). *Current concepts.* New York: Upjohn.

Herjanic, B., & Reich, W. (1983). Diagnostic interview for children and adolescents (DICA). Copies available from Washington University School of Medicine, 4940 Audubon Avenue, St. Louis, MO 63110, Attention: Dr. Reich.

Hodges, K., McKnew, D., Cytryn, L., Stern, L., & Kline, J. (1982). The child assessment schedule (CAS) diagnostic interview: A report on reliability and validity. *Journal of the American Academy of Child Psychiatry, 21,* 468–473.

Kastrup, M. (1976). Psychic disorder among pre-school children in a geographically delimited area of Aarhus County, Denmark. *Acta Psychiatrica Scandinavia, 54,* 29–42.

Klein, D. F. (1981). Anxiety reconceptualized. In D. F. Klein and J. G. Rabkin (Eds.), *Anxiety: New research and changing concepts.* New York: Raven.

Kovacs, M. (1978). Interview schedule for children. Available from Dr. Kovacs, Western Psychiatric Institute, Pittsburgh, PA 15213.

Lader, M. H., & Marks, I. M. (1971). *Clinical anxiety.* London: Heinemann Medical.

Lapouse, R., & Monk, M. A. (1958). An epidemiologic study of behavior characteristics in children. *American Journal of Public Health, 48,* 1134–1144.

Lapouse, R., & Monk, M. A. (1959). Fears and worries in a representative sample of children. *American Journal of Orthopsychiatry, 29,* 803–818.

Last, C. G., Hersen, M., Kazdin, A. E., Finkelstein, R., & Strauss, C. C. (1987). Comparison of DSM-III separation anxiety and overanxious disorders: Demographic characteristics and patterns of comorbidity. *Journal of the American Academy of Child and Adolescent Psychiatry, 26*(4), 527–531.

Lewis, M. (1986). Principles of intensive individual psychoanalytic psychotherapy for childhood anxiety disorders. In R. Gittelman (Ed.), *Anxiety disorders of childhood* (pp. 233–256). New York: Guilford.

Marks, I. M. (1969). *Fears and phobias.* New York: Academic.

Myers, J. K., Lindenthal, J. J., & Pepper, M. P. (1975). Life events, social integration, and psychiatric symptomatology. *Journal of Health and Social Behavior, 16,* 421–427.

Nesse, R. M., Cameron, O. G., Curtis, G. C., McCann, D. S., & Huber-Smith, M. J. (1984). Adrenergic function in patients with panic anxiety. *Archives of General Psychiatry, 41,* 771–776.

Offord, D. R. (1985). Child psychiatric disorders: Prevalence and perspectives. *Psychiatric Clinics of North America, 8,* 632–652.

Orvaschel, H. (1985). Psychiatric interviews suitable for use in research with children and adolescents. *Psychopharmacology Bulletin, 21,* 737–746.

Orvaschel, H., & Weissman, M. M. (1986). Epidemiology of anxiety disorders in children: A review. In R. Gittelman (Ed.), *Anxiety disorders of childhood* (pp. 58–72). New York: Guilford.

Pitts, F. N., & McClure, J. (1967). Lactate metabolism in anxiety neurosis. *New England Journal of Medicine, 277,* 1329–1336.

Quay, H. C., & Peterson, D. R. (1983). *Manual for the revised behavior problem checklist.* Available from the senior author, Box 248074, University of Miami, Coral Gables, FL 33124.

Rainey, J. M., & Nesse, R. M. (1985). Psychobiology of anxiety and anxiety disorders. *Psychiatric Clinics of North America, 8,* 133–144.

Rapoport, J., Elkins, R., Langer, D. H., Sceery, W., Bushsbaum, M. W., Gillin, J. C., Murphy, D. L., Zahn, T. P., Lake, R., Ludlow, C., & Mendelson, W. (1981). Childhood obsessive-compulsive disorder. *American Journal of Psychiatry, 138,* 1545–1554.

Rapoport, J., Elkins, R., & Mikkelsen, E. (1980). Clinical controlled trial of chlorimipramine in adolescents with obsessive-compulsive disorder. *Psychopharmacology Bulletin, 16,* 61–63.

Rickels, K. (1981). Recent advances in anxiolytic therapy. *Journal of Clinical Psychiatry, 42,* 40–44.

Robins, L. N. (1966). *Deviant children grown up: A sociological and psychiatric study of sociopathic personality.* Baltimore: Williams & Wilkins.

Robins, L. N. (1978). Sturdy childhood predictors of adult antisocial behavior. Replications from longitudinal studies. *Psychological Medicine, 8,* 611–622.

Rutter, M. (1985). Psychopathology and development: Links between childhood and adult life. In M. Rutter and L. Hersov (Eds.), *Child and adolescent psychiatry: Modern approaches* (2nd ed.) (pp. 720–742). Oxford: Blackwell.

Rutter, M., & Garmezy, N. (1983). Developmental psychopathology. In P. H. Mussen (Ed.), *Handbook of child psychology* (pp. 775–911). New York: Wiley.

Schaefer, C. E., & Millman, H. L. (1981). *How to help children with common problems.* New York: Van Nostrand Reinhold.

Schuckit, M. A. (1981). Current therapeutic options in the management of typical anxiety. *Journal of Clinical Psychiatry, 42,* 15–26.

Shaffer, D. (1986). Learning theories of anxiety. In R. Gittelman (Ed.), *Anxiety disorders of childhood* (pp. 157–166). New York: Guilford.

Silva, P. A., Justin, C., McGee, R., & Williams, S. M. (1984). Some developmental and behavioral characteristics of seven-year-old children with delayed speech development. *British Journal of Disorders of Communication, 19,* 147–154.

Simeon, J. G., & Ferguson, H. B. (1985, May). Effectiveness of drug treatment in childhood anxiety disorders. Presented at University of Minnesota Conference on Anxiety Disorder, Cape Cod, MA.

Spitzer, R., & Endicott, J. (1978). Schedule for affective disorders and schizophrenia. New York: New York State Psychiatric Institute.

Spitzer, R. L., Endicott, J. E., & Robins, E. (1978). Research diagnostic criteria. *Archives of General Psychiatry, 35,* 773–782.

Trautman, P. D. (1986). Psychodynamic theories of anxiety and their application to children. In R. Gittelman (Ed.), *Anxiety disorders of childhood* (pp. 168–187). New York: Guilford.

Ulenhuth, E. H. (1981). Specific anxiety syndromes: Current therapeutic options. *Journal of Clinical Psychiatry, 42,* 27–34.

Weissman, M. M. (1985). The epidemiology of anxiety disorders: Rates, risks, and familial patterns. In A. H. Tuma, & J. D. Maser (Eds.), *Anxiety and the anxiety disorders* (pp. 389–402). NJ: Erlbaum.

Weissman, M. M., Leckman, J. F., Merikangas, K. R., Gammon, G. D., & Prusoff, B. A. (1984). Depression and anxiety disorders in parents and children. *Archives of General Psychiatry, 41,* 845–852.

Weissman, M. M., Myers, J. K., & Harding, P. S. (1978). Psychiatric disorders in U.S. urban community, 1975–1976. *American Journal of Psychiatry, 135,* 459–462.

Werry, J. S. (1986). Diagnosis and assessment. In R. Gittelman (Ed.), *Anxiety disorders of childhood* (pp. 73–100). New York: Guilford.

Wolkowitz, O. M., & Paul, S. M. (1985). Neural and molecular mechanisms in anxiety. *Psychiatric Clinics of North America, 8,* 145–159.

Zeitlin, H. (1983). The natural history of psychiatric disorder in childhood. M.D. Thesis, University of London.

CHAPTER TEN

Affective Disorders

Michael Strober
James McCracken
Gregory Hanna

The idea that psychic "turmoil" is a universal feature of normal adolescence has had great historical attraction, figuring prominently in many representative essays on adolescent development and heavily influencing clinical issues (Blos, 1967; Freud, 1958). Because it was held to be incontrovertible, clinicians doubted that a reliable and pragmatically useful nosology of adolescent mental disorders was feasible and broadly criticized Kraepelinian diagnostic concepts as fundamentally incompatible with a developmental orientation to problems of this age.

Without ignoring the importance of developmental and psychoanalytic inquiries, a substantial body of epidemiological data from North America and Great Britain have proved these notions misleading (Douvan & Adelson, 1966; Offer, 1969; Offer & Offer, 1975; Offer, Sabshin, & Marcus, 1965; Rutter, Graham, Chadwick, & Yule, 1976). Although studies show that feelings of alienation and self-doubt are highly characteristic of adolescents in the community, they give no evidence of the preponderance of emotional upheaval predicted by traditional theories or the blurring of boundaries between normal reaction patterns and psychopathology. Rather, symptomatic measures during adolescence tend to be strongly associated either with onset of handicapping psychiatric disturbance or behavioral problems and adverse family experiences that have persisted since middle childhood (Rutter, Tizard, Yule, Graham, & Whitmore, 1976). Simply put, research has been unable to demonstrate any robust effect of developmental "turmoil" as either cause or precipitant of psychiatric disturbance in adolescence. Moreover, the concept does not hold up as a standard against which to measure the reliability or validity of psychiatric diagnosis in this age group.

Clinical studies of adolescent patients also indicate that, in general, their symptom patterns are not dissimilar to those of seriously ill adults (Graham & Rutter, 1985). The feasibility of applying the same diagnostic inclusion and exclusion criteria developed for use with adults to the classification of adolescent disorders was first noted by Hudgens (1974) in a detailed study of 110 patients, ranging in age from 12 to 19 at the time of their psychiatric hospitalization. Based on review of their hospital course and information from a structured interview which probed current and past symptoms, early history, and social functioning, each was diagnosed using criteria established by Feighner (Feighner et al., 1972) for conditions recognized as valid nosological entities. Although the number of undiagnosable cases was two times more common in this sample than among adult patients in the same facility, it was still possible to assign Feighner diagnoses in nearly 75%.

In a more recent study, Strober, Green, and Carlson (1981a) examined the reliability of Axis I and Axis II DSM-III (APA, 1980) diagnoses made independently by two clinicians in 95 consecutively hospitalized adolescent patients. A broad range of disturbance was noted, comprising 13 major diagnostic categories. The differentiation of schizophrenia, major depression, and manic illness was found to be highly reliable, the kappa coefficients ranging from 0.75 to 0.82. In all, agreement on the primary diagnosis was reached in 77 of the 95 patients (kappa = 0.74).

Longitudinal follow-up studies of treated samples have also produced relevant data on developmental continuities. This literature has been reviewed thoroughly by Robins (1979), Graham and Rutter (1985), and Rutter and Garmezy (1983), the conclusion being that major psychiatric illness arising in adolescence runs true to form and is strongly predictive of similar adult disturbance if symptoms persist or recur. Further evidence of these linkages and the importance of developmental factors in the precipitation of psychiatric disorders is found in the marked acceleration of first onsets of schizophrenia (Slater & Cowie, 1971), major depression (Lewinsohn, Duncan, Stanton, & Hautzinger, 1986), manic-depressive illness (Loranger & Levine, 1978; Winokur, Clayton, & Reich, 1969), and anxiety disorders (Thyer, Parish, Curtis, Nesse, & Cameron, 1985) at the time of puberty.

Similar parallels in theory development and conceptualization have defined the last two decades of research and speculation on the nature and form of adolescent depression. Until the late 1970s, prominent authorities argued forcefully that adult-type depressive conditions in which guilt, retardation, and morbid delusions were main features were rare in adolescence (Toolan, 1962; Weiner, 1970). Rather, teenagers were said to be naturally predisposed to express depression in forms that were not referable to the usual signs and symptoms of depression in adults. The implication was that no single, coherent definition of affective disturbance could be applied to adolescence and that practitioners would need to make allowance for the wide range of possible diagnostic manifestations in young patients. As a result, through much of the 1960s and 1970s the concepts of "masked depression" and "depressive equivalents" were invoked haphazardly and unquestioningly to infer affective disturbance in adolescents whose presenting symptoms extended the full range of psychopathology, from antisocial behavior and school failure to psychosomatic complaints and general malaise.

From a clinical standpoint, these notions proved unhelpfully vague because rules governing their application and assessment of validity were never spelled out. Consequently, by the late 1970s, the quest for new empirical finding and theoretical concepts was beginning to draw heavily upon innovations in adult psychiatry, in particular the development of structured interviews for assessing and quantifying psychopathological symptoms, agreement on operational criteria for diagnoses, interest in family-genetic risk factors and developmental precursors of serious mental illness, and the advent of more effective pharmacological and psychosocial treatment methods (Klerman, 1986a). Although the appropriateness of DSM-III for child and adolescent psychiatry has been questioned (Rutter & Shaffer,

1980), most authorities now agree that use of specific descriptive criteria to diagnose affective disorders in adolescents establishes a common framework for implementing research on the phenomenology, course, epidemiology, family history, biology, and treatment of these conditions.

Advances in these areas will, of course, bear the influence of prevailing theories of the major etiologic determinants of affective disorders. Historically, three causal models have predominated: psychodynamic, behavioral, and biological. The principal difference among these approaches is the assumed locus of etiology and pathogenesis.

Intrapsychic interpretations of depression have historically stressed dynamic sources within the individual and are rooted in Abraham's seminal theory of retroflexed anger directed at an internalized object that is both loved and hated for frustrating a desire for nurturance and dependency. Subsequent revisions of Abraham's instinct theory have placed greater emphasis on the centrality of object loss in predisposing to deficits in self-esteem and major depressive reactions brought on by later separation experiences or interpersonal disappointments. While there is some empirical support for a link between early object loss and adult onset of depression, the association is a statistically modest one at best (Whybrow, Akiskal, & McKinney, 1984).

More recvntly, cognitive-behavioral models of depression have received considerable attention. They represent a theoretically significant departure from traditional formulations in emphasizing the essential importance of both cognitive and situational contributions to depressive states. Rooted in the theories of Beck and Seligman, this approach traces the most immediate cause of depression to certain prepotent and more or less stable negative attributions of self-worth and self-control that bias and distort the individual's everyday perceptions. Empirically, the evidence is conflicting; some studies confirm the persistence of negative cognitions in depressed patients even in the remitted state (Eaves & Rush, 1984; Dobson & Shaw, 1986), while others suggest that negative cognitions are merely epiphenomena of depression itself (Hamilton & Abramson, 1983; Simons, Garfield, & Murphy, 1984).

Also of relatively recent origin, biological theories of affective disorder today stimulate burgeoning interest and research efforts in view of strong evidence for the involvement of genetic factors in their etiology. This interest is further stimulated as techniques for measuring brain function become increasingly sophisticated and precise. Most hypotheses in this area have focused on changes in monoamine neurotransmission (with noradrenergic, serotonergic, and cholinergic systems emphasized to a greater or lesser degree), adrenocortical function, or receptor responsiveness, all of which are associated with depressive and manic states. However, in spite of the numerous studies of monoamine and steroid levels in body fluids, our understanding of biological abnormalities associated with depression and mania remains incomplete. Though the original catecholamine hypothesis (relating depression to lower than optimal amine levels and mania to an excess of amine) established a heuristically valuable framework for biological research, it has proven too narrow and simplistic. Because the affective disorders are phenotypically diverse and evidence favors greater genetic heterogeneity than previously suspected, a variety of genetic-biologic abnormalities must be considered. For this reason, most contemporary researchers now believe that the pathophysiology of affective disorders is less a matter of simple increases or decreases in amine levels than the relative balance among different neurotransmitter systems and their dynamic regulation (Siever & Davis, 1985).

The pitfalls of viewing the etiology of affective disorders from a single conceptual frame of references are all too obvious and must be avoided as research on adolescent populations progresses. The evidence seems incontrovertible that depressive and manic states represent the final common pathway for a variety of interacting developmental, psychosocial, and biological processes (Whybrow et al., 1984).

DIAGNOSIS AND DEVELOPMENTAL CONSIDERATIONS

Epidemiology

Conventional wisdom has long held that rates of depression increase steadily with advancing age. However, recent epidemiologic research indicates that the proportion of cases with onset in adolescence may be increasing. As part of the National Institute of Mental Health Collaborative Program on the Psychobiology of Depression, rates of depression were determined among over 2200 first-degree relatives of 523 adult probands with major depressive disorder (Klerman et al., 1985). All relatives were interviewed directly using the Schedule for Affective Disorders and Schizophrenia (SADS) and diagnosed by Research Diagnostic Criteria (RDC). For purposes of data analysis, relatives were aggregated into six strata (before 1910; 1910–1919; 1920–1929, etc.), and life table statistics were used to estimate age-specific cumulative probabilities of onset within each of the six birth cohorts up to the time of interview. The findings of particular importance were as follows: (1) risk for depression increased significantly in successive cohorts, the most dramatic rise occurring in individuals born after World War II; (2) first onsets of disorder were occurring earlier in the life span in later birth cohorts; and (3) in younger individuals, differences between males and females in rates of depression were decreasing. These secular trends were found to be robust even when analyses were restricted only to relatives under age 50 and more stringent criteria for diagnosis were employed, for example, somatic treatment, hospitalization, and greater duration of symptoms (Klerman, 1986b).

There is no unequivocal explanation of why the incidence of depression in youth might be increasing. Nonetheless, these findings raise broader questions of the distribution of depressive disorders in the adolescent population and the nature of developmental influences that shape both continuities and discontinuities in their psychopathological expression.

Population studies of depressive disorder in adolescence employing advanced methods of case ascertainment and diagnosis are still scant. In the Isle of Wight study of 10-year-old children, Rutter et al. (1976) found a prevalence of only 0.14 per 100; 9 cases of depressive disorder were identified when this cohort was reexamined at age 14, and an additional 26 were found with mixed anxiety and depressive features. Overall, new onsets at age 14 were more common in females than in males.

Two recent studies in the United States were concordant with the Isle of Wight findings in two respects: both found an increase in the prevalence of depression marking the transition from childhood to adolescence, and both found a change in sex ratio after puberty with a predominance of females among new cases compared with male and female rates of roughly the same order during childhood. Cohen, Velez, and Garcia (1985) carried out independent parent and child diagnostic interviews in 757 families randomly selected from two counties in New York. Children ranged in age from 9 to 18 at the time of interview. For the total sample, the prevalence of major depression was 1% when diagnoses were based on information given by mothers and 1.7% when based on interviews of the children themselves; the prevalence of past episodes of major depression, by the child's report, was estimated at 4.5%. There were no cases of depression among females prior to age 13, whereas depression among males in the cohort was predominantly prepubertal. Age-specific rates of disorder increased steadily in females, from 1% at age 13 to 7% at age 19. A high proportion of the cases of major depression in this cohort also displayed nonaffective symptoms, including oppositional behavior, conduct disturbance, and anxiety.

Kashani and colleagues (Kashani et al., 1986) estimated the prevalence of major depression among 150 adolescents, 14 to 16 years of age, representing 7% of all adolescents attending public schools in Columbia, Missouri. Diagnoses based on DSM-III criteria were derived from structured interviews conducted separately with the adolescent and his or her parents, with the additional provision that symptoms were judged sufficiently handicapping to warrant treatment. Of the 150 subjects, 7 (4.7%) met criteria for current or past major depression and an additional 5 (3.3%) met criteria for dysthymic disorder. Ten of the 12 cases were female, and, as in the cohort studied by Cohen et al. (1985), anxiety, conduct, and oppositional disorder were frequent concomitants of depression in this small sample.

The literature on the epidemiology of self-assessed depressive *symptoms* in adolescence is larger by comparison, although prevalence figures vary by method of assessment and cutoff score used in designating symptom severity. A detailed review of this work can be found elsewhere (Schoenbach, Garrison, & Kaplan, 1984).

In the Isle of Wight sample of 14-year-olds, nearly 50% reported feelings of misery and depression upon direct interview, 20% acknowledged self-denigrating ideas, and 7% admitted to suicidal ideation—the rates of each being nearly equal among males and females (Rutter, Graham, Chadwick, & Yule, 1976). Some 20% of the males and females of this sample also reported feelings of misery and sleep difficulties on a self-report measure of general malaise. In four studies (Albert and Beck, 1975; Kaplan, Hong, & Weinhold, 1984; Schoenbach, Kaplan, Wagner, Grimson, & Miller, 1983; Teri, 1982), cutoff scores on self-report rating scales (Beck Depression Inventory; Center for Epidemiologic Studies of Depression Scale) indicative of at least moderate levels of depressive symptomatology in the general adult population have been used to estimate the prevalence of depressive symptoms among adolescents in the community; these figures range from 8% to 50%. By contrast, assessments of this kind in adults have produced lower prevalence rates—6% to 13% in males and 11% to 24% in females (Boyd & Weissman, 1981).

The most extensive and best designed examination of this issue has been carried out by Kandel and Davies (1982). Depression severity was measured by six items selected from the previously developed depression subscale of the Symptom Checklist-90 and independently validated on a small clinical sample including adolescents with a diagnosis of primary major depressive disorder. The scale was administered to some 8000 13- to 18-year-old students in upstate New York, and, in a subset, to their parents as well. Nearly 20% of the cohort were found to have scores equal to or greater than the mean scale score obtained by affectively ill adolescents in the clinical validation sample. Mean levels of depression were higher in females than in males from age 14 on, and scores were higher among the adolescents than among their parents. Higher levels of depression were predicted by delinquent behavior, low self-esteem, and alienation from parents. A more recently published (Kandel & Davies, 1986) 9-year follow-up of 1000 members of this original cohort revealed that high levels of depression had continuity into early adult life and were also moderately associated with increased liability to later psychiatric disturbance (among females only) and poorer social adjustment.

Concerning bipolar illness, we are unaware of any systematically collected population figures on its lifetime prevalence, annual incidence, or annual rate of hospitalization in adolescence, despite evidence of the greatly increased frequency of bipolar conditions following puberty (Loranger & Levine, 1978; Winokur, Clayton, & Reich, 1969). Comparable data on the epidemiology of bipolar illness in adults can be found in Boyd and Weissman (1981).

In sum, the epidemiology of depression and depressive disorders in adolescence requires further comprehensive study. Although current data are still too fragmentary to allow unequivocal estimates of prevalence or incidence at this age, tentative conclusions may be drawn on some key issues. Clearly, there is a substantial increase during adolescence in a variety of depressive phenomena. Onsets of major depression are markedly more frequent after age 14, at which time it becomes (like unipolar depression in adults) more common among females. Major depression is not an adolescent phenomenon per se, however, as prevalence rates continue to rise after puberty until peaking in early adulthood. On the other hand, self-report data suggest depressive symptoms to be much more common in adolescents than in adults. Perhaps for this reason, its significance as a risk factor for later affective morbidity is unclear. For instance, in adults, high levels of self-reported depressive symptomatology may increase subsequent risk of full-blown major depressive episodes by as much as threefold (Weissman, Myers, Thompson, & Belanger, 1986). Whether these linkages also hold true during adolescence is not known, although the finding of Kandel and Davies (1986) that depressive symptoms in some adolescents persist into the 20s and impact adversely on certain aspects of social and psychological adaptation is suggestive.

Of course, underlying these issues is the critically important question of why depressive phenomena of one sort or another become more evident during adolescence. The expression of genetic risk, shifts in hormonal function, changes in cognitive capacity and self-awareness, and ambiguities in role expectations have all been mentioned as having important causal effects (Rutter, 1986) although their significance remains largely unproven.

Clinical Phenomenology

There is good clinical evidence that adolescents who fit criteria for major depression exhibit the same spectrum and relative frequency of symptoms found in adults. In addition, there is evidence that phenomenological assessments of younger patients can be performed reliably.

Inamdar, Siomopoulos, Osborn, and Bianchi (1979) examined the frequency of depressive symptoms in a hospital sample of 30 adolescents, in whom "depressed mood" was a primary aspect of the presenting picture. Interviews lasting from 50 to 90 minutes were conducted using a semistructured format that covered 50 operationally defined items. Common to the sample were symptoms of diminished interest, loss of pleasure, suicidal thought, impaired concentration, self-depreciation, social withdrawal, insomnia, and morning fatigue.

Strober, Green, and Carlson (1981b) investigated the frequency and interrater reliabilities of depressive symptoms and RDC subtypes in 40 hospitalized adolescents with a DSM-III diagnosis of major depressive episode. Each was examined jointly by two experienced clinicians using the SADS in an interviewer/observer format. Interrater reliabilities were, on average, satisfactory, the coefficients ranging from 0.51 to 0.95. The sample portrayed a wide range of depressive characteristics; symptoms with the highest frequency included depressed mood, loss of interest, impaired concentration, suicidal ideation, anorexia, low self-esteem, sleep disturbance, lack of specific concern, guilt, anergia, discouragement, and distinct quality of mood. Depressive syndromes further distinguished by retardation and morbid delusions were also present in a subgroup of patients; the subtypes of endogenous, retarded, and psychotic depression were also found to be reliably classified in this sample, the kappa coefficients similar to values reported on adult depressives.

Using very similar methods, Friedman, Hurt, Clarkin, Corn, and Aronoff (1983) compared symptom profiles among 26 adolescents and 27 adults, all hospitalized with a DSM-III and RDC diagnosis of major depression. The percentages of adolescents fitting RDC for endogenous and psychotic subtypes were 77 and 23%, respectively; corresponding rates in adults were 93 and 22%, respectively. Correlating the rank order of symptom frequencies in this sample with the adolescent sample reported by Strober et al. (1981b) produced a coefficient 0.75; likewise, the rank order coefficient of symptom frequencies among the adolescent and adult patients was 0.94.

Additional information on the reliability of affective symptom ratings is provided by Chambers and colleagues (Chambers et al., 1985) in a study of 52 patients, 6 to 17 years of age, who were interviewed with the Kiddie-SADS in a test-retest format. Acceptable levels of reliability were obtained for 12 of the 14 symptoms rated, the exceptions being pathological guilt and impaired concentration. Except for these same two items, correlations between separate parent and child interview ratings were also satisfactory. On balance, reliabilities of composite depression scale scores were higher than constituent items (intraclass coefficients 0.63 to 0.81), and kappa values for the diagnoses of major depression, endogenous subtype, and chronic minor depressive disorder were satisfactory (0.54 to 0.70).

Since sex differences in depression become evident following puberty, it is necessary to ask the broader question of whether affective symptom profiles vary across adjacent developmental periods. Ryan and his colleagues (Ryan et al., 1987) compared symptom frequencies and RDC subtype rates in a consecutive series of 95 children and 92 adolescents who met RDC criteria for major depression. On balance, the depressive syndromes in the children and adolescents had comparable features.

Principal components analyses carried out separately in the child and adolescent samples yielded similar clinically interpretable endogenous and anxious-somatic factor structures. The two groups also had roughly equal rates (50%) of endogenous subtype depression, although psychotic subtype was somewhat more frequent among children (39% versus 24%). There were, however, age related differences in the prominence of particular symptoms. Occurring more frequently in the prepubertal children were symptoms of depressed appearance, agitation, somatic complaints, and depressive hallucinations, whereas adolescent depressives were more likely to exhibit hopelessness, hypersomnia, and weight change. Similarly, other reports have indicated that when psychosis is present in depressed children it is reflected mainly in auditory hallucinations, whereas the depressive psychoses arising in adolescence are distinguished mainly by classic adult-type delusions of sin, guilt, or persecution (Chambers & Puig-Antich, 1982; Strober et al., 1981b).

Also in question is whether other psychopathological symptoms are reliably associated with depression in adolescents—more so than in children or adults. The data on hand are still limited and equivocal. As noted, examination of adolescents selected in epidemiological studies (Cohen et al., 1985; Kashani et al., 1986) shows that depression is often coupled with other behavioral symptoms during the active clinical phase, particularly disobedience, anxiety, and oppositional tendencies. More or less the same pattern holds true for children. However, Strober et al. (1981b) found premorbid or comorbid symptoms of aggression, sexual misconduct, substance abuse, and general somatic complaints to be rare among hospitalized adolescent depressives, especially those with endogenous subtypes of illness. Likewise, two other studies (Geller, Chestnut, Miller, Price, & Yates, 1985; Ryan et al., 1987) reported that anxiety symptoms and conduct disturbance were significantly more frequent among children with major depression than among adolescents with major depression.

In all three of these studies, nonaffective features arose in most patients at the time of or following onset of depressive symptoms, suggesting they are unlikely to represent direct, influencing causes of affective illness. However, some empirical data suggest the possible heuristic merit of distinguishing between adolescents who exhibit comorbid features during an active phase of depression and those with "pure" depression. In a study of psychiatric disorders in the 6- to 17-year-old children of adults with primary major depression, anxiety disorder and depression were significantly more prevalent in offspring of probands with accompanying panic or agoraphobia (Weissman, Leckman, Merikangas, Gammon, & Prusoff, 1984a). It seems reasonable to infer on the basis of these findings that genetic influences may be important in determining risk to simultaneous symptoms of anxiety and depression, although effects of personality style, coping mechanisms, early life experiences, and other relevant risk and protective factors cannot be discounted.

Clinical data on the phenomenology of bipolar illness in adolescence are disappointingly sparse, and opinion is divided on whether problems of differential diagnosis and classification are any greater at this age than in adulthood. For example, several workers (Ballenger, Reus, & Post, 1982; Landolt, 1957; Olsen, 1961) have suggested that schizophrenic-like symptoms and other atypical features are more likely to be present when mania arises in adolescence, thereby obscuring early recognition of the illness. In contrast, however, others (Carlson & Strober, 1978; Coryell & Norten, 1980; Hassanyeh & Davison, 1980; Horowitz, 1977; Hsu & Starzynski, 1986) have described the same range of symptomatology and cyclicity of episodes in adolescent manics as in adults.

In sum, existing evidence points to greater continuity than discontinuity of depressive syndromes across age periods, although some changes in symptom patterns do occur. Anxiety, somatic complaints, and depressive hallucinations are somewhat more frequent in children with affective disorder than in adolescents, whereas manic states, hopelessness, anhedonia, hypersomnia, depressive delusions, and appetite disturbance become increasingly common after puberty. Although it seems intuitively likely that the phenomenology of affective symptoms acquired in adolescence is effected, to a greater or lesser extent, by intrinsic maturational influences, the possibility cannot be ruled out that symptomatic differences of this sort are due, at least in part, to age-specific psychosocial or biological dysfunctions.

Course and Outcome

As far as follow-up and natural history are concerned, the evidence from several studies is that affective disorders in adolescence are highly predictive of recurrences in adults. A study by Welner, Welner, and Fishman (1979) described the course of 28 adolescents 10 years after hospitalization for primary depression or bipolar illness. At follow-up, 3 of 12 bipolar patients had committed suicide, and the remaining patients were chronically ill with poor social and vocational adjustment. Of the 16 nonbipolar depressives, 11 had episodic courses, and 5 had single episodes from which they recovered and remained well. However, other reports (Carlson, Davenport, & Jamison, 1977; Hsu & Starzynski, 1986) gave no evidence of any greater morbidity, mortality, or social impairment in adolescent versus adult onset bipolar illness.

Three recent naturalistic prospective studies were conducted with broadly comparable findings: one in which depressed or dysthymic children first seen between 8 and 13 years of age were followed into adolescence (Kovacs, Feinberg, Crouse-Novak, Paulauskas, & Finkelstein, 1984; Kovacs et al., 1984) and two in which adolescents with a diagnosis of nonbipolar major depression were followed up 3 to 4 years later (Akiskal et al.,

1983; Strober & Carlson, 1982). The results of particular importance were (1) the diagnosis of affective disorder showed very strong temporal stability, and (2) relapse rates were high. Also worth noting is that the mean duration of episodes and rates of chronicity found in these juvenile samples are remarkably similar to figures reported for adults (Keller, Shapiro, Lavori, & Wolfe, 1982).

Given the therapeutic importance of differentiating unipolar and bipolar subtypes of affective disorder, attempts have been made at identifying clinical, genetic, and pharmacological precursors of manic outcome in adolescents presenting initially with a diagnosis of major depression. In two large studies (Akiskal et al. 1983; Strober & Carlson, 1982), teenagers whose illness pursued a bipolar course at outcome were more likely to have delusions and psychomotor retardation during their index episodes, increased rates of familial bipolar illness, and a somewhat greater susceptibility to tricyclic induced hypomania than were teenagers with unipolar outcomes. The specificities of these variables were high, ranging from 83 to 100%. Predictive values in the cohort studied by Strober and Carlson (1982) ranged from 42 to 100%, and 72 to 100% in the cohort studied by Akiskal et al. (1983). Also significant is the fact that in neither study was a single case of schizophrenic outcome observed. This fact reinforces the idea that schizophrenia and manic-depressive illness can be differentiated in adolescence when careful attention is paid to patterns of premorbid adjustment, symptom phenomenology and course over time, quality of inter-episode functioning, and type of psychiatric illness in biological relatives (Bowden & Sarabia, 1980; Carlson & Strober, 1978).

PHARMACOLOGICAL AND BIOLOGICAL APPROACHES

Family-Genetic Studies

Studies of familial concordance in adolescents with affective disorders have used two parallel methodologies. One involves the ascertainment of psychiatric disorders in relatives of adolescent probands and nonaffectively ill, psychiatric controls; the other involves the study of psychiatric disorder in adolescent offspring of adult probands and normal controls.

In an initial study of familial illness in the adult relatives of 35 adolescent probands with nonbipolar major depression (Strober, 1984), a particularly high lifetime prevalence of affective disorder was found in the mothers of probands (25.7/100). In all, there were 108 cases of diagnosable illness among 348 first- and second-degree relatives, of which 69% were comprised of affective disorder or alcoholism. In a more recent blind family study of first-degree relatives of depressed, manic, and schizophrenic adolescent probands (Strober et al., in preparation), we found a nearly fourfold higher rate of affective illness in relatives of depressed and manic probands than in relatives of schizophrenic probands, whereas schizophrenic conditions aggregated mainly in relatives of the same diagnosis. A significant aggregation of bipolar illness in relatives of adolescent manics also has been reported (Strober & Carlson, 1982).

By and large, studies of the young offspring of affectively ill parents, who in most studies ranged from 6 to 18 years of age, showed that rates of affective disorder and the total prevalence of general psychopathology are higher than in offspring of control probands (Beardslee, Keller, & Klerman, 1985; Conners, Himmelhoch, Goyette, Ulrich, & Neil, 1979; Decina et al., 1983; Gershon et al., 1985; Greenhill & Shopsin, 1979; Klein, Depue, & Slater, 1985; Kuyler, Rosenthal, Igel, Dunner, & Fieve, 1980; McKnew, Cytryn, Efron, Gershon, & Bunney, 1979; O'Connell, Mays, O'Brien, & Mirsheidaie, 1979; Orvaschel, Weissman, Padian, & Lowe, 1981; Rutter & Quinton, 1984; Weissman, Prusoff, et al., 1984b; Welner, Welner, McCrary, & Leonard, 1977). However, it is not possible to fix any stable estimate of affective risk in this population since the studies differed so widely in instruments used, source of data, and diagnostic criteria.

A further point of theoretical note is that onsets of disorder in adolescence may have a more appreciable genetic component. In a family study of 133 probands with major depression and 1500 of their first-degree relatives, Weissman and her colleagues (Weissman, Wickramaratne, et al., 1984c) found a significant inverse relationship between age of onset of depression in probands and risk of major depression in relatives. Specifically, the proportion of relatives affected was greatest in probands whose onsets occurred prior to age 20, and decreased linearly as age of onset in the proband increased. If it is true that differences in age of onset reflect greater or lesser degrees of genetic loading, the study of adolescent patients and their relatives may shed new light on the nature of predisposing genetic effects, their pathophysiological expression, and the contributions made by environmental factors to symptom development.

Laboratory Studies

At present, laboratory studies of depression in adolescents lag far behind analogous research on adult and prepubertal depressives. An extensive review of this area can be found in Ryan and Puig-Antich (1985) and Puig-Antich (1986).

Disturbances of hypothalamic pituitary adrenal axis (HPAA) regulation have been studied extensively in adult depression for two decades. Hypersecretion of cortisol, disrupted diurnal pattern, resistance to suppression by dexamethasone, and hyporesponsiveness of the axis to corticotropin releasing factor (CRF) have been reported (Carroll et al., 1981; Gold et al., 1984; Sachar et al., 1973). The most commonly used laboratory measures of HPAA activity are mean level of 24-hour urinary free cortisol excretion and the dexamethasone suppression test (DST). The DST has received greater attention to date due to its simplicity of administration and the suggestion that it served as a sensitive and specific state marker of endogenous depression.

While initial estimates of moderate sensitivity and high specificity have been disputed by recent research, nonsuppression and high post-dexamethasone plasma cortisol values continue to be found significantly more often among depressed than among nondepressed controls (Arana, Baldessarini, & Ornsteen, 1985; Coppen et al., 1983; Kasper & Beckmann, 1983; Rubin & Poland, 1984) and are usually correlated positively with episode severity and endogenicity. Coupled with the finding that continued nonsuppression may be associated with higher risk of relapse (Holsboer, Steiger, & Maier, 1983; Yerevanian et al., 1983), the DST may have clinical application as an ancillary monitor of treatment response. This awaits further research verification and standarization, as some studies found only moderate overlap between the DST and urinary free cortisol values (Brown, Keitner, Qualls, & Haier, 1985), casting uncertainty over its validity and what level of feedback regulation it reflects.

The DST is the only measure of HPAA activity studied in adolescence with some consistency (Doherty et al., 1986; Extein, Rosenberg, Pottash, & Gold, 1982; Ha, Kaplan, & Foley, 1984; Hsu et al., 1983; Klee & Garfinkel, 1984; Robbins, Alessi, Yanchyshyn, & Colfer, 1983; Strober, 1983; Targum & Capodanno, 1983). In spite of diverse patient groups and differences in methodology, the ability of the DST to identify adolescents with severe depression is comparable to its application in adults. Sensitivity values have ranged from 35 to 64% in adolescents with major depressive disorder, and specificity is high. Although these studies are preliminary, they seem to show that neuroendocrine dysregulations found in adults also exist in a subgroup of adolescents with severe depression. However, the small numbers of patients in these studies limit the generality of conclusions regarding DST associations with endogenicity, primary subtypes, suicidality, and symptom profiles.

Studies of the response of growth hormone (GH), an anterior pituitary hormone whose release is modulated by a variety of neurotransmitters, to various provocative stimuli were pursued recently in both adults and children. Studies in adults were in agreement that GH response to clonidine, insulin-induced hypoglycemia, and desipramine is significantly blunted in major depressives compared to controls (Checkley, Slade, & Shur, 1981; Sachar, Finkelstein, & Hellman, 1971; Siever et al., 1984).

Puig-Antich and colleagues in a series of reports (Puig-Antich et al., 1981; Puig-Antich et al., 1984a), documented similar blunting of GH release in response to insulin-induced hypoglycemia in a sample of endogenously depressed prepubertal children compared to nonendogenous depressed children and neurotic controls. Upon recovery and while drug-free, depressed children continued to show blunting of GH release to insulin challenge. This finding seems to suggest that blunting of GH release is a marker of endogenous depression, a past episode of depression, or affective vulnerability, although such conclusions remain tentative pending further investigation.

No completed studies of GH release in depressed adolescents have been published, however Puig-Antich (1986) notes that an ongoing study has found no difference in the release of GH to insulin-induced hypoglycemia between endogenously depressed versus nonendogenously depressed teenagers. Puig-Antich hypothesizes that higher estrogen levels during puberty, which augment GH responsiveness, may override neuroregulatory differences among groups at this age.

Changes in sleep-related GH release also have been studied in a small number of adults and prepubertal children, but no completed study of depressed adolescents has been reported. Puig-Antich (1986) notes that adolescents may hyposecrete GH during sleep, although data are sketchy. Because the majority of GH release during a 24-hour period occurs at night in synchrony with slow wave sleep, studies utilizing indwelling catheters for all night sampling may reveal altered secretory patterns of GH that reflect changes in regulatory systems, which are distinct from those involved in the response to provocative tests (Hindmarsh, Smith, Taylor, Pringle, & Brook, 1985). Preliminary data seem to show that prepubertal depressives and adults may have opposite nighttime secretory patterns, with depressed children showing hypersecretion (Puig-Antich et al., 1984b; Puig-Antich et al., 1984c).

Sleep electroencephalogram (EEG) studies of depressed adults have yielded fairly robust findings of decreased first rapid eye movement (REM) period latency, decreased delta sleep, decreased sleep efficiency, and increased REM density (Gillin et al., 1984). While REM sleep parameters normalize in many patients upon recovery, some demonstrate polysomnographic abnormalities even in the recovered, drug-free state (Rush et al., 1986). Therefore, it is unclear whether these measures constitute markers of state, trait, or past episode. The persistence of polysomnographic findings may indicate less than complete remission of episode, emerging relapse, high risk for relapse, or enduring biological states, in particular cholinergic supersensitivity.

Two controlled studies of prepubertal children indicated there are no significant sleep EEG abnormalities during an episode of major depression (Puig-Antich et al., 1982; Young, Knowles, MacLean, Boag, & McConville, 1982). Few studies of sleep EEG measures in depressed adolescents have been reported. Lahmeyer, Poznanski, and Bellur (1983) found evidence of shortened REM latency and increased REM density in 13 late adolescents with major depression, although patient-control differences in mean latency values were not as dramatic as those found with adult depressives. However, a more detailed sleep study of 49 adolescents with major depression and 40 normal controls found no group differences in REM sleep parameters (Goetz et al., 1986).

It would appear then that the characteristic alterations in polysomnographic measures found in older adult depressives are absent in prepubertal and adolescent patients. This may be due to a "masking" of sleep changes during affective episodes by the natural prominence of REM sleep and longer REM latencies during childhood and early adolescence, which itself may reflect maturational effects on the balance of cholinergic, noradrenergic, and serotonergic systems (Puig-Antich, 1986). Further studies using sensitive pharmacologic probes of cholinergic mechanisms regulating REM sleep may be useful in investigating with greater precision the neurochemical underpinnings of these developmental effects.

In sum, relatively little is known about the role played by abnormal biological processes in the genesis of adolescent affective disorders, although adult studies provide useful leads for future inquiry. It is not unreasonable to suppose that the pathophysiology of conditions arising in adolescence is markedly different from those developing later in adulthood. In this vein, Post, Rubinow, and Ballenger (1986) have hypothesized that with recurrences of illness and eventual chronicity, individuals accrue greater propensity for biological dysregulation coupled with lower thresholds for the precipitation of new episodes. If this is so, cross-sectional and longitudinal studies beginning in adolescence may reveal new insights into the course and progression of these pathophysiological mechanisms and possible protective factors.

On the other hand, adolescents may reveal fewer robust biological findings because of lesser exposure to noxious influences (e.g., stressors, drugs, toxins) that conceivably alter responsivity to provocative test stimuli. Conversely, abnormalities found in adolescence may be more proximal to the causal pathophysiology of affective illness rather than epiphenomena of aging or external influences. Therefore, only by integrating findings from child, adolescent, and adult studies will the salience and developmental significance of pathogenic biological factors be fully understood.

Pharmacotherapy

Clinical studies of antidepressant medication in adolescent major depression are few, and the results are difficult to interpret. One double-blind placebo-controlled study found no difference between amitriptyline hydrochloride at 200 mg/day and placebo given for 6 weeks in hospitalized adolescents with a diagnosis of major depression (Kramer & Feiguine, 1983). However, the study was marred by several shortcomings: first, there was no placebo washout period, which may well account for the 75%

rate of improvement found in both groups; second, drug dosage was fixed and plasma levels were not obtained; and last, the small size of each group would have allowed only a large treatment effect to achieve statistical significance.

Ryan and his colleagues (Ryan et al., 1986a) found that only 15 of 34 adolescents (44%) with major depression responded to imipramine hydrochloride during a 6 week-trial in which dosage was titrated to 5.0 mg/kg/day unless limited by side effects. Patients achieved a mean dose of 243 mg/day and a mean imipramine plus desipramine plasma level of 284 ng/ml. No linear or curvilinear relationship was found between plasma level and clinical response; predictors of poor drug response included separation anxiety, being female, endogenous subtype, and high plasma imipramine level. Ryan and Puig-Antich (1985) have hypothesized that the relationship between plasma levels and clinical response may be particularly weak in adolescence because of the effects of high gonadotropins levels on the pharmacodynamics of tricyclic drugs.

Geller and colleagues described in several reports the pharmacokinetics of nortriptyline in children and adolescents with major depression. Similar to adults, its elimination in children and adolescents has apparently first order kinetics with a logarithmically linear rate of disappearance (Geller, Cooper, Chestnut, Abel, & Anker, 1984). The mean half-life for the adolescent group was 27.1 ± 17.1 hours, which indicates that a once a day dosage usually would be sufficient. However, the wide range of values (14.1 to 76.2 hours) suggests that some adolescents would require twice a day dosage for optimal plasma level control. It was also found (Geller et al., 1985) that sampling 24 hours after a single fixed dose of nortriptyline could be used to predict steady state plasma levels and suggested therapeutic dose, and that nortriptyline plasma levels in children and adolescents are as stable over time as they are in adults (Geller, Cooper, & Chestnut, 1985).

Finally, these workers found that adolescents with delusional depression who received a combination of nortriptyline and chlorpromazine required significantly lower nortriptyline doses than did adolescents with nondelusional major depression who received nortriptyline alone to obtain equivalent mean steady state plasma levels (Geller, Cooper, Farooki, & Chestnut, 1985). Taken together, these findings indicate that the pharmacology of nortriptyline in adolescents differs little from its action in adults.

Preliminary data from open trials of nontricyclic antidepressants in adolescent major depression have been reported recently. Simeon and Ferguson (1986) treated nine adolescents with fluoxetine in an open trial, seven of whom improved markedly. Ryan, Puig-Antich, Rabinovitch, Fried, & Dachille (1986b) described a series of 20 adolescents with either unipolar or bipolar depression who were refractory to tricyclic antidepressants who subsequently had robust responses during open trials with monoamine oxidase inhibitors.

Use of lithium carbonate in the treatment of adolescent mania has been described (Horowitz, 1977; Steinberg, 1985; Hsu & Starzynski, 1986; Youngerman & Canino, 1979). However, controlled studies of its effectiveness do not exist.

In sum, while pharmacological interventions obviously deserve serious consideration in the treatment of severely depressed and bipolar adolescents, the question of whether they achieve the same effectiveness as in adults remains unresolved.

BEHAVIORAL AND PSYCHODYNAMIC APPROACHES

There is considerable evidence that behavioral and cognitive therapies are at least as effective as tricyclic antidepressants in the treatment of nonbipolar, nondelusional major depression in adults (Beckham & Leber, 1985). These therapies have as their starting point a clearly articulated set of intervention strategies whose goals are the attainment of self-reinforcing behavioral and interpersonal competencies and the direct modification of certain negative cognitions believed to lie at the core of depressive states.

Although similar deficits have been invoked in the causation of child and adolescent depression (Dweck, 1977; Petti, 1983), these issues have been elaborated mainly in laboratory studies of prepubertal children (Dweck, 1975; Dweck & Repucci, 1973; Kaslow, Tanebaum, Abramson, Peterson, & Seligman, 1983; Lefkowitz & Testiny, 1980; Moyal, 1977; Schwartz, Friedman, Lindsay, & Narrol, 1982). These studies indicate that higher levels of self-reported depressive symptoms tend to be associated with poorer performance on problem-solving tasks, external attributions of control of positive events, and lower self-esteem. An association between depressive symptoms and "depressogenic" attributional style in which failure and unpleasant events are attributed to internal, stable, and global causes has not yet shown relevance, etiologically or therapeutically, to any form of clinical depression in this age group.

Given its promise in the treatment of adult depression, cognitive therapy also has been proposed as a beneficial treatment for adolescent depressives (Emery, Bedrosian, & Garber, 1983). However, we know of no published studies in which the applicability, efficacy, or limitations of this modality in clinical samples have been assessed empirically under controlled conditions. Moreover, it seems likely, to us at least, that these techniques will have to be modified and specially tailored to the unique treatment needs of depressed adolescents, since cognitive processes at this age are not at all congruent with those operating in adults.

Much the same can be said of psychoanalytic theories and clinical approaches. Although they have strongly influenced accounts of the nature and developmental origins of depression since the writings of Freud and

Abraham, studies of the effectiveness of psychoanalytic therapies in adult depression are sparse, and the data are equivocal (Bellack, 1985; Rosenberg, 1985). Nonetheless, psychoanalytic notions can enrich and extend our understanding of clinical observational material.

Bemporad (1978) has commented astutely on how aspects of psychic organization and defensive style in adolescence effect the reaction to depressive states at this age. He suggests that because of the adolescent's cognitive egocentrism and normal dependence on the environment for narcissistic equilibrium, feelings of despair, hopelessness, and inferiority are felt with greater intensity and construed as permanent features of their psychological makeup. In this light, contemporary psychoanalytic concepts can serve as valuable aids in understanding the psychological dynamics in which depressive symptoms take root and the particular constellations of defense adolescents use to ameliorate their effects.

CLINICAL PROBLEMS

It cannot be assumed by any means that differential diagnosis in adolescent patients is always a straightforward task. Indeed, the problems can be quite formidable and of a different kind than those faced with children or adults. Although the techniques of diagnostic interviewing are the same, teenagers often devalue exploration of sensitive feelings and are deeply ambivalent about acknowledging distress or uncertainty. Consequently, some will disguise, block, or explain away symptomatic behavior out of shame or embarrassment, whereas others challenge the most skilled interviewer with denial, anger, or outright defiance.

It is not surprising in this regard that studies of parent-adolescent agreement on the presence of affective symptomatology generally reveal low levels of concordance (Chambers et al., 1985; Cohen et al., 1985; Moretti, Fine, Haley, & Marriage, 1985; Kashani et al., 1986). By the same token, use of self-report instruments to measure degree of depressive symptomatology in individual patients will rarely give data that are of sufficient quality or validity for differential diagnosis (Ryan & Puig-Antich, 1985). Thus on the surface, neither the parents' failure to note indicators of a depressive condition nor the teenager's denial of symptoms constitutes grounds for rejecting the presence of illness.

Obviously, knowledge of interview techniques that help set patients and families at ease greatly increases the likelihood that reliable information will be elicited, especially when the purpose and use made of the interview is described honestly. There is, of course, no substitute for skilled observation and knowledge of psychopathology, both of which imply the ability to infer special meaning from phenomena described by informants. The use of structured diagnostic interviews such as the SADS or

Kiddie-SADS can greatly assist this process in that by their very nature they help structure the informant's perception of possibly relevant changes in behavior, the onset of these changes, and their temporal and situational stability. Furthermore, clinicians should never ignore the possible effects of the circumstances under which the interview is conducted on the depth and quality of information obtained. As a general rule of thumb, diagnostic appraisals are most reliable when data are pooled from interviews conducted jointly with the family as well as individually with each family member.

A second practical difficulty arises when evaluating depressive manifestations superimposed on chronic personality difficulties and family turmoil. In such cases, cross-sectional assessments do not readily allow for clear-cut distinctions between patients with early onset of subaffective dysthymic symptoms and patients whose dysphoric symptoms reflect sequelae of chronic life stressors, traumatic experiences, or nonaffective character pathology. In adults, attempts have been made to subdivide the broader group of chronic depressions into the primary affective type and the character-spectrum type on the basis of comparative genetic, biological, descriptive data. The results of this work have been helpfully summarized by Akiskal and Simmons (1985). In the primary type: family history is frequently positive for unipolar or bipolar illness; there are more frequent episodes of an endogenous type; susceptibility to pharmacologically induced hypomania is greater; REM latencies are often within the range reported for primary unipolar depression; and premorbid personality is introverted and obsessive. In contrast, character-spectrum patients are distinguished by: high rates of familial alcoholism; personality disorder marked by histrionic, dependent, and unstable traits; normal REM latency values; and a high frequency of developmental antecedents, such as object loss, neglect, and other adverse family experiences. As this scheme rests largely on data from older patients, further study is required to test its validity in adolescence.

Differential diagnosis also proves difficult in patients whose symptoms have not reached full syndromal intensity. Even as teenagers progress from a prodromal to acutely symptomatic state, the diagnostic picture may remain ambiguous (Fard, Hudgens, & Welner, 1978). Conversely, many adolescent patients who present initially with intermittent dysphoric symptoms associated with neurotic or characterologic disturbance exhibit frank affective illness at a later point in time (Akiskal, Bitar, Puzantian, Rosenthal, & Walker, 1978). The point is that even with adherence to specific diagnostic criteria, the interpretation of clinical data in many cases remains unclear.

Interestingly, both Kraepelin and Bleuler noted the frequency with which certain abnormalities in behavior and temperament in childhood and adolescence seemed to presage later schizophrenic and affective psychoses. Confirming these early speculations, studies of high-risk populations and follow-back studies examining the premorbid adolescent adjustment of already ill individuals indicate that in some 30 to 50% of cases (especially in males), adult onset schizophrenia is preceded by withdrawal, oddities in social relating, emotional volatility, anhedonia, and solitary acts of antisocial conduct (for review, see Rutter & Garmezy, 1983).

Likewise in the case of affective illness, several studies (Weissman et al., 1984b; Akiskal et al., 1985; Klein, Depue, & Slater, 1985) indicate that certain temperamental abnormalities originally considered by Kraepelin to be on a genetic continuum with severe manic-depressive illness (i.e., dysthymia, hyperthymia, cyclothymia) are significantly more prevalent in the adolescent offspring of adults with affective disorders than in controls. One implication of these findings is that combining assessment of family history with closer scrutiny of premonitory signs of illness within the psychotic and affective spectrum might have utility in differentiating varying levels of predisposition to later, full-blown disorder. Of course, the validity of such a taxonomy has not yet been tested.

There are also numerous practical problems in the treatment of adolescent depression. Despite the lack of systematic studies, there are hints that even under ordinary conditions of psychopharmacological management with good compliance, adequate blood levels, and certainty of diagnosis, adolescents respond less favorably to tricyclic antidepressant drugs than adults (Ryan et al., 1986a). In adults, a variety of strategies is available to potentiate antidepressant effects in tricyclic nonresponders, including the addition of triiodothyronine, lithium carbonate, and monoamine oxidase inhibitors. Their utility in treating adolescents who are refractory to standard antidepressant therapy is not known, though each deserves consideration.

Resistance to pharmacological intervention also arises in the treatment of adolescents with bipolar illness. Although clinical experience shows clearly that lithium carbonate ameliorates acute symptoms of mania in many, we have found lithium resistance to be particularly common in a subgroup with familial loading of bipolar illness and symptoms of persistent hyperactivity and impulsive behavior dating back to early childhood (Strober, Morrell, Burroughs, Lampert, Danforth, & Freeman, in press). The presence of mixed episodes, in which manic and depressive symptoms occur simultaneously, also has been linked to greater lithium resistance (Himmelhoch & Garfinkel, 1986) and reflects the need for aggressive intervention with other potential antimanic compounds, such as carbamazepine, clonidine, clonazepam, and calcium channel blockers. However, even when adequate pharmacological control is achieved, the outcome of these patients often remains precarious.

Finally, mention must be made of treatment complications arising from the multifaceted nature of stressors, both individual and familial, that occur in association with depression in adolescents. Probably, on the whole, therapeutic management is more difficult in younger patients because of the greater variability and immaturity of their adaptive coping responses and because of the potentially adverse effects of depression on the teenager's self-esteem, identity formation, school functioning, and interpersonal competencies. Each requires attention, as does the patient's family, as influences in the home environment (e.g., disharmonious interactions and rejecting or critical attitudes toward the identified patient) may predispose to future relapses, although no data are presently available on how frequently this occurs in adolescents with major affective disorders. Of course, special preventive measures are needed to manage suicidal crises precipitated by chronic depressive or bipolar conditions in this population, an issue reviewed more completely elsewhere (Shaffer, 1985).

The treatment of affective disorders in adolescent patients will involve, by necessity, a multiplicity of approaches, including continuing psychotherapy to help master the self-perpetuating cycle of doubt and insecurity which often follows resolution of acute symptoms. Thus clinicians must remain alert to the pitfalls of treatment that is too one-sided, and they must use each method flexibly in taking a broad view of the patient's needs.

SUMMARY

This review portrays the affective disorders of adolescence as areas of immense scientific and clinical importance. Informative data on diagnostic prevalence and phenomenology, family history, and course over time point up the continuity of affective syndromes in adolescence and adulthood, although the significance of social and biological risk factors has yet to be determined. The potentially chronic, recurring nature of affective disorders and their adverse effects on adolescent identity and self-esteem indicate that questions of treatment response and long-term prevention must now be aggressively pursued through well-controlled randomized clinical trials that are modeled after adult studies.

REFERENCES

Akiskal, H. S., Bitar, A. H., Puzantian, V. R., Rosenthal, T. L., & Walker, P. W. (1978). The nosological status of neurotic depression: A prospective three-to-four year examination in light of the primary-secondary and unipolar-bipolar dichotomies. *Archives of General Psychiatry, 35,* 756–766.

Akiskal, H. S., Downs, J., Jordan, P., Watson, S., Daughterty, D., & Pruitt, D. B. (1985). Mode of onset of affective disturbances in the children and younger siblings of manic depressives: A prospective study. *Archives of General Psychiatry, 42,* 996–1003.

Akiskal, H. S., & Simmons, R. C. (1985). Chronic and refractory depressions: Evaluation and management. In E. E. Beckham & W. R. Leber (Eds.), *Handbook of depression* (pp. 587–605). Homewood, IL: Dorsey.

Akiskal, H. S., Walker P., Puzantian, V. R., King, D., Rosenthal, T. L., & Dranon, M. (1983). Bipolar outcome in the course of depressive illness: Phenomenologic, familial, and pharmacologic predictors. *Journal of Affective Disorders, 5,* 115–128.

Albert, N., & Beck, A. T. (1975). Incidence of depression in early adolescence: A preliminary study. *Journal of Youth and Adolescence, 4,* 301–306.

American Psychiatric Association (1980). Diagnostic and statistical manual of mental disorders (3rd ed.). Washington, D.C.: Author.

Arana, G. W., Baldessarini, R. J., & Ornsteen, M. (1985). The dexamethasone suppression test for diagnosis and prognosis in psychiatry: Commentary and review. *Archives of General Psychiatry, 42,* 1193–1204.

Ballanger, J. C., Reus, V. I., & Post, R. M. (1982). The "atypical" clinical picture of adolescent mania. *American Journal of Psychiatry, 139,* 602–606.

Beardslee, W. R., Keller, M. B., & Klerman, G. L. (1985). Children of parents with affective disorder. *International Journal of Family Psychiatry, 6,* 283–299.

Beckham, E. E., & Leber, W. R. (1985). The comparative efficacy of psychotherapy and pharmacotherapy for depression. In E. E. Beckham & W. R. Leber (Eds.), *Handbook of depression* (pp. 316–342). Homewood, IL: Dorsey.

Bellack, A. S. (1985). Psychotherapy research in depression: An overview. In E. E. Beckham & W. R. Leber (Eds.), *Handbook of depression* (pp. 204–219). Homewood, IL: Dorsey.

Bemporad, J. (1978). Psychodynamics of depression and suicide in children and adolescents. In S. Arieti & J. Bemporad (Eds.), *Severe and mild depression* (pp. 185–210). New York: Basic Books.

Blos, P. (1967). The second individuation process of adolescence. *Psychoanalytic Study of the Child, 22,* 162–186.

Bowden, C. L., & Sarabia, F. (1980). Diagnosing manic-depressive illness in adolescence. *Comprehensive Psychiatry, 21,* 263–269.

Boyd, J. H., & Weissman, M. M. (1981). The epidemiology of affective disorders. *Archives of General Psychiatry, 38,* 1039–1047.

Brown, W. A., Keitner, G., Qualls, C. B., & Haier, R. (1985). The dexamethasone suppression test and pituitary-adrenocortical function. *Archives of General Psychiatry, 42,* 121–123.

Carlson, G. A., Davenport, Y. B., & Jamison, K. (1977). A comparison of outcome in adolescent and late onset bipolar manic-depressive illness. *American Journal of Psychiatry, 134,* 919–922.

Carlson, G. A., & Strober, M. (1978). Manic-depressive illness in early adolescence: A study of clinical and diagnostic characteristics in six cases. *Journal of the American Academy of Child Psychiatry, 17,* 138–153.

Carroll, B. J., Feinberg, M., Greden, J. F., Tarika, J., Albala, A., Haskett, R., James, N., Kronfol, Z., Lohr, N., Steiner, M., deVigne, J. P., & Young, E.

(1981). A specific laboratory test for the diagnosis of melancholia. *Archives of General Psychiatry, 38,* 15–23.

Chambers, W. J., & Puig-Antich, J. (1982). Psychotic symptoms in prepubertal major depressive disorder. *Archives of General Psychiatry, 39,* 921–927.

Chambers, W. J., Puig-Antich, J., Hirsch, M., Paez, P., Ambrosini, P. J., Tabrizi, M. A., & Davies, M. (1985). The assessment of affective disorders in children and adolescents by semistructured interview. *Archives of General Psychiatry, 42,* 696–702.

Checkley, S. A., Slade, A. P., & Shur, E. (1981). Growth hormone and other responses to clonidine in patients with endogenous depression. *British Journal of Psychiatry, 138,* 51–55.

Cohen, P., Velez, C. N., & Garcia, M. (1985). The epidemiology of childhood depression. Presented at the annual meeting of the American Academy of Child Psychiatry, San Antonio, TX.

Conners, C. K., Himmelhoch, J., Goyette, C. H., Ulrich, R., & Neil, J. F. (1979). Children of parents with affective illness. *Journal of the American Academy of Child Psychiatry, 18,* 600–607.

Coppen, A., Abou-Saleh, M., Millin, P., Metcalfe, M., Harwood, J., & Bailey, J. (1983). Dexamethasone suppression test in depression and other psychiatric illness. *British Journal of Psychiatry, 142,* 498–504.

Coryell, W., & Norten, S. G. (1980). Mania during adolescence. *Journal of Nervous and Mental Disease, 168,* 611–613.

Decina, P., Kestenbaum, C. J., Farber, S., Kron, L., Gargan, M., Sackeim, H. A., & Fieve, R. R. (1983). Clinical and psychological assessment of children of bipolar probands. *American Journal of Psychiatry, 140,* 548–553.

Dobson, K. S., & Shaw, B. F. (1986). Cognitive assessment with major depressive disorders. *Cognitive Therapy and Research, 10,* 13–29.

Doherty, M. B., Madansky, D., Kraft, J., Carter-Ake, L. L., Rosenthal, P. A., & Coughlin, B. F. (1986). Cortisol dynamics and test performance of the dexamethasone suppression test in 97 psychiatrically hospitalized children aged 3–16 years. *Journal of the American Academy of Child Psychiatry, 25,* 400–408.

Douvan, E., & Adelson, J. (1966). *The adolescent experience.* New York: Wiley.

Dweck, C. S. (1975). The role of expectations and attributions in the alleviation of learned helplessness. *Journal of Personality and Social Psychology, 31,* 674–685.

Dweck, C. S. (1977). Learned helplessness: A developmental approach. In J. Schulterbrandt & A. Raskin (Eds.), *Depression in childhood: Diagnosis, treatment and conceptual models* (pp. 135–138). New York: Raven.

Dweck, C. S., & Repucci, N.D. (1973). Learned helplessness and reinforcement responsibility in children. *Journal of Personality and Social Psychology, 25,* 109–116.

Eaves, G., & Rush, A. J. (1984). Cognitive patterns in symptomatic unipolar major depression. *Journal of Abnormal Psychology, 93,* 31–40.

Emery, G., Bedrosian, R., & Garber, J. (1983). Cognitive therapy with depressed children and adolescents. In D. P. Cantwell & G. A. Carlson (Eds.), *Affective disorders in childhood and adolescence: An update* (pp. 445–472). New York: Spectrum Publications.

Extein, I., Rosenberg, G., Pottash, A. L. C., & Gold, G. (1982). The dexamethasone suppression test in depressed adolescents. *American Journal of Psychiatry, 139,* 1617–1619.

Fard, I., Hudgens, R. W., & Welner, A. (1978). Undiagnosed psychiatric illness in adolescents: A prospective and 7-year follow-up. *Archives of General Psychiatry, 35,* 279–282.

Feighner, J. P., Robins, E., Guze, S. B., Woodruff, R., Winokur, G., & Munoz, R. (1972). Diagnostic criteria for use in psychiatric research. *Archives of General Psychiatry, 26*, 57–63.

Freud, A. (1958). Adolescence. *Psychoanalytic Study of the Child, 13,* 255–278.

Friedman, R. C., Hurt, S. W., Clarkin, J. F., Corn, R., & Aronoff, M. S. (1983). Symptoms of depression among adolescents and young adults. *Journal of Affective Disorders, 5,* 37–43.

Geller, B., Chestnut, E. C., Miller, M., Price, D. T., & Yates, E. (1985). Preliminary data on DSM-III associated features of major depressive disorder in children and adolescents. *American Journal of Psychiatry, 142,* 643–644.

Geller, B., Cooper, T. B., & Chestnut, E. C. (1985). Serial monitoring and achievement of steady state nortriptyline plasma levels in depressed children and adolescents: Preliminary data. *Journal of Clinical Psychopharmacology, 5,* 213–216.

Geller, B., Cooper, T. B., Chestnut, E., Abel, A. S., & Anker, J. A. (1984). Nortriptyline pharmakinetic parameters in depressed children and adolescents: Preliminary data. *Journal of Clinical Psychopharmacology, 4,* 265–269.

Geller, B., Cooper, T. B., Chestnut, E. C., Anker, J. A., Price, D. T., & Yates E. (1985). Child and adolescent nortryptyline single dose kinetics predict steady state plasma levels and suggested dose: Preliminary data. *Journal of Clinical Psychopharmacology, 5,* 154–158.

Geller, B., Cooper, T. B., Farooki, Z. Q., & Chestnut, E. C. (1985). Dose and plasma levels of nortriptyline and chlorpromazine in delusionally depressed adolescents. *American Journal of Psychiatry, 142,* 336–338.

Gershon, E. S., McKnew, D., Cytryn, L., Hamovit, J., Schreiber, J., Higgs, E., & Pellegrini, D. (1985). Diagnosis in school-age children of bipolar affective disorder patients and normal controls. *Journal of Affective Disorders, 8,* 283–291.

Gillin, J. C., Sitaram, N., Wehr, T., Duncan, W., Post, R., Murphy, D. L., Mendelson, W. B., Wyatt, R. J., & Bunney, W. E. (1984). Sleep and affective illness. In R. M. Post & J. C. Ballenger (Eds.), *Neurobiology of Mood Disorders* (pp. 157–189). Baltimore: Williams & Wilkins.

Goetz, R. R., Puig-Antich, J., Ryan, N. D., Rabinovich, H., Ambrosini, P. J., Nelson, B., & Krawiec, V. (1986). Electroencephalographic sleep of adolescents with major depression and normal controls. *Archives of General Psychiatry, 44,* 61–68.

Gold, P. W., Chrousos, G., Kellner, C., Post, R., Roy, A., Augerinos, P., Schulte, H., Oldfield, E., & Loriaux, D. L. (1984). Psychiatric implications of basic and clinical studies with corticotropin-releasing-factor. *American Journal of Psychiatry, 141,* 619–627.

Graham, P., & Rutter, M. (1985). Adolescent disorders. In M. Rutter & L. Herson (Eds.), *Child and adolescent psychiatry* (pp. 351–367). London: Blackwell.

Greenhill, L. L., & Shopsin, B. (1979). Survey of mental disorders in the children of patients with affective disorders. In J. Mendlewicz & B. Shopsin (Eds.), *Genetic aspects of affective Illness* (pp. 75–92). New York: Spectrum Publications.

Ha, H., Kaplan, S., & Foley, C. (1984). The dexamethasone suppression test in adolescent psychiatric patients. *American Journal of Psychiatry, 141,* 421–423.

Hamilton, E. W., & Abramson, L.Y. (1983). Cognitive patterns and major depressive disorders: A longitudinal study in the hospital setting. *Journal of Abnormal Psychology, 92,* 173–184.

Hassanyeh, F., & Davison, K. (1980). Bipolar affective psychosis with onset before age 16: Report of 10 cases. *British Journal of Psychiatry, 137,* 530–539.

Himmelhoch, J. M., & Garfinkel, M. E. (1986). Sources of lithium resistance in mixed mania. *Psychopharmacology Bulletin, 22,* 613–620.

Hindmarsh, P. C., Smith, P. J., Taylor, B. J., Pringle, P. J., & Brook, C. G. D. (1985). Comparison between a physiological and a pharmacological stimulus of growth hormone secretion: Response to stage IV sleep and insulin induced hypoglycemia. *Lancet,* 1033–1035.

Holsboer, F., Steiger, A., & Maier, W. (1983). Four cases of reversion to abnormal dexamethasone suppression test response as indicator of clinical relapse. *Biological Psychiatry, 18,* 911–916.

Horowitz, M. M. (1977). Lithium and the treatment of adolescent manic-depressive illness. *Diseases of the Nervous System, 38,* 480–483.

Hsu, L. K. G., Molcan, K., Cashman, M. N., Lee, S., Lohr, J., & Hindmarsh, D. (1983). The dexamethasone suppression test in adolescent depression. *Journal of the American Academy of Child Psychiatry, 22,* 470–473.

Hsu, L. K. G., & Starzynski, J. M. (1986). Mania in adolescence. *Journal of Clinical Psychiatry, 47,* 596–599.

Hudgens, R. W. (1974). *Psychiatric disorders in adolescence.* Baltimore: Williams & Wilkins.

Inamdar, S., Siomopoulos, G., Osborn, M., & Bianchi, E. C. (1979). Phenomenology associated with depressed moods in adolescents. *American Journal of Psychiatry, 136,* 156–159.

Kandel, D. B., & Davies, M. (1986). Adult sequelae of adolescent depressive symptoms. *Archives of General Psychiatry, 43,* 255–264.

Kandel, D. B., & Davis, M. (1982). The epidemiology of depressed mood in adolescents: An empirical study. *Archives of General Psychiatry, 39,* 1205–1212.

Kaplan, S. L., Hong, G. K., & Weinhold, C. (1984). Epidemiology of depressive symptomatology in adolescents. *Journal of the American Academy of Child Psychiatry, 23,* 91–98.

Kashani, J. H., Carlson, G. A., Beck, N. C., Hoeper, E. W., McAllister, J. A., Corcoran, C. M., Fallahi, C., Rosenberg, T. K., & Reid, J. C. (1986). Depression, depressive symptomatology, and depressed mood among a community sample of adolescents. Manuscript submitted for publication.

Kaslow, N. J., Tanebaum, R. C., Abramson, L. Y., Peterson, C., & Seligman, M. E. P. (1983). Problem solving deficits and depressive symptoms among children. *Journal of Abnormal Child Psychology, 11,* 497–502.

Kasper, S., & Beckmann, H. (1983). Dexamethasone suppression test in a pluridiagnostic approach: Its relationship to psychopathological and clinical variables. *Acta Psychiatrica Scandinavica, 68,* 31–37.

Keller, M. B., Shapiro, R. W., Lavori, P. W., & Wolfe, N. (1982). Recovery in major depressive disorder: Analysis with life table and regression models. *Archives of General Psychiatry, 39,* 905–910.

Klee, S. H., & Garfinkel, B. D. (1984). Identification of depression in children and adolescents: The role of the dexamethasone suppression test. *Journal of the American Academy of Child Psychiatry, 23,* 410–415.

Klein, D. N., Depue, R. A., & Slater, J. F. (1985). Cyclothymia in the adolescent offspring of parents with bipolar affective disorder. *Journal of Abnormal Psychology, 94,* 115–127.

Klerman, G. L. (1986a). Historical perspectives on contemporary schools of psychopathology. In T. Millon & G. L. Klerman (Eds.), *Contemporary directions in psychopathology: Toward the DSM-IV* (pp. 3–28). New York: Guilford.

Klerman, G. L. (1986b). Evidence for increase in rates of depression in North America and Western Europe in recent decades. In H. Hippius, G. L. Klerman, N. Matussek (Eds.), *New results in depression research* (pp. 7–15). Berlin: Springer-Verlag.

Klerman, G. L., Lavori, P. W., Rice, J., Reich, T., Endicott, J., Andreasen, N. C., Keller, M. B., & Hirschfield, R. M. A. (1985). Birth-cohort trends in rates of major depressive disorder among relatives of patients with affective disorder. *Archives of General Psychiatry, 42,* 689–695.

Kovacs, M., Feinberg, T. L., Crouse-Novak, M., Paulauskas, S. L., & Finkelstein, R. (1984). Depressive disorders in childhood: I. a longitudinal prospective study of characteristics and recovery. *Archives of General Psychiatry, 41,* 229–237.

Kovacs, M., Feinberg, T. L., Crouse-Novak, M., Paulauskas, S. L., Pollock, M., & Finkelstein, R. (1984). Depressive disorders in childhood. II. A longitudinal study of risk for a subsequent major depression. *Archives of General Psychiatry, 41,* 643–649.

Kramer, A. D., & Feiguine, B. A. (1983). Clinical effects of amitryptyline in adolescent depression. *Journal of the American Academy of Child Psychiatry, 20,* 636–644.

Kuyler, P. L., Rosenthal, L., Igel, G., Dunner, D. L., & Fieve, R. R. (1980). Psychopathology among children of manic-depressive patients. *Biological Psychiatry, 15,* 589–597.

Lahmeyer, H. W., Poznanski, E. O., & Bellur, S. N. (1983). EEG sleep in depressed adolescents. *American Journal of Psychiatry, 140,* 1150–1153.

Landolt, A. B. (1957). Follow-up studies on circular manic-depressive reactions occurring in the young. *Bulletin of the New York Academy of Medicine, 33,* 65–73.

Lefkowitz, M. M., & Testiny, E. P. (1980). Assessment of childhood depression. *Journal of Consulting and Clinical Psychology, 48,* 43–50.

Lewinsohn, P. M., Duncan, E. M., Stanton, A. K., & Hautzinger, M. (1986). Age at first onset for nonbipolar depression. *Journal of Abnormal Psychology, 95,* 378–383.

Loranger, A. W., & Levine, P. M. (1978). Age of onset of bipolar illness. *Archives of General Psychiatry, 35,* 1345–1348.

McKnew, D. H., Cytryn, L., Efron, A. M., Gershon, E. S., & Bunney, W. E. (1979). Offspring of patients with affective disorders. *British Journal of Psychiatry, 134,* 148–152.

Moretti, M. M., Fine, S., Haley, G., & Marriage, M. B. (1985). Childhood and adolescent depression: Child-report versus parent-report information. *Journal of the American Academy of Child Psychiatry, 24,* 298–302.

Moyal, B. R. (1977). Locus of control, self esteem, stimulus appraisal, and depressive symptoms in children. *Journal of Consulting and Clinical Psychology, 45,* 951–952.

O'Connell, R. A., Mays, J. A., O'Brien, J. D., & Mirsheidaie, F. (1979). Children of bipolar manic-depressives. In J. Mendlewicz & B. Shopsin (Eds.), *Genetic aspects of affective illness* (pp. 75–92). New York: Spectrum Publications.

Offer, D. (1969). *The psychological world of the teenager.* New York: Basic Books.

Offer, D., & Offer, J. L. (1975). *From teenager to young manhood.* New York: Basic Books.

Offer, D., Sabshin, M., & Marcus, D. (1965). Clinical evaluation of normal adolescents. *American Journal of Psychiatry, 121,* 864–872.

Olsen, T. (1961). Follow-up study of manic-depressive patients whose first attack occurred before the age of 19. *Acta Psychiatrica Scandanavica* (suppl.), *162,* 45–51.

Orvaschel, H., Weissman, M. M., Padian, N., & Lowe, T. L. (1981). Assessing psychopathology in children of psychiatrically disturbed parents: A pilot study. *Journal of the American Academy of Child Psychiatry, 20,* 112–122.

Petti, T. A. (1983). Behavioral approaches in the treatment of depressed children. In D. P. Cantwell, & G. A. Carlson (Eds.), *Affective disorders in childhood and adolescence: An update* (pp. 417–444). New York: Spectrum Publications.

Post, R. M., Rubinow, D. R., & Ballenger, J. C. (1986). Conditioning and sensitization in the longitudinal course of affective illness. *British Journal of Psychiatry, 149,* 191–201.

Puig-Antich, J. (1986). Psychobiological markers: Effects of age and puberty. In M. Rutter, C. E. Izard, & P. B. Read (Eds.), *Depression in young people* (pp. 341–381). New York: Guilford.

Puig-Antich, J., Davies, M., Novacenko, H. Tabrizi, M. A., Ambrosini, P., Goetz, R., Bianca, J., & Sachar, E. J. (1984a). Growth hormone secretion in prepubertal major depressive children. III. Response to insulin induced hypoglycemia in a drug-free, fully recovered clinical state. *Archives of General Psychiatry, 41,* 471–475.

Puig-Antich, J., Goetz, R., Davies, M., Fein, M., Hanlon, C., Chambers, W. J., Tabrizi, M. A., Sachar, E. J., & Weitzman, E. D. (1984b). Growth hormone secretion in prepubertal major depressive children. II. Sleep related plasma concentrations during a depressive episode. *Archives of General Psychiatry, 41,* 463–466.

Puig-Antich, J., Goetz, R., Davies, M., Tabrizi, M. A., Novacenko, H., Hanlon, C., Sachar, E. J., & Weitzman, E. D. (1984c). Growth hormone secretion in prepubertal major depressive children. IV. Sleep related plasma concentrations in a drug-free, fully recovered clinical state. *Archives of General Psychiatry, 41,* 479–483.

Puig-Antich, J., Goetz, R., Hanlon, C., Tabrizi, M. A., Davies, M., & Weitzman, E. D. (1982). Sleep architecture and REM sleep measures in prepubertal major depressives during an episode. *Archives of General Psychiatry, 39,* 932–939.

Puig-Antich, J., Tabrizi, M. A., Davies, M., Chambers, W., Halpern, F., & Sachar, E. J. (1981). Prepubertal endogenous major depressives hyposecrete growth hormone in response to insulin-induced hypoglycemia. *Biological Psychiatry, 16,* 801–818.

Robbins, D. R., Alessi, N. E., Yanchyshyn, G. W., & Colfer, M. V. (1983). The dexamethasone suppression test in psychiatrically hospitalized adolescents. *Journal of the American Academy of Child Psychiatry, 22,* 467–469.

Robins, L. (1979). Follow-up studies. In H. C. Quay & J. S. Werry (Eds.), *Psychopathological disorders of childhood* (2nd ed.) (pp. 483–513). New York: Wiley.

Rosenberg, S. E. (1985). Brief dynamic psychotherapy for depression. In E. E. Beckham & W. R. Leber (Eds.), *Handbook of depression* (pp. 100–123). Homewood, IL: Dorsey.

Rubin, R. T., & Poland, R. E. (1984). The dexamethasone suppression test in depression: Advantages and limitations. In G. D. Burrows, T. R. Norman, & K. P. Maguire (Eds.), *Biological psychiatry: Recent studies* (pp. 76–83). London: John Libbey.

Rush, A. J., Erman, M. K., Giles, D. E., Schlesser, M. A., Carpenter, G., Vasavada, N., & Roffwarg, H. P. (1986). Polysomnographic findings in recently drug-free and clinically remitted depressed patients. *Archives of General Psychiatry, 43,* 878–884.

Rutter, M. (1986). The developmental psychopathology of depression: Issues and perspectives. In M. Rutter, C. E. Izard, & P. B. Read (Eds.), *Depression in Young People: Developmental and Clinical Perspectives* (pp. 3–30). New York: Guilford.

Rutter, M., & Garmezy, N. (1983). Developmental psychopathology. In P. H. Mussen (Ed.), *Handbook of child psychology: Volume IV. Socialization, personality, and social development* (pp. 776–991). New York: Wiley.

Rutter, M., Graham, P., Chadwick, O. F. D., & Yule, W. (1976). Adolescent turmoil: Fact or fiction. *Journal of Child Psychology and Psychiatry, 17,* 35–56.

Rutter, M., & Quinton, D. (1984). Parental psychiatric disorder: Effects on children. *Psychological Medicine, 14,* 853–880.

Rutter, M., & Shaffer, D. (1980). DSM-III: A step forward or back in terms of the classification of child psychiatric disorder? *Journal of the American Academy of Child Psychiatry, 19,* 371–394.

Rutter, M., Tizard, J., Yule, W., Graham, P., & Whitmore, K. (1976). Isle of Wight Studies 1964–1974. *Psychological Medicine, 6,* 313–332.

Ryan, N. D., & Puig-Antich, J. (1985). Affective illness in adolescence. In A. F. Frances & R. E. Hales (Eds.), *Psychiatry Update: American Psychiatric Association annual review, Volume 5* (pp. 420–450). Washington, DC: American Psychiatric Press.

Ryan, N. D., Puig-Antich, J., Ambrosini, P., Rabinovitch, H., Robinson, D., Nelson, B., Iyengar, S., & Twomey, J. (1987). The clinical picture of major depression in children and adolescents. *Archives of General Psychiatry, 44,* 854–861.

Ryan, N. D., Puig-Antich, J., Cooper, T., Rabinovich, H., Ambrosini, P., Davis, M., King, J., Torres, D., & Fried, J. (1986a). Imipramine in adolescent major depression: Plasma level and clinical responses. *Acta Psychiatrica Scandanavica, 73,* 275–288.

Ryan, N., Puig-Antich, J., Rabinovich, H., Fried, J., & Dachille, S. (1986b). MAOI treatment of adolescent major depression unresponsive to tricyclic antidepressants. Presentation at the annual meeting of the American Academy of Child and Adolescent Psychiatry, Los Angeles, CA.

Sachar, E. J., Finkelstein, J., & Hellman, L. (1971). Growth hormone responses in depressive illness: Response to insulin tolerance test. *Archives of General Psychiatry, 25,* 263–269.

Sachar, E. J., Hellman, L., Roffwarg, H. P., Halpern, F. S., Fukushima, D. K., & Gallagher, R. F. (1973). Disrupted 24-hour patterns of cortisol secretion in psychotic depression. *Archives of General Psychiatry, 28,* 19–24.

Schoenbach, V. J., Garrison, C. Z., & Kaplan, B. H. (1984). Epidemiology of adolescent depression. *Public Health Review, 12,* 159–189.

Schoenbach, V. J., Kaplan, B. H., Wagner, E. H., Grimson, R. C., & Miller, F. T. (1983). Prevalence of self-reported depressive symptoms in young adolescents. *American Journal of Public Health, 73,* 1281–1287.

Schwartz, M., Friedman, R., Lindsay, R., & Narrol, H. (1982) The relationship between conceptual tempo and depression in children. *Journal of Consulting and Clinical Psychology, 50,* 488–490.

Shaffer, D. (1985). Depression, mania and suicidal acts. In M. Rutter & L. Herson (Eds.), *Child and adolescent psychiatry* (pp. 698–719). London: Blackwell.

Siever, L. J., & Davis, K. L. (1985). Toward a dysregulation hypothesis of depression. *American Journal of Psychiatry, 142,* 1017–1031.

Siever, L. J. Uhde, T. W., Jimerson, D. C., Post, R. M., Lake, C. R., & Murphy, D. L. (1984). Plasma cortisol responses to clonidine in depressed patients and controls. *Archives of General Psychiatry, 41,* 63–71.

Simon, J. G., & Ferguson, H. B. (1986). Efficiency and safety of fluoxetine in the treatment of depressive disorders in adolescents. Presentation at the annual meeting of the American Academy of Child Psychiatry, Los Angeles, CA.

Simons, A. D., Garfield, S. L., & Murphy, G. E. (1984). The process of change in cognitive therapy and pharmacotherapy of depression: Changes in mood and cognition. *Archives of General Psychiatry, 41,* 22–28.

Slater, E., & Cowie, V. (1971). *The genetics of mental disorders.* London: Oxford University Press.

Steinberg, D. (1980). Use of lithium carbonate in adolescence. *Journal of Child Psychology and Psychiatry, 21,* 263–271.

Strober, M. (1983). Clinical and biological perspectives on depressive disorders in adolescence. In D. P. Cantwell & G. A. Carlson (Eds.), *Affective disorders in childhood and adolescence* (pp. 97–103). New York: Spectrum Publications.

Strober, M. (1984). Familial aspects of depressive disorder in early adolescence. In E. B. Weller & R. A. Weller (Eds.), *Major Depressive disorders in children* (pp. 38–48). Washington DC: American Psychiatric Press.

Strober, M., & Carlson, G. (1982). Bipolar illness in adolescents: Clinical, genetic and pharmacologic predictors in a three- to four-year prospective follow-up. *Archives of General Psychiatry, 39,* 549–555.

Strober, M., Green, J., & Carlson, G. A. (1981a). Reliability of psychiatric diagnosis in hospitalized adolescents: Inter rater agreement using DSM-III. *Archives of General Psychiatry, 38,* 141–145.

Strober, M., Green, J., & Carlson, G. A. (1981b). Phenomenology and subtypes of major depressive disorder in adolescents. *Journal of Affective Disorders, 3,* 281–290.

Strober, M., Morrell, W., Burroughs, J., Lampert, C., Danforth, H., & Freeman, R. (in press). A family study of bipolar I disorder in adolescence: Early onset of symptoms linked to increased familial loading and lithium resistance. *Journal of Affective Disorders.*

Strober, M., Salkin, B., Burroughs, J., Green, J., Lampert, C., & Danforth, H. A family interview study of affective illness and schizophrenia in adolescence. Manuscript in preparation.

Targum, S. D., & Capodanno, A. E. (1983). The dexamethasone suppression test in adolescent psychiatric patients. *American Journal of Psychiatry, 140,* 589–591.

Teri, L. (1982). The use of the Beck Depression Inventory with adolescents. *Journal of Abnormal Child Psychology, 10,* 277–284.

Thyer, B. A., Parrish, R. T., Curtis, G. C., Nesse, R. M., & Cameron, O. G. (1985). Ages of onset of DSM-III anxiety disorders. *Comprehensive Psychiatry, 85,* 113–122.

Toolan, J. M. (1962). Depression in children and adolescents. *American Journal of Orthopsychiatry, 32,* 404–415.

Weiner, I. B. (1970). *Psychological disturbance in adolescence.* New York: Wiley.

Weissman, M. M., Leckman, J. E., Merikangas, K. R., Gammon, G. D., & Prusoff, B. A. (1984a). Depression and anxiety disorders in parents and children. *Archives of General Psychiatry, 41,* 845–852.

Weissman, M. M., Myers, J. K., Thompson, W. D., & Belanger, A. (1986). Depressive symptoms as a risk factor for mortality and for major depression. In L. Erlenmeyer-Kimling & N. E. Miller (Eds.), *Life span research on the prediction of psychopathology* (pp. 251–260). Hillsdale, NJ: Erlbaum.

Weissman, M. M., Prusoff, B. A., Gammon, G. D., Merikangas, K. R., Leckman, J. F., & Kidd, K. K. (1984b). Psychopathology in the children (ages 6–18) of depressed and normal parents. *Journal of the American Academy of Child Psychiatry, 23,* 78–84.

Weissman, M. M., Wickramaratne, P., Merikangas, K. R., Leckman, J. F., Prusoff, B. A., Caruso, K. A., Kidd, K. K., & Gammon, G. D. (1984c). Onset of major depression in early adulthood: Increased family loading and specificity. *Archives of General Psychiatry, 41,* 1136–1143.

Welner, A., Welner, Z., & Fishman, R. (1979). Psychiatric adolescent inpatients: A 10-year follow-up. *Archives of General Psychiatry, 36,* 698–700.

Welner, Z., Welner, A., McCrary, M. D., & Leonard, M.A. (1977). Psychopathology in children of inpatients with depression: A controlled study. *Journal of Nervous and Mental Disease, 164,* 408–413.

Whybrow, P. C., Akiskal, H. S., & McKinney, W. T. (1984). *Mood disorders: Toward a new psychobiology.* New York: Plenum.

Winokur, G., Clayton, P. J., & Reich, T. (1969). *Manic-depressive illness.* St. Louis: C.V. Mosby.

Yerevanian, B. I., Olafsdottor, H., Milanese, E., Russotto, J., Mallon, P., Baciewicz, G., & Sagi, E. (1983). Normalization of the dexamethasone suppression test at discharge from hospital. *Journal of Affective Disorders, 5,* 191–197.

Young, W., Knowles, J., MacLean, A., Boag, L., & McConville, B. J. (1982). The sleep of childhood depressives: Comparison with age matched controls. *Biological Psychiatry, 17,* 1163–1168.

Youngerman, J., & Canino, I. A. (1979). Lithium carbonate use in children and adolescents: A survey of the literature. *Archives of General Psychiatry, 34,* 216–224.

CHAPTER ELEVEN

Attention Deficit Disorder

Debra A. Murphy
William E. Pelham

Although the literature regarding attention deficit disorder (ADD) in childhood is considerable, very few studies have been conducted to investigate ADD in adolescence. One reason for this is the traditional belief that children outgrow the hyperactive syndrome at puberty. However, as Gittelman and Mannuzza (1985) have noted, this view of ADD is clearly outdated. The persistence of ADD into adolescence and adulthood for a large number of children diagnosed during their childhood has been documented in a number of studies (e.g., Borland & Heckman, 1976; Mendelson, Johnson, & Stewart, 1971; Satterfield, Hoppe, & Schell, 1982; Weiss & Hechtman, 1986).

Hyperactivity or ADD (terms that will be used interchangeably when the diagnostic category is being discussed) is one of the most commonly reported clinical problems of childhood. Children with this disorder comprise the largest category of child referrals to child and family outpatient treatment clinics (Ross & Ross, 1982). More than 2% of the elementary school children in North America, approximately 600,000 children, receive psychostimulant medication for the treatment of ADD (Lambert, Sandoval, & Sassone, 1978; Sprague & Gadow, 1976). Even if only 50 to 75% of these children continue to exhibit ADD symptomatology through adolescence—and these are the estimates of persistence of the disorder into adolescence found in a number of follow-up studies—the number of ADD adolescents is extremely high compared to what was once believed.

The purpose of this chapter is to review briefly what is know about the symptomatology, treatment, and prognosis of ADD in adolescence. Because so much more has been written regarding ADD in prepubertal children (see for comprehensive discussions, Barkley, 1981; Campbell, 1985; Pelham, 1982), we will at times draw from that literature in our discussion of ADD in adolescence. In addition, especially with regard to behavioral treatment, we will draw from methods that have been used to treat delinquency and other externalizing disorders of adolescence, as it is likely that a substantial number of the adolescents treated in these studies would have been diagnosed as ADD in childhood. In the course of the review, some reasons for past beliefs regarding adolescent ADD will be suggested, and directions for future research will be delineated.

DIAGNOSTIC AND DEVELOPMENTAL CONSIDERATIONS

It is important to note at the outset that the disorder of ADD in adolescents is different from most other adolescent psychiatric disorders. All of the studies that have investigated ADD in adolescence are follow-up studies; that is, all of the adolescents studied were diagnosed as ADD when they were children. ADD is a diagnosis given in childhood, and adolescents with the diagnosis are those individuals in whom the disorder has persisted. It is quite rare for an adolescent without a childhood history of ADD to receive an ADD diagnosis. Therefore, in studies reported here, the term *ADD adolescents* will refer to adolescents who were diagnosed in childhood as having ADD.

The diagnostic picture of adolescent ADD is complicated by the fact that ADD with hyperactivity is defined in the DSM-III (APA, 1980) in terms of developmentally inappropriate levels of inattention, impulsivity, and hyperactivity. Because children's attention span, impulse control, and control over activity level improve dramatically with age, children with these problems appear to improve as they become adolescents. The same *absolute* levels of these symptoms that would warrant an ADD diagnosis in a child would rarely if ever be found in an adolescent. For example, because of developmental changes in activity level, DSM-III included a diagnosis of ADD, residual type, for individuals who no longer showed signs of hyperactivity but whose symptoms of inattention and impulsivity had persisted. Deficits in attention, impulse control, and subtle forms of excessive activity continue to exist in adolescents with ADD, although identifying those deficits is considerably more complicated than it is in children. These issues—(1) that the primary diagnostic criteria for ADD are relatively more difficult to identify in the adolescent than in younger children and (2) that a childhood history of ADD must be verified retrospectively to make the diagnosis in adolescence—complicate the diagnosis of ADD in adolescents.

Definition of ADD

A consensus definition of ADD has never been developed. For clinical purposes, the definitions that have been most widely used are those provided in the DSM-III and its revision, DSM-III-R (APA, 1987). The DSM-III defined ADD in terms of developmentally inappropriate degrees of inattention, impulsivity, and hyperactivity. In DSM-III behavioral descriptors of these three core symptoms are listed (e.g., "often fails to finish things he or she starts" is a descriptor of the core symptom of inattention), and in order for the presence of a core symptom to be verified, suspected cases must exhibit a specified number of these descriptors (e.g., three inattention descriptors) to a degree that is developmentally inappropriate.

The definition of ADD has been changed in the DSM-III-R (where it has been renamed Attention-deficit Hyperactivity Disorder [ADHD]), but the changes are somewhat controversial, and it is not clear whether the revised definition will gain widespread acceptance. The requirement that a child exhibit each of the three core symptoms has been dropped. Instead, all of the behavioral descriptors have been listed as a group, and a child can be diagnosed if any combination of 8 of the 13 symptoms is present to a developmentally inappropriate degree. For both the DSM-III and the DSM-III-R definitions, the particular difficulty in making a diagnosis of ADD in an adolescent comes in determining the degree to which the symptoms are present to a developmentally inappropriate degree. We shall discuss that process later.

As noted, the DSM definitions are the most commonly used for clinical purposes. The current research conceptualization of ADD is consistent with DSM-III and DSM-III-R definitions in some ways. One of the most influential researchers has described ADD as a constitutional predisposition toward deficits in four major areas: (1) impaired ability to invest, organize, and maintain attention and effort; (2) deficits in the inhibition of impulsive responding; (3) problems in modulation of arousal levels to meet situation demands; and (4) a strong inclination to seek immediate reinforcement (Douglas, 1983). In contrast, Barkley (1982) has defined ADD as a significant deficiency in age-appropriate attention, impulse control, and rule-governed behavior.

Whatever the definition, across all of the shifts in thinking regarding salient features of ADD and throughout its various labels (e.g., hyperkinetic-impulse disorder, minimal brain dysfunction, hyperkinesis, hyperactivity, ADD with or without hyperactivity, and attention-deficit/hyperactivity disorder), two conclusions drawn by Douglas (Douglas & Peters, 1979) have consistently been supported by research and appear in the DSM-III and DSM-III-R definitions. These are that ADD children have an inability to: (1) sustain attention, and (2) inhibit responding in task situations requiring focused, directed, and organized effort. Because of these deficits in attention and impulse control, ADD children have difficulty in tasks and social situations that require organized, planful, and strategic behavior that is consistent with social norms. These symptoms of ADD thus result in deficits in a number of areas of functioning, such as academic performance; relationships with parents, teachers, peers, and siblings; and self-concept. In childhood, these problems are manifested in lower grades and more retentions than expected, given the ADD child's intelligence. Further, prepubescent ADD children exhibit high levels of noncompliance to adult requests and commands; as a result, teachers and parents have a larger number of controlling negative interactions with ADD children than with controls (Barkley & Cunningham, 1979). These problems in the social sphere are especially obvious in the area of peer relations. Teachers, mothers, and peers report severe disturbances in ADD children's peer relations. Particularly salient are peer ratings, which have revealed ADD children to be intensely disliked (Pelham & Bender, 1982) and which have been confirmed in observational studies (Milich & Landau, 1982; Pelham & Milich, 1984). No doubt as a result of their repeated failure in academic and social spheres, ADD children have very low levels of self-esteem.

Given the problems exhibited by prepubertal ADD children, one of the questions that remains is whether the symptomatology for adolescents is the same as, or at least similar to, that for ADD children. This question is of primary importance, because it leads to the second question of interest: Should measures used for childhood diagnoses be used for adolescent diagnosis? In order to formulate a tentative answer to the first question, a review of the available studies regarding the nature of the disorder in adolescents is necessary.

CLINICAL PROBLEMS

As noted, the symptoms of ADD lead to difficulties for prepubertal children in a number of functional areas, including academic performance and social relationships. For adolescents, the number of areas affected by ADD symptomatology broadens. This is not surprising given that the social environment of an adolescent extends far beyond the single classroom and nuclear family settings that younger children experience. For example, a young ADD boy who impulsively pockets a candy bar in the mother's company at the grocery store and is caught is chastised by this mother or the clerk and punished at home. In contrast, an adolescent ADD child who impulsively pockets a cassette at the record store and is caught comes into contact with the legal authorities for shoplifting. Similarly, a second grader who talks back to the teacher may be kept in at recess and receive a note to his or her mother. In contrast, a 10th grader who talks back to a teacher is likely to be suspended or, if the student talks back repeatedly, expelled. In the follow-up studies in the following sections, therefore, we shall discuss not only cognitive and academic functioning and social relationships, but also concordance with societal norms, which will include findings regarding ADD adolescents' rates of school dropout, criminal offenses, referrals for psychiatric care, and rates of institutionalization for delinquency or psychopathology.

Cognitive and Academic Deficits

As previously noted, the core cognitive deficits of prepubescent ADD children are inattention and impulsivity. These difficulties have been identified on laboratory tasks that tap vigilance or sustained attention and impulse control (Douglas, 1983; Milich & Kramer, 1984, for reviews). ADD children have great difficulty performing a vigilance task that requires them to attend to a task for a period of time and to respond to the presence of infrequent targets. Their impulsivity is shown on tasks as an inability to withhold response to a target stimulus or acting before fully understanding a problem or before giving adequate time to a possible solution. These well-documented deficits in young ADD children have been little studied in adolescents, and an important question has been whether these core deficits improve with age.

In an early study, the cognitive styles of 13- to 16-year-old teenagers (who 5 years previously had been diagnosed as hyperactive) were investigated (Cohen, Weiss, & Minde, 1972) to determine if subjects exhibited a style characterized by impulsivity and inattention compared to normal controls of similar age and intelligence. ADD adolescents exhibited a similar pattern of inefficient approaches to problem-solving situations as did hyperactive children. They took less time than control subjects in reflecting over problem solutions when numerous alternative solutions were available and therefore showed a greater number of impulsive errors. Hyperactives also took a longer time to correctly find figures embedded in a complex background. The authors suggested that adolescent hyperactives were not impaired in their ability to perform tasks involving highly overlearned abilities even under distracting conditions but that they did show deficiencies on more complex tasks that had a greater degree of response uncertainty. Consistent with these findings is Nuechterlein's (1983) report that hyperactive young adolescents were not different from controls on a *d'* measure of performance on a vigilance task—presumably their ability to sustain attention had improved with age—but that they had greater difficulty than controls inhibiting responses to perceptually degraded stimuli.

In another report from the Canadian investigators, adolescents diagnosed as hyperactive 5 years previously were compared to a control group on 11 cognitive tests measuring sustained attention, visual-motor skills, abstraction, reading ability, self-esteem, activity level, social functioning, academic status, and career aspirations (Hoy, Weiss, Minde, & Cohen, 1979). The ADD adolescent group performed more poorly on the sustained attention, visual-motor, and motor tasks, and on two of four reading tests. In addition, they had lower ratings of self-esteem and sociability on self-report measures.

Other studies of cognitive functioning in adolescent hyperactives have reported that problems in attention and impulse control continue, as measured on a variety of psychological tasks or as reflected in electrophysiological measures such as evoked potentials (Loiselle, Stamm, Maitinsky, & Whipple, 1980; Satterfield & Braley, 1977; White, Barratt, & Adams, 1979). However, the pattern of ADD-control differences is neither as consistent nor as dramatic as is obtained with younger children. Why the ADD-control differences appear to be less in adolescents than in younger children is not yet clear. Whether the core cognitive deficits of the ADD children have improved to the point where the adolescents perform as well as normals on some cognitive tasks or whether the tasks that are being used to compare them to controls are too easy to discriminate true differences between groups is unclear at this point.

That this latter explanation may account for the lack of clear findings on laboratory tasks is supported by studies investigating self-reported cognitive deficits of ADD adolescents. These studies have shown that the adolescents clearly continue to exhibit the core symptoms of inattention, impulsivity, and restlessness. For example, Stewart, Mendelson, and Johnson (1973) interviewed a group of 81 adolescents ages 12 to 16 who had been diagnosed as hyperactive 2 to 5 years earlier. Most subjects reported that they were restless, impulsive, and easily upset. Nearly half of the subjects reported that they had difficulty concentrating and finishing tasks. Sixty-seven percent of the subjects indicated that they said things without thinking, had a quick temper, and were irritable. Similarly, in a more recent follow-up study, restlessness and hyperactivity, inattention, and impulsivity were all reported by 19-year-old formerly diagnosed adolescents to continue to be problems (Gittelman & Mannuzza, 1985).

Cognitive and behavioral deficits such as those reported appear to take their toll in the area of academic performance. Two-thirds of ADD adolescents are serious discipline problems in school, with high rates of school suspensions and expulsions found (Mendelson, Johnson, & Stewart, 1971; Weiss & Hechtman, 1986). Fifty to 70% of adolescent hyperactives have average failing grades in high school and have failed at least one grade in school; half of these failed two grades (Dykman & Ackerman, 1980; Hussey & Cohen, 1976; Weiss, Hechtman, Perlman, Hopkins, & Wener, 1979; Weiss, Minde, Werry, Douglas, & Nemeth, 1971). Hyperactive children followed up for 10 years, until they were age 17 to 24, were rated by teachers and employers (Weiss, Hechtman, & Perlman, 1978). Hyperactive subjects were rated by employers as functioning as competently at work as do normals. Teachers, however, saw the hyperactives during their final year of high school as performing significantly less well on a number of variables compared to matched normal controls.

In addition to noting cognitive and academic deficits, follow-up studies have also focused on the percentages of adolescents still needing treatment, rates of school dropout and criminal offenses, and rates of later referral for psychiatric care or institutionalization for delinquency or psychopathology. Estimates as to the percentages of adolescents who still experience difficulty after having had a childhood diagnosis of hyperactivity have been offered by Lambert, Hartsough, Sassone, and Sandoval (1987). One hundred-seventeen boys, identified from an epidemiological sample as hyperactive 3 to 4 years prior to the time of the study, were followed to a minimum age of 12 (mean age = 14). Twenty percent of the sample showed no evidence of problems at follow-up; that is, they were not considered to be still hyperactive by parents, teachers, or physicians. Thirty-seven percent were no longer under treatment, but were reported to still be experiencing residual problems. Forty-three percent were still being treated and exhibited learning and behavior problems.

These figures are consistent with the much earlier studies of clinical cases previously cited (Stewart et al., 1973; Mendelson et al., 1971). In the Mendelson et al. study, formerly diagnosed children were evaluated at the ages of 12 to 16. Five percent of the mothers interviewed reported no signs of hyperactivity or other problems at follow-up; an additional 5% said their children were well-adjusted as long as their stimulant medication regimen was maintained; 55% of the children were said to be improved relative to the initial contact but still exhibiting problems; and the remaining 35% were seen by their mothers as unchanged or worse. The major referral complaints were overactivity, poor school performance, and behavior problems at home and school. At follow-up, 74% were still reported to be defiant and hard to discipline; 56% exhibited temper tantrums; and 40 to 50% had feelings of rejection from peers, failure in school, and low self-confidence. Police contact had occurred among 59% of the children, and the psychiatric interviewer found that 22% were exhibiting antisocial behavior and predicted that a diagnosis of sociopathy in adulthood would be likely.

A more recent follow-up of adolescent ADD children found the poorest outcome for ADD children that has yet been reported (Satterfield et al., 1982). These investigators followed 110 boys (who had been referred to an outpatient clinic for hyperactive children) and a group of matched controls. At the time of follow-up, the mean age of the ADD adolescents was 17.3 (range 14 to 21). Arrest for serious crimes (robbery, burglary, grand theft automobile, and assault with a deadly weapon) was the measure of interest. Rates of both single and multiple arrests were significantly higher for the ADD group, as was the rate of institutionalization for delinquency. For lower, middle, and upper socioeconomic classes, the rates of at least one arrest were 58, 36, and 52% for the ADD children, respectively; and 11, 9, and 2% for the matched controls. Twenty-five percent of the ADD adolescents had been institutionalized compared to 1% of the controls. These disturbing figures indicate that ADD children, especially those from upper SES families, are at a high risk compared to controls for serious criminal behavior in late adolescence. It should be emphasized that these data were obtained directly from courts rather than subject's report.

In contrast to the findings of Satterfield et al., Weiss and colleagues (1979) reported a more benign outcome for ADD children. Their hyperactive subjects, 17- to 24-years old at the time of a 10-year follow-up evaluation, were found to have less education, a history of more motor vehicle accidents, and more geographical moves than matched controls. However, only a small percentage of the hyperactive group were still exhibiting antisocial behavior or severe psychopathology. More frequent diagnoses of impulsive and immature personality trait disturbances were found among the hyperactive subjects. In addition, there was a trend for more hyperactive subjects to have had one or more court referrals in the 5 years prior to the follow-up, but not in the year immediately prior to the follow-up. This same pattern was found for use of drugs, mainly hashish and marijuana.

Some researchers have suggested that early and middle adolescence is the most problematic development period for previously diagnosed hyperactive boys, and therefore outcomes at that time may not represent a clear picture of their long-term risk for maladjustment (Gittelman, Mannuzza, Shenker, & Bonagura, 1985). In a study of 101 male adolescents who had been diagnosed as hyperactive when children, Gittelman et al. reported that 31% of the probands' attention deficit disorder with hyperactivity (ADD-H) persisted when they were followed up at age 16 to 23, compared to 3% of the control group. Their results indicated a reduction in functional problems for the hyperactive group across the ages 13 to 18. However, two variables that distinguished the hyperactive group from the control group were conduct disorder and substance abuse, which were more prevalent among the probands with ADD-H. They concluded that the continuance of ADD-H symptomatology indicates risk for the development of concurrent drug use and conduct disorder. Others also have reported that hyperactive children have been found to be at higher risk for teenage alcohol use than children who have school difficulties but are not hyperactive (Blouin, Bornstein, & Trites, 1978).

Although this discussion has shown that many if not most ADD children continue to exhibit serious problems in adolescence, the studies we have reviewed differ dramatically in their rates of adolescent problems. Not all of the children continue to have difficulties, and a critical question has been whether predictors of adolescent continuance can be identified. Given that many of the problems noted in these studies have been typically subsumed under the diagnosis of conduct disorder, it should not be surprising that childhood aggressiveness has been implicated as a good predictor of adolescent outcome among ADD children. Milich and Loney (1979) were the first to note that the presence of concurrent aggression appeared to place ADD children at great risk for continued problems, and their conclusions have been validated in a number of recent studies (Loney, Kramer, & Milich, 1981; August, Stewart, & Holmes, 1983; Johnston & Pelham, 1986).

Unfortunately, aggression was typically not measured systematically in early studies, and much of the data used to predict outcome is inferential. For example, Douglas (1985) has noted that she believes the difference between findings of the Montreal follow-up studies and Satterfield's Los Angeles studies resulted from the fact that the Montreal researchers made a systematic effort to exclude children with concurrent aggression. One adolescent outcome study that subgrouped their sample into "pure" hyperactive versus hyperactive and aggressive groups was conducted by August et al. (1983). Their sample consisted of pure hyperactives and hyperactive, unsocialized-aggressive males followed up 4 years after their original diagnosis. Subjects previously diagnosed as purely hyperactive showed little evidence of aggressive or antisocial behaviors at follow-up, in spite of the fact that inattention and impulsivity were still significant problems for this group. Overactivity was rated as less of a problem than it had been when they were children. On the other hand, hyperactive boys who had problems with aggression at the time of diagnosis continued to be inattentive, impulsive, and overactive. In addition, a significant proportion of the hyperactive boys who exhibited concurrent aggression continued to have conduct disorder problems; August et al. diagnosed 37% of this group as having major aggressive conduct disorder. They concluded that hyperactivity in children does not lead to major behavior problems in adolescence—that while inattention and impulsivity remain stable cognitive styles, antisocial and delinquent behaviors in adolescence depend on the early presence of aggression. As noted, this is the only subgrouping study reported here.

A multivariate model of the relationship between the hyperactive child and environmental variables and adolescent outcome variables has been developed by Loney, Kramer, and Milich (1981). Their data also suggest that aggression and hyperactivity have different consequences. Anticipated links between childhood hyperactivity and adolescent delinquency were not found. The single significant predictor of aggressive interpersonal behavior at adolescence was child aggression at referral, while predictors of hyperactive symptoms at follow-up included hyperactivity, lower socioeconomic status, child aggression, and perinatal complications.

A slightly different picture has emerged from the Cambridge study in delinquent development of boys from London (Farrington, Loeber, & van Kammen, 1987). In this epidemiological study, subjects were classified as hyperactive-impulsive-attention deficit or conduct problems at the ages of 8 to 10. The hyperactive group tended to be convicted of a crime at an early age and tended to become juvenile delinquents and chronic offenders, while the conduct problem group also tended to become chronic offenders, but convictions occurred at all ages. For example, the percentages of juvenile (ages 10 to 16) convictions for the normal control quartile of the sample, for the conduct problem group, for the hyperactive quartile, and for the quartile that exhibited both hyperactivity and conduct problems were 12.6, 35, 23.5, and 45.8, respectively. In summary, this study indicates that hyperactivity alone may predict juvenile delinquency problems.

An important question that has not been addressed in the majority of follow-up studies thus far is whether *treatment* influences the course of prognosis. Hechtman, Weiss, and Perlman (1984) followed up children diagnosed through adolescence and young adulthood who received 3 years of sustained stimulant medication between the ages 6 to 12. The drug was discontinued when the children had begun their growth spurt or when subjects were thought to be sufficiently improved. The normal control group consisted of former classmates of the stimulant-treated hyperactives who had experienced no significant problems academically or behaviorally in school. Another group of hyperactives, that did not receive stimulant medication, was also used as a control condition. Several findings are noteworthy. There were a few areas in which the treated hyperactives showed a better outcome than the untreated hyperactives, including: fewer car accidents, remembering their childhood more positively, less stealing throughout elementary school, fewer problems with aggression, less need for current psychiatric treatment, and better social skills and self-esteem. At the time of follow-up, the use of alcohol did not differ for all of the groups. However, more untreated hyperactives were involved with heroin. The investigators concluded that their findings supported other results indicating that there does not appear to be an association between stimulant treatment and increased use of nonmedical drugs. Overall, they concluded that stimulant treatment in childhood probably does not eliminate later adjustment problems in the areas of education, occupation, and personal situations, but it may result in less social ostracism and better self-esteem.

Comments. It is apparent from the studies reviewed here that ADD adolescents show some of the deficits also found in ADD children. These deficits may include continued attentional problems, impulsivity, inefficient approaches to problem solving, oppositional behavior, delinquency, and continued problematic levels of overactivity or restlessness. The percentage of adolescents who were diagnosed as hyperactive when they were children and continued to experience problems and the nature of the problems they experienced varied somewhat across studies. There is a consensus that the majority of children diagnosed as ADD will continue to have problems into their adolescence, with percentages of ADD children who continue to experience problems at adolescence ranging from 50 to 80%, although the severity of these problems varies across outcome studies to some extent. One major predictor for a poorer prognosis appears to be concurrence of childhood aggression. Those ADD children who are also aggressive appear to be at much greater risk for continuing to have serious problems in adolescence than those who are not. However, the Satterfield study, the Loney findings, and the Farrington et al. conclusions are somewhat discrepant regarding whether aggression alone is predictive of later juvenile delinquency problems or whether hyperactivity alone is also predictive. In the Farrington et al. study, the sample size was small and consisted of lower-class, intercity boys. Further investigation and replication of all of these findings is necessary.

It has been suggested by a number of investigators (Cantwell, 1979; Clampit & Pirkle, 1983; Wender, 1983) that for many ADD adolescents, some of the salient characteristics of childhood ADD, such as overactivity, may decline in adolescence, with other symptoms becoming primary. Cognitive dysfunction, antisocial behavior, underachievement, depression, learning disabilities, and low self-esteem have all been shown to become predominant in ADD adolescents. As this review has shown, school failure and antisocial behavior clearly are present in a number of ADD children followed to adolescence.

DIAGNOSIS OF ADD ADOLESCENTS

Methods of obtaining information for diagnosis of ADD children have included parent, teacher, and self-rating scales, diagnostic interview, observational data, laboratory measures, or a combination of these methods. The rationale and studies of the use of these methods for the diagnosis of ADD in adolescence will be reviewed here.

Parent, Teacher, and Self-Rating Scales

Numerous standardized parent and teacher rating scales have been used as diagnostic instruments for ADD with children, such as the parent-teacher Abbreviated Conners Ratings Scale and the full Conners Teacher and Parent Rating Scales (Conners, 1969; Goyette, Conners, & Ulrich, 1978); the IOWA Conners Teacher Rating Scale (Loney & Milich, 1982; Murphy, Pelham, & Milich, 1985); the Child Behavior Checklist (CBCL) for parents and teachers (Achenbach, 1978; Achenbach & Edelbrock, 1979); the revised Behavior Problem Checklist (Quay & Peterson, 1983); the ADD-H Comprehensive Teacher's Rating Scale (Ullman, Sleator, & Sprague, 1985); and the Swanson, Nolan, and Pelham (SNAP) Rating Scale (Pelham, Atkins, Murphy, & Swanson, 1985). Teacher and parent rating scales have been found to be extremely helpful in the assessment of childhood ADD. They discriminate well between diagnosed children and normals and between stimulant treated and untreated children. For most of these checklists, however, normative data are available only for elementary-age children. The Behavior Problem Checklist has norms through the eighth grade; however, the numbers of seventh and eighth grade students in the normative sample are too small to provide helpful information. The CBCL has norms up through 16 years of age and is the only rating scale that can be used currently for gathering information for diagnosis of adolescent ADD. However, the CBCL does not have items or factors that are tied directly to DSM-III or DSM-III-R. It needs to be determined if the other rating scales should be adapted for adolescents, and if so, normative studies need to be conducted to obtain data on adolescent populations.

Adolescents' teachers may prove to be less useful informants than children's teachers, because at higher grade levels, teachers have much less contact with their students (Klorman, 1985). Therefore, collecting ratings from a number of teachers should be considered. In addition, Klorman has suggested that elevated ratings by a majority of teachers, but not all teachers, may be all that is required for diagnosis of ADD, in conjunction with parent report.

When rating scale information is gathered on prepubescent children, parents and teachers are the raters. Self-ratings by children age 6 to 9 do not correlate significantly with adult ratings and are thus thought to be invalid (Edelbrock, Costello, Dulcan, Kalas, & Conover, 1985). Given that adolescents are more cognitively mature and possibly able to self-monitor better than children, a question related to collecting rating scale information to diagnose adolescent ADD is whether the client should complete self-ratings. Klee and Garfinkel (1983) asked 27 boys (mean age 17.4) formerly diagnosed and treated for ADD with stimulant medication to complete two versions of a modification of the Conners Behavior Rating Scale that had questions regarding current and past functioning. Subjects also underwent an interview by a psychiatrist. Subjects were divided into residual and nonresidual groups. One-third of the former ADD children were diagnosed as having residual ADD. Residual subjects more frequently were involved in family therapy and had a record of poorer academics and of more grades repeated than did the nonresidual group. However, these investigators found that on self-report, residual and nonresidual groups did not differentiate themselves.

Diagnostic Interviews

Gittelman and Mannuzza (1985) interviewed 86 children formerly diagnosed as hyperactives and 95 of their parents, in addition to control children and their parents. Subjects were ages 16 to 23 at the time of the interview. The interview consisted of questions from standard teenager and parent interview schedules and were tailored to meet DSM-III criteria of ADD. Information both on the presence of attention deficit, impulsivity, and hyperactivity, and on the severity of each symptom was obtained. Twenty-four percent of the probands had all three symptoms of ADD-H (attention deficit, impulsivity, and hyperactivity), compared to 3% of the control group. It appeared that more valid diagnostic information was obtained from parental reports. Gittelman and Mannuzza concluded that diagnosis of ADD adolescents can be conducted using interviews but it is important to obtain clinical information from parents, as is the case with diagnosis of childhood ADD.

Comments. In summary, procedures for diagnosing ADD adolescents require extensive research. Regarding the rating scales, the items for adolescents need investigation, as many child rating scale items will not be applicable for adolescents. In addition, when this first step has been undertaken, normative data on adolescent ages are needed for the majority of ADD parent and teacher rating scales, and collection of such data will be a major undertaking. A similar amount of research is needed in the area of diagnostic interviews with adolescents. Apparently, questions remain as to the value of obtaining self-reports from adolescents. However, it does seem clear that rating scales and parent interviews similar to those used for the diagnosis of children are useful and that the triad of inattention, impulsivity, and overactivity should remain as the major variables of interest.

Brown and Borden (1986) have suggested that, for purposes of research, it would be best to use similar assessment instruments for diagnosis of childhood and adolescent ADD in order to allow comparisons of reports across different age cohorts. However, this may neither be feasible nor useful. New measures developed specifically for an adolescent's environment are needed, so that multiassessment approaches to diagnosis in childhood can be used with adolescents. For example, an important question that was not addressed in this section due to the lack of empirical investigation on the topic was that of direct observation and laboratory measures for diagnosis of ADD adolescents. Work on the efficacy of direct observation of ADD children for diagnosis is currently being conducted, but procedures have not been developed to the extent that they can be used in purely clinical settings. Some dependent variables used for children, such as fidgeting, out-of-seat behavior, and calling out in class, may not be relevant for adolescents. Observational coding systems, such as comprehension tests after lectures are presented, amount of note taking, and other measures more specific to an adolescent's environment, may be more useful than trying to rely or expand on measures employed with ADD children.

While the work continues in the area for ADD children, new work needs to begin regarding ADD adolescents. Similarly, although laboratory measures such as continuous performance tasks have proven useful in group studies to determine information processing deficits among ADD children and adolescents, they also are not sufficiently developed to diagnose individual cases (Milich, Pelham, & Hinshaw, 1986).

PHARMACOLOGICAL APPROACHES

Despite the fact that it is very common for children who have been diagnosed as ADD to be treated with stimulant medication, clinical tradition has been that such treatment should not be used for adolescents. Although this view is widespread, there are no empirical data to support it. In fact, as will be seen later in this section, recent studies have reported results that support the opposite view—that stimulant treatment is appropriate and effective for at least a portion of ADD adolescents.

As Klorman (1986) has noted, it has been known for some time that stimulants affect normal adults, normal children, and ADD children in the same way (Rapoport et al., 1980). It would indeed be surprising if ADD adolescents were affected differently. How did the belief that stimulant medication should not be used with ADD adolescents become so widespread and entrenched? Clampit and Pirkle (1983) have offered a list of possible reasons why psychostimulants are thought to be an effective treatment only until a child reaches adolescence. The first factor that they cite as a possible cause concerns psychostimulant dosage levels. Clampit and Pirkle suggest that dosages insufficient to maintain improvements that were found in childhood may be administered to adolescents, thereby falsely supporting the belief that this treatment stops working at the onset of adolescence. A child who has been receiving a given dose of psychostimulant and has shown a clinically efficacious response to that dosage may not show an efficacious response if he or she increases in body weight.

The second hypothesis offered by Clampit and Pirkle as to why psychostimulants are not used for ADD adolescents is that the majority of adolescents' academic study time may be during hours when they are not medicated. This fact leads to the appearance that medication has ceased to have benefits on academic work. That is, in middle schools or junior high schools, much academic work is done during afternoon or evening homework sessions and on weekends. If medication is still given at breakfast and at noon, as is typical, there will be no medication effect for the majority of the time adolescents spend on academic work.

The third and perhaps most influential reason that psychostimulants have not been widely used with adolescents is that many professionals believe ADD goes away during adolescence and stimulants are no longer necessary (Cantwell, 1979; Klorman, 1986). As we discussed earlier, however, the core symptoms of ADD improve in *absolute* levels as children mature, and although these improvements may give the *appearance* that many adolescents have outgrown their problems, the disorder does not remit for a large percentage of these children. Cognitive dysfunction in the form of inattention and impulsivity continues to be a serious problem associated with ADD during adolescence. Therefore, although the topography of symptoms may change, problems still exist that may be amenable to treatment by psychostimulants.

Pharmacotherapy with ADD Adolescents

Possibly due to the traditional beliefs surrounding the use of psychostimulants with ADD adolescents, few studies investigating medication trials with this population have been conducted. However, of the few studies that have been conducted, a consensus seems to be building that stimulant drug therapy can be efficacious for ADD adolescents. For example, in an early series of case studies, Safer and Allen (1975) reported the effect of psychostimulant treatment on the classroom behavior of 38 ADD subjects treated with stimulants between 1969 and 1974. They compared drug responsiveness in three groups of children: (1) those who took stimulants only as children; (2) those who took stimulants as adolescents; and (3) those who were medicated from childhood through adolescence. They found a very high rate of positive drug response across all three groups. Therefore, ADD adolescents achieved the same clinical benefit judged by teacher ratings as did ADD children. Improvement in academic grades also has been used as a measure of the effectiveness of psychostimulant treatment with adolescents (Mackay, Beck, & Taylor, 1973). Subjects showed increased competence in school performance on medication ranging from small, significant advances to extreme improvement.

Similar findings were reported in a double-blind, placebo-controlled, crossover study with 22 adolescents age 13 to 18, all of whom had been diagnosed as attention deficit disorder, hyperactive, or minimal brain dysfunctioned at some time and had been noted to be stimulant responders (Varley, 1983). Adolescents with a concurrent conduct disorder by DSM-III criteria were excluded. Subjects received 0.15 mg/kg methylphenidate, 0.3 mg/kg methylphenidate, or placebo for 1 week each. Seventy-two percent of the subjects continued to show improvement on the Conners Abbreviated Parent/Teacher Questionnaire and on daily narratives regarding the subjects' behavior and school performance completed by their teachers. The investigators concluded that there was evidence of persistence of both symptoms and drug effect among their adolescent subject group.

A recent study has extended these findings by broadening the range of measures of drug effect (Coons, Korman, & Borgstedt, 1987; Klorman, Coons, & Borgstadt, 1987). Nineteen ADD adolescents were evaluated in a blind, crossover with placebo and 40 mg/day methylphenidate (15 mg with breakfast and lunch and 10 mg at 4:00 P.M.). Both clinical measures (Conners rating scales completed by parents and teachers) and laboratory measures (e.g., continuous performance task and measures of cortical evoked potential during task performance) were taken. Parents rated 56% of the adolescents as improved on medication weeks, an evaluation agreed with by 35% of the adolescents themselves. In contrast, teacher ratings revealed only weak effects of medication. The laboratory measures showed significant effects of methylphenidate that were as substantive as those that have been obtained with ADD children.

Thus an uncontrolled trial reported in the 1970s and two recent controlled trials show that psychostimulant medication appears to continue to exert the same effect on ADD adolescents as it does on ADD children. However, numerous issues regarding the suitability of stimulant treatment for adolescents remain unresolved. For example, the Varley (1983) study, using subjects previously identified as responders to stimulants, reported the same rate of medication response, approximately 70%, that is commonly cited for stimulant response in ADD children (Cantwell & Carlson, 1978; Gittelman & Kanner, 1986). In contrast, Klorman et al. medicated adolescents unselected for response to stimulants and reported only a 50% response rate. It appears that the proportion of ADD adolescents who respond to stimulants may be lower than that which responds in childhood.

This would be consistent with findings for stimulant treatment of adults, which report improvement rates of only 40% (Mattes & Gittelman, 1981). Further, Varley's findings imply that 30% of ADD children who show a positive response to stimulants will no longer show a positive response as adolescents.

Some of the factors that Clampit and Pirkle cited as reasons why stimulants may not have been used with adolescents may contribute to a reduced rate of medication response. For example, doses typically used with adolescents may be too low. It is the norm for an ADD child who is medicated to require higher doses of stimulant as weight increases. This leads to the prediction that higher doses will be needed by adolescents. Indeed, the doses employed in both controlled studies were relatively low, between 0.15 and 0.3 mg/kg, and nonresponders may have been simply children whose doses were insufficient. It is also the case, however, that adults cannot tolerate as high doses of stimulants as children (Cantwell & Carlson, 1978). This suggests that adolescents may *not* need higher doses to respond. It is not clear where ADD adolescents fall on this spectrum. Do they need increased doses because their weight is increasing, or do they need decreased doses because their bodies begin to metabolize medication as adults? Clearly, dosage is a variable that has been little studied in adolescents, and additional research is warranted.

As previously discussed, a second factor limiting ADD adolescents' response to stimulants may be the lack of overlap between medication time and study time. We have speculated that failure to demonstrate beneficial effects on academic tasks in ADD children may result in part from lack of overlap between the time when the children perform their academic tasks and the time of peak medication effectiveness (Pelham, 1983). Further, not only the timing of stimulant administration but also the nature of the academic task appears to be a critical determinant of whether drug effects will be obtained on academic performance (Pelham, 1986).

For example, the classroom measures on which clearly beneficial stimulant effects have been reported for ADD children have been daily measures of accuracy and productivity on teacher-supervised reading and math tasks and on teacher-supervised seatwork (Pelham, Bender, Caddell, Booth, & Moorer, 1985; Pelham & Hoza, 1987; Pelham et al., 1987). These effects may be mediated by stimulant effects on sustained attention (Pelham, 1986). Mainstreamed children in junior high school typically engage in different kinds of tasks, however. Adolescent schoolroom tasks typically involve listening to lectures, watching educational films, taking notes, and taking tests. Sustained attention may not be the key stage of information processing that mediates performance in such tasks. In any case, studies of stimulant effects on these types of academic tasks have not been conducted, and it is therefore unclear whether stimulants will improve performance on typical academic tasks in ADD adolescents.

In addition to task variables, the effects of stimulant therapy are in part a function of concurrent environmental conditions (Pelham, 1983, 1986; Whalen, Henker, Collins, McAuliffe, & Vaux, 1979). Stimulant effects in school depend in part on the structure that the teacher establishes in the classroom and the contingencies that he or she arranges to encourage the students to complete assigned tasks. In junior high school, these concurrent environmental conditions may be dramatically different from those that exist in elementary school, in that less structure and fewer contingencies may be present. For example, an adolescent changes classes and teachers every 45 to 60 minutes. Different teachers dealing with different subjects almost certainly have different rules and different expectations of the children, yielding a less consistent environment than would typically be present for an elementary-age ADD child with one teacher in one classroom for the entire day. Further, teachers in middle school settings typically place a great deal of responsibility on the students to organize and complete their own work. This contrasts with grade school teachers who constantly monitor and prompt children's performance. All of these differences between grade schools and junior high or middle schools may decrease stimulant effects (see also Clampit & Pirkle, 1983).

Compliance with a medication regimen may be a major treatment consideration with ADD adolescents. Lack of compliance is a clear limiting factor in medicating ADD children, particularly those from disrupted families, who tend to be ADD children with concurrent problems of conduct. Many ADD children dislike taking medication and may actively avoid doing so (Sleator, Ullman, & von Neumann, 1982). When these children become adolescents, they are likely to be especially noncompliant with a medication regimen. It may be necessary with such cases to establish behavioral programs that focus on getting the adolescents to take their medication (see following discussion).

Beyond these factors that may limit response to stimulants in adolescents, two other concerns of clinicians regarding psychostimulant treatment of ADD adolescents are later drug abuse and physical growth. Each of these concerns will be briefly addressed here. It has been found that both the use and the duration of the use of stimulant medication are not associated with subsequent drug abuse at adolescence (Kramer & Loney, 1981). In fact, Loney, Kramer, and Milich (1981) have data suggesting that a positive response to methylphenidate may be associated with a lower probability of drug abuse, a finding that has been suggested by other investigators (Beck, Langford, Mackay, & Sum, 1975). Beck et al. found that drug abuse use was more prevalent among 14- to 19-year-old adolescents in their control group than in their group of adolescents who had a history of pharmacotherapy treatment with methylphenidate.

Hechtman, Weiss, and Perlman (1984) compared stimulant-treated hyperactive children, untreated hyperactive children, and a control group on their amount of drug use in young adulthood. They concluded that stimulant-treated hyperactives did not later abuse most of a variety of illicit drugs or alcohol, but they also reported that their stimulant-treated group did show a trend toward greater use of stimulants such as cocaine. Hartsough and Lambert (1987) investigated the pattern and progression of drug use across a 1-year interval for 54 hyperactive and 47 control adolescents. The ADD adolescents had all been treated with stimulants as children. A self-report instrument querying use of a variety of drugs revealed only that there was a higher initiation and use rate of cigarettes among the hyperactive group.

Though the prognosis for hyperactive children who have not received treatment presents a slightly different picture, the overall findings for subsequent drug abuse among children who have been treated with psychostimulants do not indicate that such children are more likely to abuse drugs when they are adolescents. However, it should be noted that all of the studies reported here consisted of subject groups that had received stimulants only during childhood. Whether this finding would hold for later adult abuse of drugs by ADD *adolescents* treated with psychostimulants is not yet answered and obviously is an important question.

A second medical concern regarding treatment with psychostimulants of ADD adolescents is that of growth in height. This question has been directly addressed by Beck et al. (1975). They compared 30 adolescents ages 14 to 19 who had a childhood history of pharmacotherapy with an equal number of adolescents who were comparable in age, sex, and socioeconomic background who had been surgical inpatients. The control group had no previous psychiatric history. Findings were that methylphenidate had no perceptible effect on physical growth as measured by height.

In the study described earlier, Hechtman et al. (1984) followed up children who received 3 years of sustained stimulant medication between the ages 6 to 12, a second group of hyperactives who did not receive stimulant medication, and two control groups. No differences between the stimulant-treated hyperactives, the untreated hyperactives, or their control groups were found on physiological measures of height, weight, blood pressure, and pulse. It was concluded that stimulant treatment had not significantly affected growth or cardiovascular status. Similar results have been reported in other studies (Beck et al., 1975). We should emphasize, however, that no studies have evaluated the effects of stimulant treatment throughout childhood and adolescence on adult height. Since the suppressant effects of stimulants in growth appear to be a function of the total amount taken, stimulant treatment that occurs *throughout* childhood and adolescence might well be expected to reduce a treated child's eventual height. In this case, the risk of the lost stature needs to be compared against the benefits of long-term medication use.

Finally, we should emphasize that compared to the volume of studies of stimulant effects in childhood, only two controlled studies in adolescence constitute a very limited data base for decision making regarding such pharmacological treatment of adolescence. Of particular concern is that the range of dependent measures used by Varley and by Klorman et al. was quite narrow. Effects were shown on the Conners Teacher Rating Scale, global ratings of improvement, and CPT tasks. These measures provide only the crudest measure of stimulant effects, and they are only slightly correlated with other measures that reflect improvement in the natural environment (Pelham & Milich, 1987). It has only been in the past few years that the response to stimulants of ADD children has been comprehensively described on ecologically critical measures (see for example, Whalen et al., 1979; Pelham et al., 1985). From these studies, we have a good descriptive data base regarding stimulant effects on ADD children. These effects include improvement in on-task behavior and disruptive behavior in the classroom, increased productivity and accuracy on academic tasks, improved social interactions with other children in play settings, and improved compliance with adult requests. We do not know whether stimulants exert effects on such measures in adolescents.

We have gathered data on a small number of adolescents on these measures, and as a case example, we present one medication evaluation here. We have developed what we believe to be an assessment that measures most of the relevant aspects of a child's response to stimulants that we conduct in our summer day treatment program (Pelham & Hoza, 1987). The assessment includes direct measures of classroom behavior and academic performance measures; both prosocial and antisocial interactions with peers and adults; laboratory measures of information processing; ratings completed by teachers, parents, and others working with the children; and evaluations of medication side effects. Table 11.1 shows the data obtained on Bob, a 14-year-old ADD adolescent treated in one of our recent programs. Bob is a large boy (weight = 71.8 kgs.) who had a long history of ADD, conduct disorder, and some symptoms of depression. He had been treated with a variety of medications over the years, beginning with Ritalin and including imipramine, and lithium. He was receiving 112.5 mg Cylert q.a.m. prior to entry into the program. In conjunction with his referring psychiatrist, we decided to evaluate him on that dose of Cylert and a comparable dose of slow-release Ritalin (two slow-release tablets q.a.m.).

As the medication summary table indicates, Bob generally showed a good response to medication. This included decreases in negative verbalizations and noncompliance and improvement in on-task behavior and teacher ratings in the classroom. On the measures of seatwork in the classroom as well as on the measure of timed reading, he showed positive effects of different types (productivity or accuracy) to different medications. In

Table 11.1. **Medication Assessment Results for Bob by Dependent Variable and Medication Type**

Variable Measured	Placebo (9 Days) Avg.	SD	SR 20 mg Ritalin q.a.m. (3 Days) Avg.	SD	% Change from PL	SR 20 mg Ritalin 2 q.a.m. (6 Days) Avg.	SD	% Change from PL
Daily frequencies:								
% Following rules	82	7.99	84	14	2.42	99	10	20.72
Noncompliance	2.66	2	2	1	−24.83	1.5	1.37	−43.61
Positive peer								
behaviors	185.11	29.13	161	54.23	−13.04	228.5	52.32	23.43
Conduct problems	.55	.72	0	0	−100	0	0	−100
Negative								
verbalizations	4.1	2.03	2	1	−51.35	.83	.75	−79.82
Time outs:								
Number per day	.65	.7	0	0	−100	0	0	−100
Minutes per day	7.76	9.71	0	0	−100	0	0	−100
Average minutes								
per time out	11	2.23	—	—	—	—	—	—
Classroom:								
% On task	76.33	25.61	100	0	31	100	0	31
% Following rules	93.33	7.41	97.65	4.26	4.63	98.83	2.99	5.89
Timed math:								
Number attempted	30.32	6.27	38.32	7.05	26.36	26.5	5.6	−12.63
Percentage correct	89	13	90	15	1.12	96	5	7.85
Timed reading:								
Number attempted	16.1	11.53	26.65	9.1	65.47	16	7.4	−.69
Percentage correct	44	12	39	10	−11.38	65	14	47.71
Seatwork:								
% Completion	54	36	55	20	1.85	78	30	44.43
% Correct	59	30	82	9	38.98	80	20	35.59
Teacher rating								
(Conners short form)	8.25	6.39	1.5	2.12	−81.82	1	1	−87.88
Counselor rating	109.27	14.32	112.12	5	2.59	97.83	6.11	−10.47
Pos. daily report card								
(% of days received)	57	53	100	0	75.43	100	0	75.43
Observed interactions:								
Positive peer	99.87	1.45	100	0	.11	100	0	.11
Negative peer	.1	.32	0	0	−100	0	0	−100
No interactions	0	0	0	0	—	0	0	—

Table 11.1. *Medication Assessment Results for Bob by Dependent Variable and Medication Type (continued)*

Variable Measured	Placebo (9 Days)		56.25 mg Cylert q.a.m. (2 Days)			112.5 mg Cylert q.a.m. (4 Days)		
	Avg.	SD	Avg.	SD	% Change from PL	Avg.	SD	% Change from PL
Daily frequencies:								
% Following rules	82	7.99	87	13	6.08	93	14	13.41
Noncompliance	2.66	2	2	1.41	−24.83	.5	1	−81.22
Positive peer behaviors	185.11	29.13	175.5	27.57	−5.2	189.5	56.79	2.37
Conduct problems	.55	.72	0	0	−100	0	0	−100
Negative verbalizations	4.1	2.03	1.5	.69	−63.52	.75	.94	−81.76
Time outs:								
Number per day	.65	.7	0	0	−100	.25	.5	−62.13
Minutes per day	7.76	9.71	0	0	−100	2.5	5	−67.84
Average minutes per time out	11	2.23	—	—	—	10	0	−9.11
Classroom:								
% On task	76.33	25.61	100	0	31	100	0	31
% Following rules	93.33	7.41	100	0	7.14	96.75	6.5	3.66
Timed math:								
Number attempted	30.32	6.27	37.5	7.76	23.63	32.5	8.69	7.15
Percentage correct	89	13	91	17	2.24	82	21	−7.87
Timed reading:								
Number attempted	16.1	11.53	21.5	3.53	33.45	12.75	5.05	−20.86
Percentage correct	44	12	71	14	61.35	57	29	29.53
Seatwork:								
% Completion	54	36	86	19	59.25	70	37	29.61
% Correct	59	30	89	15	50.84	60	22	1.68
Teacher rating (Conners short form)	8.25	6.39	2	0	−75.76	5.5	.69	−33.35
Counselor rating	109.27	14.32	129.5	26.15	18.5	101	7.41	−7.58
Pos. daily report card (% of days received)	57	53	100	0	75.43	75	50	31.57
Observed interactions:								
Positive peer	99.87	1.45	100	0	.11	99.75	.5	−.15
Negative peer	.1	.32	0	0	−100	.25	.5	127.27
No interactions	0	0	0	0	—	0	0	—

addition, he had a very large increase in the number of days he received a positive daily report card when medicated as compared to placebo. In contrast to the measures taken during the day, however, measures of side effects completed by Bob's mother showed that he had a severe rebound in the evenings on days on which he received doses of Cylert; he consistently became moody, irritable, noncompliant, and disruptive. In addition, he had great difficulty sleeping on nights when he had received Cylert. Because the evaluation was double-blind and included placebo as well as another medication, it was very clear that this parent-reported rebound effect in Bob was a real one. Therefore, although he had been medicated with 112.5 mg Cylert prior to entering into the program, it was not recommended in his future treatment. When Bob's rebound to Cylert became apparent, the evaluation was modified to allow assessment of a lower dose of Cylert and a lower dose of slow-release Ritalin. Although he showed less of a rebound to the low dose of Cylert, he still consistently became worsened in the evenings on which he received Cylert.

When the two doses of Ritalin are compared in the medication summary table, it is clear that the lower dose has better effects on some measures and the higher dose has better effects on others. Because the major difficulties with Bob were his noncompliant and disruptive behavior, and because on his classroom teacher's rating, on his daily report card evaluation, and on measures of noncompliance and negative verbalizations, the low dose appeared to be as effective as the higher, it was recommended for his future treatment. The recommendation, of course, was that Bob receive medication in conjunction with a powerful behavior modification program. He was enrolled in a special school where such a program was in effect. The recommendation also allowed for an increase in medication to two tablets of slow-release Ritalin, should that become necessary.

This evaluation showed that teacher ratings, individualized targets on a daily report card, academic performance in the classroom, and direct observational measures of a variety of disruptive behaviors all showed improvement with medication. Studies that evaluate the effects of psychostimulants on adolescents that utilize a wide variety of ecologically valid measures such as these are needed before we have a comprehensive picture of the effects of stimulants in adolescence.

Comments. Even though there are numerous unresolved questions regarding stimulant therapy for ADD adolescents, the evidence indicates that ADD in some adolescents may be efficaciously treated with psychostimulants. Cantwell's (1979) advice therefore seems appropriate. He recommends that if a clinician has an adolescent client who manifests the classical clinical picture of ADD as a child and who still has psychiatric symptoms— even if not the typical childhood ADD symptoms—a trial of stimulant medication may be appropriate. He concludes that stimulants should be stopped only when evaluation shows that they are no longer effective, and not because a certain age has been reached (see also, Pelham, 1986). Cantwell goes through a number of guidelines for evaluating the effectiveness of psychostimulant administration, which can also be found in detail elsewhere (e.g., Pelham & Hoza, 1987). However, one important point he does note that is specific to adolescents with ADD is that the client should be involved in the treatment process to a greater extent than an ADD child. One reason this may be integral to treatment with adolescents is that they are of an age where they may be noncompliant to their medication regimen, and therefore involving them in the treatment process may elicit their cooperation. In addition, the potential usefulness of obtaining ADD adolescents' self-reports of mood fluctuations on psychostimulants and their perceptions of the efficacy of drug treatment has not been studied at this time but may lead to important new ways of assessing psychostimulant response.

It appears that pharmacotherapy often may be the treatment of choice for ADD adolescents. However, not all ADD children respond to psychostimulant treatment, and this appears also to be the case for adolescents, given the reports of the studies reviewed here. A second treatment often used with ADD children is that of behavioral management, often referred to in the literature as behavior modification or behavior therapy. This may prove to be a fruitful area of study for ADD adolescents as well.

While other types of drugs have been used for the treatment of ADD (see Gittelman & Kanner, 1986, for a review), there is little research yet to support their use. For example, lithium has been reported to improve aggressivity in children, but the current knowledge regarding the use of this drug with children is not strong enough to suggest definite indications for therapy (Lena, 1979). Similarly, antidepressants have been used in the treatment of ADD. While a few studies have reported positive effects of imipramine on ADD symptoms (e.g., Rapoport, Quinn, Bradbard, Riddle, & Brooks, 1974), the magnitude of the effects have not been impressive. Even where imipramine has had some beneficial effects, they tend to be short-lived (Gittelman & Kanner, 1986). It appears that at this time psychostimulants are the drug of choice for pharmacotherapy, both with ADD children and with ADD adolescents.

Behavioral Approaches

As previously noted, few studies on treatment of ADD adolescents have been conducted. Those that have been conducted have concentrated on pharmacotherapy as the treatment method. Future studies need to investigate behavior therapy with ADD adolescents, as it has become the treatment for childhood ADD with the greatest promise as an alternative to medication (Conners & Wells, 1987; Pelham, 1986; Pelham & Murphy, 1986; Wells, 1986). The rationale for using behavior therapy with ADD adolescents is that it has been shown to be a very effective approach for children. Some ADD children treated with behavior therapy show the same degree of improvement on standard teacher rating scales as children on low to moderate doses of medication (O'Leary & Pelham, 1978; Pelham, 1977). Behavior management techniques have been shown to improve children's on-task behavior in the classroom and to decrease disruptive behavior to the same extent as medication (Ayllon, Laymen, & Kandell, 1975; Rapport, Murphy, & Bailey, 1980). In addition, behavioral intervention has been shown to increase ADD children's academic productivity (Ayllon et al., 1975).

Behavioral management intervention has been conducted with adolescents, albeit not with ADD adolescents, and has been found to be effective (Ross, 1981). In a case study investigating behavioral contracting in the family of a delinquent, Stuart (1971) reported that contracting not only served to change the subject's behavior through the contingencies set up in the contract, but it also served to provide a way of interacting constructively for the adolescent and her parents. Kifer, Lewis, Green, and Phillips (1974) reported teaching parents and their adolescents negotiation responses to hypothetical conflict situations and using behavioral rehearsal and social reinforcement; these responses then generalized to actual conflict situations in the subjects' home settings. Marlowe, Madsen, Bowen, Reardon, and Logue (1978) found that teacher attention, consisting of approval for appropriate social behavior and good academic performance, was highly effective in reducing adolescents' off-task behavior. This effect was increased when teacher praise was paired with delivery of tokens. The adolescents, age 12 to 16 years, reduced their off-task behavior more quickly than adolescents in the other treatment groups, who had been assigned to a client-centered counseling condition and a no-contact control condition.

A great deal of work on behavioral intervention in families of delinquents has been conducted by Alexander and his colleagues (Alexander, Barton, Schiavo, & Parsons, 1976; Alexander & Parsons, 1973). Their short-term family intervention program is built around the principle of contingency contracting. In their training paradigm, therapists model, prompt, and reinforce family members for clear communication of messages and feeling and clear presentation of demands and alternative solutions. Families that received this intervention significantly differed from a comparison control group that had been exposed to client-centered family group therapy on a number of process measures. In addition, at follow-up, which occurred 6 to 18 months after treatment, juvenile court records were reviewed to ascertain the number of adolescents who had records since treatment. The adolescents who had received the short-term behavioral family treatment had a significantly lower recidivism rate than both adolescents from a nontreated control group and adolescents who had received other types of family therapy.

Cognitive-behavioral interventions have not been particularly successful for ADD children (Abikoff, 1985), although cognitive-behavioral treatment may exceed the cognitive capabilities of that age group. Brown and Borden (1986) have suggested that cognitive-behavioral training programs will be more successful for ADD adolescents, given their more advanced cognitive functioning. However, given that there has been no demonstration that cognitive training without operant behavioral treatment is effective, this speculation should be treated with caution.

Treatment studies that have been conducted with parent and non-ADD adolescents in conflict situations indicate that some cognitive behavioral techniques, in conjunction with behavioral techniques, can be used effectively with adolescents. For example, Robin, Koepke, and Nayar (1986) have developed an intervention that includes problem solving, communication training, and cognitive restructuring for parent-adolescent conflict. Skills are taught to families through modeling, behavioral rehearsal, feedback, and correction techniques. The effectiveness of this treatment package has been evaluated in four investigations that have been conducted throughout a 10-year period. Overall, intervention with the training package was found to ameliorate specific disputes in families, reduce general conflict, and increase the acquisition of positive problem-solving communication behavior. However, there was large variability in the degree of and consistency of change across the investigations.

Comments.   In summary, there is evidence that both pharmacotherapy and behavioral management techniques are very effective for ADD children and that behavioral management techniques have been used successfully for parent-adolescent conflict. Studies need to be conducted specifically to investigate the use of behavioral management techniques with ADD adolescents. However, that will only be the first step of many that need to be taken before the multiple questions regarding treatment of ADD adolescents can even begin to be addressed. Many years of studies on behavioral management with ADD children, pharmacotherapy with ADD children, and a combination of these treatments are needed before some consensus can be reached regarding appropriate assessment and treatment of ADD children. Similar work needs to be conducted for adolescents.

It has been found repeatedly in recent research that for most ADD children a combined psychosocial and pharmacological treatment "package" is the most effective, strongest intervention, providing levels of change that cannot be obtained with medication or behavior therapy alone (Pelham & Murphy, 1986). Given the increasingly serious nature of the symptomatology displayed with age, especially those for whom aggression is a concurrent problem, this will probably be even more true for ADD adolescents.

ADULT PROGNOSIS

The prognosis of ADD children when they reach adolescence has in a sense been reviewed in this chapter throughout the section on the nature of the disorder in adolescents. What is the prognosis of ADD children and adolescents when they reach adulthood? The findings in this area have been expanding as more and more follow-up studies have reached their conclusive years. Extremely comprehensive reviews are available (Wallander & Hubert, 1985; Weiss & Hechtman, 1986). A brief summary of the adult prognostic literature will be reviewed here.

Borland and Hechtman (1976) examined adult adjustment in a group of 20 men who had been seen at a child guidance clinic 25 years earlier and retrospectively diagnosed as hyperactive. In cases selected, the target hyperactive adult had a living brother with whom a comparison could be made. Percentages of probands and their brothers who reported the following psychological problems were, respectively: nervousness, 60 and 20%; restlessness, 60 and 0%; difficulty with temper, 60 and 15%; impulsiveness, 40 and 10%; and lack of friends, 40 and 10%. Twenty percent of the targets were diagnosed as sociopathic, and 25% reported that they had sought professional help in the past. None of the comparison group was given a diagnosis or reported ever having sought professional help. Although the rates of adjustment problems in this study are high for the hyperactive group, their rate of serious psychopathology is fairly low. Results similar to Borland and Hechtman have been reported in a prospective study conducted by Weiss et al. (1979). Hyperactives were found to have a variety of adjustment difficulties, but the majority did not exhibit serious psychopathology.

In the vocational domain, hyperactive adults also have been found to have adjustment problems. A summary of studies on the work record of hyperactive adults reported in Weiss and Hechtman's book (1986) concluded that hyperactive adults were laid off and quit jobs more frequently than controls. They also reported more difficulties in carrying out assigned tasks at work.

The Borland and Hechtman (1976) and Weiss et al. (1979) studies indicate that hyperactive adults—while exhibiting a range of mild to serious adjustment problems—may not be at risk for as serious psychopathology as the Satterfield studies cited earlier suggest. However, in a recent prospective follow-up of 15 years, Weiss, Hechtman, Milroy, and Perlman (1985) reported much bleaker findings. Eighty-three percent of the ADD subjects who had been evaluated 5 years previously were followed-up, along with a control group matched for IQ and SES. The age range of the ADD and control groups was 21 to 33, with a mean of 25 at follow-up. Among the ADD group, 31% had failed to graduate from high school, compared to 10% of the controls. A significantly greater number of the ADD group reported problems with restlessness, distractibility, impulsivity, and a variety of psychological difficulties including sexual, neurotic, interpersonal, and psychotic problems compared to the control group. Over half the ADD group (52%) received a DSM-III diagnosis, and two-thirds of this group received multiple diagnoses. Twenty-three percent of the ADD group were given a diagnosis of antisocial personality disorder versus 2% of the controls.

It is somewhat difficult to summarize and make generalizations because of the differences among the prognostic studies. Some are retrospective, and sample inclusion criteria differ, as do the informants. A plausible summary of studies conducted thus far is that hyperactive children have a possibility for one of three adult outcomes, each being approximately equally probable. Approximately one-third of hyperactive children may be essentially normal as adults, one-third may exhibit signs of mild to moderate adjustment difficulties that may interfere with their interpersonal and vocational adjustment, and one-third are likely to be diagnosed as having serious psychopathology or serious trouble with legal authorities.

SUMMARY

The persistence of ADD into adolescence and adulthood for large numbers of children diagnosed during their childhood has been documented, with percentages of children diagnosed as ADD continuing to experience problems during their adolescence ranging from approximately 50 to 80%. The diagnostic picture of ADD is complicated by two factors: (1) ADD is defined in terms of developmentally inappropriate levels of inattention, impulsivity, and hyperactivity, and these symptoms are relatively more difficult to identify in adolescents; and (2) a childhood history of ADD must be verified to make a diagnosis of ADD for an adolescent.

ADD adolescents show the same core deficits as ADD children, and they begin to exhibit a variety of related problems such as low self-esteem, peer relationship problems, restlessness, learning disabilities, parent-adolescent conflict, school dropout, and delinquency. A major predictor of poor prognosis is concurrent aggression in childhood.

There are no adequate standardized diagnostic instruments available for ADD adolescents. Parent and teacher rating scales with appropriate item content and norms are needed as well as appropriate laboratory measures of attention and direct observational systems relevant to adolescents' school behaviors.

A small number of current studies reviewed indicates that some ADD adolescents may be efficaciously treated with psychostimulants. Adolescents who present with a clinical picture of ADD as a child and who still are experiencing problems may be appropriate for a stimulant medication trial. The efficacy of other drugs for treatment of ADD, such as lithium and imipramine, has not been yet established. In addition, given the success of behavioral intervention with non-ADD behavior-problem adolescents and parent-adolescent conflict situations, such interventions promise to be a potentially efficacious treatment for ADD adolescents and their families. Combined pharmacological and psychosocial interventions may be most appropriate for many adolescents. Further controlled studies of all treatments are needed.

REFERENCES

Abikoff, H. (1985). Efficacy of cognitive training interventions in hyperactive children: A critical review. *Clinical Psychology Review, 5,* 479–512.

Achenbach, T. M. (1978). The child behavior profile: I. Boys aged 6–11. *Journal of Consulting and Clinical Psychology, 46,* 478–488.

Achenbach, T. M., & Edelbrock, C. S. (1979). The Child Behavior Profile: II. Boys aged 12–16 and girls aged 6–11 and 12–16. *Journal of Consulting and Clinical Psychology, 46,* 223–233.

Alexander, J. F., Barton, C., Schiavo, R. S., & Parsons, B. V. (1976). Systems-behavioral intervention with families of delinquents: Therapist characteristics, family behavior, and outcome. *Journal of Consulting and Clinical Psychology, 44,* 656–664.

Alexander, J. F., & Parsons, B. V. (1973). Short-term behavioral intervention with delinquent families: Impact on family process and recidivism. *Journal of Abnormal Psychology, 81,* 219–225.

American Psychiatric Association (1987). *Diagnostic and statistical manual of mental disorders* (3rd ed., revised). (DSM-III-R). Washington, DC: Author.

American Psychiatric Association (1980). *Diagnostic and statistical manual of mental disorders* (3rd ed.). (DSM-III). Washington, DC: Author.

August, G. J., Stewart, M. A., & Holmes, C. S. (1983). A four-year follow-up of hyperactive boys with and without conduct disorder. *British Journal of Psychiatry, 143,* 192–198.

Ayllon, T., Laymen, D., & Kandell, H. (1975). A behavioral-educational alternative to drug control of hyperactive children. *Journal of Applied Behavior Analysis, 8,* 179–188.

Barkley, R. A. (1981). *Hyperactive Children: A handbook for diagnosis and treatment.* New York: Guilford.

Barkley, R. A. (1982). Guidelines for defining hyperactivity in children: Attention deficit disorders with hyperactivity. In B. B. Lahey & A. E. Kazdin (Eds.), *Advances in clinical child psychology* (Vol. 5). New York: Plenum.

Barkley, R. A., & Cunningham, C. (1979). The effects of Ritalin on mother-child interactions of hyperactive children. *Archives of General Psychiatry, 36,* 201–208.

Beck, L., Langford, W. S., Mackay, M., & Sum, G. (1975). Childhood chemotherapy and later drug abuse and growth curve: A follow-up study of 30 adolescents. *American Journal of Psychiatry, 132,* 436–438.

Blouin, A. G. A., Bornstein, R. A., & Trites, R. L. (1978). Teenage alcohol use among hyperactive children: A five year follow-up study. *Journal of Pediatric Psychology, 3,* 188–194.

Borland, B. L., & Heckman, H. K. (1976). Hyperactive boys and their brothers: A 25-year follow-up study. *Archives of General Psychiatry, 33,* 669–675.

Brown, R. T., & Borden, K. A. (1986). Hyperactivity at adolescence: Some misconceptions and new directions. *Journal of Clinical Child Psychology, 15,* 194–209.

Campbell, S. B. (1985). Hyperactivity in preschoolers: Correlates and prognostic implications. *Clinical Psychology Review, 5,* 405–428.

Campbell, S. B., & Paulauskas, S. (1970). Peer relations in hyperactive children. *Journal of Child Psychology and Psychiatry, 20,* 233–246.

Cantwell, D. P. (1979). Use of stimulant medication with psychiatrically disordered adolescents. In S. C. Feinstein & P. L. Giovacchini (Eds.), *Adolescent psychiatry: Developmental and clinical studies* (Vol. 7, pp. 375–388). New York: Basic Books.

Cantwell, D. P., & Carlson, G. (1978). Stimulants. In J. S. Werry (Ed.), *Pediatric psychopharmacology.* New York: Brunner/Mazel.

Clampit, M. K., & Pirkle, J. B. (1983). Stimulant medication and the hyperactive adolescent: Myths and facts. *Adolescence, 28,* 811–822.

Cohen, N. J., Weiss, G., & Minde, K. (1972). Cognitive styles in adolescents previously diagnosed as hyperactive. *Journal of Child Psychology and Psychiatry, 13,* 203–209.

Conners, C. K. (1969). A teacher rating scale for use in drug studies with children. *American Journal of Psychiatry, 126,* 152–156.

Conners, C. K., & Wells, K. C. (1986). *Hyperkinetic children: A neuropsychosocial approach.* Beverly Hills: Sage Publications.

Coons, H. W., Korman, R., & Borgstedt, A. D. (1987). Enhancing effects of methylphenidate on sustained attention and evoked related potentials of adolescent patients with Attention Deficit Disorder. *Psychophysiology, 21,* 573–574.

Douglas, V. I. (1983). Attention and cognitive problems. In M. Rutter (Ed.), *Behavioral syndromes of brain dysfunction in childhood,* New York: Guilford.

Douglas, V. I. (1985). The response of ADD children to reinforcement: Theoretical and clinical implications. In L. Bloomingdale (Ed.), *Attention deficit disorder: Identification, course, and rationale.* New York: Spectrum.

Douglas, V., & Peters, K. (1979). Toward a clearer definition of the attentional deficits of hyperactive children. In G. Hale & M. Lewis (Eds.), *Attention and the development of cognitive skills.* New York: Plenum.

Dykman, R. A., Ackerman, P. T. (1980). Long-term follow-up studies of hyperactive children. *Advances in Behavioral Pediatrics, 1,* 97–128.

Edelbrock, C., Costello, A. J., Dulcan, M. K., Kalas, R., & Conover, N. C. (1985). Age differences in the reliability of the psychiatric interview of the child. *Child Development, 56,* 265–275.

Farrington, D. P., Loeber, R., & van Kammen, W. B. (1987, October). *Long-term criminal outcomes of hyperactivity-impulsivity-attention deficit and conduct problems in childhood.* Paper prepared for the Society for Life History Research meeting on "Straight and Devious Pathways from Childhood to Adulthood," St. Louis, MO.

Gittelman, R., & Kanner, A. (1986). Psychopharmacotherapy. In H. Quay and J. Werry (Eds.), *Psychopathological disorders of childhood* (3rd ed.). New York: Wiley.

Gittelman, R., & Mannuzza, S. (1985). Diagnosing ADD-H in adolescents. *Psychopharmacology Bulletin, 21,* 237–242.

Gittelman, R., Mannuzza, S., Shenker, R., & Bonagura, N. (1985). Hyperactive boys almost grown up: I. Psychiatric status. *Archives of General Psychiatry, 42,* 937–947.

Goyette, C. H., Conners, C. K., & Ulrich, R. F. (1978). Normative data on revised Conners parent and teacher rating scales. *Journal of Abnormal Child Psychology, 6,* 221–236.

Hartsough, C. S., & Lambert, N. M. (1987). Pattern and progression of drug use among hyperactives and controls: A prospective short-term longitudinal study. *Journal of Child Psychology and Psychiatry, 4,* 543–553.

Hechtman, L., Weiss, G., & Perlman, T. (1984). Young adult outcome of hyperactive children who received long-term stimulant treatment. *Journal of the American Academy of Child Psychiatry, 23,* 261–269.

Hoy, E., Weiss, G., Minde, K., & Cohen, N. (1979). The hyperactive child at adolescence: Emotional, social, and cognitive functioning. *Journal of Abnormal Child Psychology, 6,* 311–324.

Huessy, M., & Cohen, A. (1976). Hyperkinetic behaviors and learning disabilities followed over seven years. *Pediatrics, 54,* 4–10.

Johnston, C. J., & Pelham, W. E. (1986). Teacher ratings predict peer ratings of aggression at 3-year follow-up in boys with attention deficit disorder with hyperactivity. *Journal of Consulting and Clinical Psychology, 54,* 571–572.

Kifer, R. E., Lewis, M. A., Green, D. R., & Phillips, E. L. (1974). Training predelinquent youths and their parents to negotiate conflict situations. *Journal of Applied Behavior Analysis, 7,* 357–364.

Klee, S. H., & Garfinkel, B. D. (1983). A comparison of residual and nonresidual attention deficit disorder in adolescents. *Psychiatric Hospital, 14,* 167–170.

Klorman, R. (1985). Some thoughts on the diagnosis of ADD/H in adolescence. *Psychopharmacology Bulletin* (Vol. 21). *4,* 913.

Klorman, R. (1986). Attention deficit disorder in adolescence. *Advances in Adolescent Mental Health, 1,* 19–62.

Klorman, R., Coons, H. W., & Borgstadt, A. D. (1987). Effects of methylphenidate on adolescents with a childhood history of attention deficit disorder: II. Information processing. *Journal of the American Academy of Child and Adolescent Psychiatry, 26,* 368–374.

Kramer, J., & Loney, J. (1981). Childhood hyperactivity and substance abuse: A review of the literature. In K. Gadow & I. Bialer (Eds.), *Advances in learning and behavioral disabilities* (Vol. 1). Greenwich, CT: JAI.

Lambert, N. M., Hartsough, C. S., Sassone, D., & Sandoval, J. (1987). Persistence of hyperactivity symptoms from childhood to adolescence and associated outcomes. *American Journal of Orthopsychiatry, 57,* 22–32.

Lambert, N. M., Sandoval, J., & Sassone, D. (1978). Prevalence of hyperactivity in elementary school children as a function of social system definers. *American Journal of Orthopsychiatry, 32,* 501–506.

Lena, B. (1979). Lithium in child and adolescent psychiatry. *Archives of General Psychiatry* (Vol. 36). 854–855.

Loiselle, D., Stamm, J., Maitinsky, S., & Whipple, S. (1980). Evoked potential and behavioral signs of attention dysfunctions in hyperactive boys. *Psychophysiology, 17,* 193–201.

Loney, J., Kramer, J., & Milich, R. S. (1981). The hyperactive child grows up: Predictors of symptoms, delinquency and achievement at follow-up. In K. D. Gadow & J. Loney (Eds.), *Psychosocial aspects of drug treatment for hyperactivity* (pp. 381–415). Boulder, CO: Westview.

Loney, J., & Milich, R. (1982). Hyperactivity, inattention, and aggression in clinical practice. In M. Wolraich & D. K. Routh (Eds.), *Advances in behavioral pediatrics* (Vol. 2). Greenwich, CT: JAI.

Mackay, M. C., Beck, L., & Taylor, R. (1973). Methylphenidate for adolescents with minimal brain dysfunction. *New York State Journal of Medicine, 73,* 550–554.

Marlowe, R. H., Madsen, C. H., Jr., Bowen, C. E., Reardon, R. C., & Logue, P. E. (1978). Severe classroom behavior problems: Teachers or counselors. *Journal of Applied Behavior Analysis, 11,* 53–66.

Mattes, J. A., & Gittelman, R. (1981). Effects of artificial food colorings in children with hyperactive symptoms. *Archives of General Psychiatry, 38,* 714–718.

Mendelson, W., Johnson, N., & Stewart, M. A. (1971). Hyperactive children as teenagers: A follow-up study. *Journal of Nervous and Mental Disease, 6,* 483–492.

Milich, R., & Kramer, J. (1984). Reflections on impulsivity: An empirical investigation of impulsivity as a construct. *Advances in Learning and Behavioral Disabilities, 3,* 57–94.

Milich, R., & Landau, S. (1982). Socialization and peer relations in hyperactive children. In K. D. Gadow & I. Bialer (Eds.), *Advances in learning and behavioral disabilities* (Vol. 3). Greenwich, CT: JAI.

Milich, R., & Loney, J. (1979). The role of hyperactive and aggressive symptomatology in predicting adolescent outcome among hyperactive children. *Journal of Pediatric Psychology, 4,* 93–112.

Milich, R., Pelham, W. E., & Hinshaw, S. (1986). Issues in the diagnosis of attention deficit disorder: A cautionary note on the Gordon Diagnostic System. *Psychopharmacology Bulletin, 22,* 1101–1104.

Murphy, D. A., Pelham, W. E., & Milich, R. S. (1985, November). Normative and validity data on the IOWA Conners Teacher Rating Scale. Paper presented at the annual meeting of the Association for Advancement of Behavior Therapy, Houston, TX.

Nuechterlein, K. H. (1983). Signal detection in vigilance tasks and behavioral attributes among offspring of schizophrenic mothers and among hyperactive children. *Journal of Abnormal Psychology, 92,* 4–28.

O'Leary, S. G., & Pelham, W. E. (1978). Behavior therapy and withdrawal of stimulant medication with hyperactive children. *Pediatrics, 61,* 211–217. (Reprinted in B. Lahey (Ed.), *Behavior therapy with hyperactive and learning-disabled children.* New York: Oxford, 1979.)

Pelham, W. E. (1977). Withdrawal of a stimulant drug and concurrent behavioral intervention in the treatment of a hyperactive child. *Behavior Therapy, 8,* 473–479. (Condensed as a Clinical Memorandum in *American Journal of Diseases of Children,* 1976, 130, 565; also reprinted in C. M. Franks & G. T. Wilson (Eds.), *Annual review of behavior therapy: Theory and practice* [Vol. 6]. New York: Brunner/Mazel, 1978.)

Pelham, W. E. (1982). Childhood hyperactivity: Diagnosis, etiology, nature, and treatment. In R. Gatchel, A. Baum, & J. Singer (Eds.), *Behavioral medicine and clinical psychology: Overlapping disciplines.* Volume 1 of A. Baum & J. Singer (Eds.), *Handbook of psychology and health.* Hillsdale, NJ: Erlbaum.

Pelham, W. E. (1983). The effects of stimulant drugs on academic achievement in hyperactive and learning-disabled children. *Thalamus, 3,* 1–47.

Pelham, W. E. (1986). The effects of stimulant drugs on learning and achievement in hyperactive and learning-disabled children. In J. K. Torgesen & B. Wong (Eds.), *Psychological and educational perspectives on learning disabilities.* New York: Academic.

Pelham, W. E., Atkins, M. S., Murphy, H. A., & Swanson, J. (1985). A teacher rating scale for the diagnosis of attention deficit disorder: Teacher norms, factor analyses, and reliability. Unpublished manuscript.

Pelham, W. E., & Bender, M. E. (1982). Peer relationships in hyperactive children: Description and treatment. In K. Gadow & I. Bailer (Eds.), *Advances in learning and behavioral disabilities* (Vol. 1). Greenwich, CT: JAI.

Pelham, W. E., Bender, M. E., Caddell, J., Booth, S., & Moorer, S. (1985). The dose-response effects of methylphenidate on classroom academic and social behavior in children with attention deficit disorder. *Archives of General Psychiatry, 42,* 948–952.

Pelham, W. E., & Hoza, J. (1987). Behavioral assessment of psychostimulant effects on ADD children in a summer day treatment program. In R. Prinz (Ed.), *Advances in behavioral assessment of children and families* (Vol. 3, pp. 3–33), Greenwich, CT.: JAI.

Pelham, W. E., & Milich, R. (1984). Peer relationships in hyperactive children. *Journal of Learning Disabilities, 17,* 560–567.

Pelham, W. E., & Milich, R. (1987). Do single measures predict ADD children's comprehensive response to psychostimulants? Presented as a poster at the annual meeting of the American Academy of Child and Adolescent Psychiatry, Washington, DC.

Pelham, W. E., & Murphy, H. A. (1986). Behavioral and pharmacological treatment of attention deficit and conduct disorders. In M. Hersen (Ed.), *Pharmacological and behavioral treatment: An integrative approach.* New York: Wiley.

Pelham, W. E., Sturges, J., Hoza, J., Schmidt, C., Bijlsma, J., & Moorer, S. (1987). The effects of sustained release 20 and 10 mg Ritalin b.i.d. on cognitive and social behavior in children with attention deficit disorder. *Pediatrics, 4,* 491–501.

Quay, H. C., & Peterson, D. R. (1983). Interim manual for the *Revised Behavior Problem Checklist.* Available from Box 248074, University of Miami, Coral Gables, FL 33124.

Rapoport, J. L., Buchsbaum, M. S., Weingartner, H., Zahn, P., Ludlow, C., & Mikkelsen, E. J. (1980). Dextroamphetamine: Cognitive and behavioral effects in normal and hyperactive boys and normal men. *Archives of General Psychiatry, 37,* 933–943.

Rapoport, J. L., Quinn, P. O., Bradbard, G., Riddle, D., & Brooks, E. (1974). Imipramine and methylphenidate treatments of hyperactive boys. *Archives of General Psychiatry, 30,* 789–793.

Rapport, M., Murphy, A., & Bailey, J. (1980). The effects of a response treatment tactic on hyperactive children. *Journal of School Psychology, 18,* 98–111.

Robin, A. L., Koepke, T., & Nayar, M. (1986). Conceptualizing, assessing, and treating parent-adolescent conflict. In B. Lahey and A. Kazdin (Eds.), *Advances in Clinical Child Psychology, 9,* 87–124.

Ross, A. O. (1981). *Child behavior therapy.* New York: Wiley.

Ross, D. M., & Ross, S. A. (1982). Hyperactivity: Research, theory, and action (2nd Ed.). New York: Wiley.

Safer, D. J., & Allen, R. P. (1975). Stimulant drug treatment of hyperactive adolescents. *Diseases of the Nervous System, 36,* 454–457.

Satterfield, J. H., & Braley, B. W. (1977). Evoked potentials and brain maturation in hyperactive and normal children. *Electroencephalography and Clinical Neurophysiology, 43,* 43–51.

Satterfield, J. H., Hoppe, C. M., & Schell, A. M. (1982). A prospective study of delinquency in 110 adolescent boys with attention deficit disorder and 88 normal adolescent boys. *American Journal of Psychiatry, 139,* 795–798.

Sleator, E. K., Ullman, R. K., & von Neumann, A. (1982). How do hyperactive children feel about taking stimulants and will they tell the doctor? *Clinical Pediatrics, 21,* 474–479.

Sprague, R. L., & Gadow, K. D. (1976). The role of the teacher in drug treatment. *School Review, 85,* 109–140.

Stewart, M. A., Mendelson, W. B., & Johnson, N. E. (1973). Hyperactive children as adolescents: How they describe themselves. *Child Psychiatry and Human Development, 4,* 3–11.

Stuart, R. B. (1971). Behavioral contracting within the families of delinquents. *Journal of Behavior Therapy and Experimental Psychiatry, 2,* 1–11.

Ullman, R. K., Sleator, E. K., & Sprague, R. L. (1985). Introduction to the use of the ACTeRS. *Psychopharmacology Bulletin, 21,* 915–916.

Varley, C. K. (1983). Effects of methylphenidate in adolescents with attention deficit disorder. *Journal of the American Academy of Child Psychiatry, 22,* 351–354.

Wallander, J. L., & Hubert, N. C. (1985). Long-term prognosis for children with attention deficit disorder with hyperactivity (ADD/H). In B. Lahey & A. Kazdin (Eds.), *Advances in Clinical Child Psychology, 8,* 114–137.

Weiss, G., & Hechtman, L. (1986). *Hyperactive children grown up.* New York: Guilford.

Weiss, G., Hechtman, L., Milroy, T., & Perlman, T. (1985). Psychiatric status of hyperactives as adults: A controlled 15-year follow-up of 63 hyperactive children. *Journal of the American Academy of Child Psychiatry, 24,* 211–220.

Weiss, G., Hechtman, L., & Perlman, T. (1978). Hyperactives as young adults: School, employer, and self-rating scales obtained during ten-year follow-up evaluation. *American Journal of Orthopsychiatry, 48,* 438–445.

Weiss, G., Hechtman, L., Perlman, T., Hopkins, J., & Wener, A. (1979). Hyperactives as young adults: A controlled prospective ten-year follow-up of 75 children. *Archives of General Psychiatry, 36,* 675–681.

Weiss, G., Minde, K., Werry, J., Douglas, V., & Nemeth, E. (1971). Studies on the hyperactive child: VIII. Five-year follow-up. *Archives of General Psychiatry, 24,* 409–414.

Wells, K. C. (1987). What do we know about the use and effects of behavior therapies in the treatment of ADD? In J. Loney (Ed.), *The young hyperactive child: Answers to questions about diagnosis, prognosis, and treatment.* New York: Haworth.

Wender, E. H. (1983). Hyperactivity in adolescence. *Journal of Adolescent Health Care, 4,* 180–186.

Whalen, C., Henker, B., Collins, B., McAuliffe, S., & Vaux, A. (1979). Peer interaction in a structured communication task: Comparisons of normal and hyperactive boys and of methylphenidate (Ritalin) and placebo effects. *Child Development, 50,* 388–401(a).

White, J., Barratt, E., & Adams, P. (1979). The hyperactive child in adolescence. *Journal of the American Academy of Child Psychiatry, 18,* 154–159.

CHAPTER TWELVE

Conduct Disorder

Michael McManus

Adolescence is viewed as a developmental stage in which experimentation with values, lifestyles, and relationships is appropriate and expected. Many adults cherish memories of misbehavior in adolescence, which in their recall contributed to their sense of autonomy and independence and increased bonds of friendship with their peers. Adolescent misbehavior is repeatedly celebrated in movies, television, and other forms of popular culture, which depict, often humorously and in highly exaggerated form, the normative adolescent urge to outwit parents, misbehave, and get away with it.

Delinquent behavior, in which legal standards rather than parental expectations are violated, also has a distinct developmental component to it. Studies in which delinquency is self-reported uniformly find that delinquent acts markedly increase in early adolescence, peak in middle adolescence, and fall off in late adolescence and early adulthood. For many adolescents, and perhaps the majority of male adolescents, some degree of involvement in or experimentation with delinquent behavior is a common developmental phenomenon.

Given this context, it is not surprising that disturbances in conduct are by far the most common reason for referral of adolescents for psychiatric evaluation. Disturbances in conduct can be divided into three general though not entirely mutually exclusive categories. The first and largest category includes adolescents whose misconduct consists of relatively minor, nonrepetitive behaviors, which fall within the spectrum of normative adolescent development. The second category is made up of adolescents who consistently violate age-expected norms of behavior, are truant from school, run away from home, and persistently bring themselves into conflict with adult authority. The third and smallest category is that group of adolescents involved in repetitive criminal offenses, some of which may lead them into violent confrontation with a victim. Adolescents in the second and third categories, in whom there is a recurrent pattern of misconduct, are those most likely to meet diagnostic criteria for conduct disorder as currently defined by DSM-III-R (APA, 1987).

Because conduct disordered behavior is a final common pathway in which a multitude of interpersonal, environmental, educational, and biologic factors converge, adolescents with conduct disorder are often more different than similar to one another. While it may be relatively straightforward to assess the significance of conduct disordered behavior at its extremes, the factors that impact on the majority of adolescents with conduct disorder are varied, multiple, and produce an array of clinical outcomes. Despite the fact that it is widely acknowledged that conduct disorder is multifactorial in nature, much of the voluminous research on the subject has had a narrow theoretical focus. This has led to a significant degree of polarization regarding the causes of conduct disordered behavior, ranging from theories that emphasize social disadvantage to those that posit genetic transmission of criminal or conduct disordered behavior.

Objections have been raised about the inclusion of conduct disorder as a psychiatric diagnosis from both within and without psychiatry. Nonpsychiatrists have argued that the causes of conduct disordered behavior, unlike other psychiatric disorders, are not "intrinsic" to the individual, but arise from social and environmental factors. From this viewpoint, attaching a psychiatric label to a basically social phenomena is not only stigmatizing, but it is also unlikely to remedy the "real" causes of conduct disorder. Many psychiatrists, on the other hand, feel that conduct disorder, with its non-specific diagnostic criteria, conveys little information to the clinician and has the potential to obscure the diagnosis of psychopathology that often underlies or accompanies symptoms of conduct disorder.

Despite these claims, there is a remarkable degree of agreement in the extensive literature on conduct disorder that aggressive, antisocial, and conduct disordered behavior in its more severe forms is an enduring symptom constellation, with clear-cut familial pattern of transmission and a highly predictable clinical course. In short, all the factors necessary to qualify conduct disorder as a psychiatric diagnosis are present. The debate about the validity and usefulness of conduct disorder as a diagnosis is likely to persist.

Despite the debate about the validity of considering conduct disorder a psychiatric diagnosis, it is clear that the role of mental health professionals in the provision of services to adolescents who are either conduct disordered or delinquent has been significant and positive. As an awareness of the developmental needs of children and adolescents has developed in this century, psychiatrists, psychologists, and social workers have insisted that social agencies and the juvenile court system reflect the needs of adolescents and their families and that they be rehabilitative rather than punitive in their approach.

Recently, however, attitudes toward conduct disordered and delinquent adolescents have become increasingly punitive. In part, this change in attitude has been an understandable reaction to a marked increase in violent juvenile crime, a situation that has led to an increasing focus on the rights of victims rather than perpetrators of crime. There is also widespread pessimism regarding the treatment of conduct disorder and delinquency which, when combined with drastic reductions in public funding of treatment programs for these disorders, creates an atmosphere of therapeutic nihilism.

Although many questions about the utility and validity of the diagnosis of conduct disorder remain to be answered, that polemical discussion about symptom constellations and diagnostic criteria are bound to flourish in an atmosphere where little treatment research is conducted and where, for the severely conduct disordered adolescent, few viable treatment options exist. The greatest current need is well-thought out, well-conducted treatment studies that seek to utilize the large body of descriptive data that has been generated in the study of conduct disorder and delinquency.

DIAGNOSTIC AND DEVELOPMENTAL CONSIDERATIONS

The current DSM-III-R criteria call for the conduct disordered child or adolescent to have a repetitive and persistent pattern of behavior in which the rights of others are violated. In the previous DSM-III (APA, 1980), conduct disorders were further categorized by parameters of socialization and aggression, creating four basic categories or types of conduct disorder in addition to the category of atypical conduct disorder. Adolescents who received a diagnosis of undersocialized conduct disorder were those lacking a normal degree of affection or empathy for others, while adolescents who received a diagnosis of aggressive conduct disorder were characterized by a repetitive pattern of direct aggression toward others. Because research has not fully supported the utility of these subcategories of conduct disorder, they have been dropped in DSM-III-R, and conduct disorder is now a single diagnosis grouped with the other externalizing or disruptive behavior disorders: attention-deficit hyperactivity disorder and oppositional defiant disorder.

Studies that have examined the prevalence of conduct disorder generally have found that conduct disorder is diagnosable in 3 to 8% of school-age children (Rutter, Tizard, & Whitemore, 1981; McGee, Williams, & Silva, 1984; Shapiro & Garfinkel, 1986). Seriously delinquent behavior has clearly been on the increase in the last several years, and it is estimated that juveniles are now involved in about 30 to 40% of violent crimes in the United States. It is well known that social and economic disadvantage, family disruption, exposure to physical abuse and emotional neglect, and a host of other adverse environmental factors are important in the genesis of conduct disorder (Glueck & Glueck, 1962; McCord & McCord, 1959).

Recent genetic studies (Bohman, Cloninger, Sigvardsson, & von Knorring, 1982; Cloninger, Sigvardsson, Bohman, & von Knorring, 1982; Mednick, Gabrielli, & Hutchings, 1984; Sigvardsson, Cloninger, Bohman, & von Knorring, 1982) indicate that hereditary factors play a role in at least some forms of criminality, particularly petty or nonviolent criminal behavior. These studies also have demonstrated close links between the transmission of criminality and alcoholism. It remains difficult at present to assess the importance of genetic factors in criminality because the relative weight of this factor in determining behavior compared with environmental or social variables is unknown.

Studies that have examined the adult outcome of conduct disorders are consistent in reporting a poor outcome (Robins, 1966, 1978; Henn, Bardwell, & Jenkins, 1980). Antisocial personality disorder is diagnosable in one-third to one-half of adults, and many of the remainder suffer a variety of negative outcomes including alcoholism, depression, and schizophrenia. Although developmental studies (Rutter, Graham, Chadwick, & Yule, 1976) indicate that for most adolescents behavior disorder peaks and declines from middle to late adolescence, adolescents who establish a persistent pattern of aggressive and antisocial behavior are likely to continue it into adulthood.

CLINICAL PROBLEMS

Substance and Alcohol Abuse

Substance abuse is ubiquitous among adolescents with conduct disorder. Numerous studies have made it clear that substance abuse is the most common psychiatric disorder to be found in association with conduct disorder and a significant factor in the commission of delinquent acts (Kraus, 1981; Kandel, 1982). There are many factors impacting on drug use among conduct disordered adolescents, ranging from peer pressure, attempts to self-medicate chronic low self-esteem and depression, or expression of a genetic/familial vulnerability. Studies that have investigated the relationship between drug use and delinquent behavior consistently have found that substance abusing adolescents are likely to commit increased numbers of delinquencies when compared with nonsubstance abusing delinquents (McManus, Alessi, Grapentine, & Brickman, 1984a; Kraus, 1981; Simonds & Kashani, 1979).

Although it has been difficult to establish a link between delinquency, substance abuse, and violent crime, it is clear that substance abuse is an important risk factor in suicidal behavior among conduct disordered adolescents. Despite the high prevalence of substance abuse among adolescents with conduct disorder, relatively little research has focused on this problem. Given what appears to be the high degree of genetic/familial vulnerability among these adolescents, more focus on this problem is needed.

Attention Deficit Disorder

In childhood, attention deficit disorder (ADD) often coexists with conduct disorder. In a large sample of nearly one thousand 7-year-old children, McGee et al. (1984) found that 3.2% were aggressive without hyperactivity, 2.7% were only hyperactive, and 4.3% were both aggressive and hyperactive (see also Shapiro & Garfinkel, 1986). Stewart, Cummings, Singer, and deBlois (1981) found that nearly one-half of a sample of prepubertal children with a diagnosis of ADD also met diagnostic criteria for an aggressive conduct disorder. Children with diagnoses of both conduct disorder and ADD are significantly more likely to have concurrent reading disability or other forms of cognitive impairment than are children with either diagnosis alone (McGee et al., 1984; Rutter et al., 1981). Family studies (Cantwell, 1972, 1978; Stewart, deBlois, & Cummings, 1980a; Stewart, deBlois,

Meardon, & Cummings, 1980b) also support a relationship between ADD and conduct disorder in that antisocial personality disorder is a significantly overrepresented diagnosis in the parents of children with ADD.

Numbers of studies have examined the adolescent outcome of childhood ADD (Gittelman, Mannuzza, Shenker, & Bonagura, 1985; Hechtman, Weiss, & Perlman, 1984; Hechtman & Weiss, 1985; Weiss, Hechtman, Milroy, & Perlman, 1985; Loney, Kramer, & Milich, 1981; Manuzza & Gittelman, 1984; Satterfield, Hoppe, & Schell, 1982). All are in agreement that childhood ADD frequently eventuates in adolescent conduct disorder. The recent studies of Gittelman et al. (1985) and Weiss et al. (1985) are the best designed studies of the adolescent outcome of ADD. Both are prospective, and both attempt to exclude children with conduct disorder from the childhood ADD group, employ comparison groups, and carry out adolescent evaluations blind to childhood diagnosis. Gittelman et al. (1985) found that 40% of the adolescents with childhood ADD retained the diagnosis in adolescence. Of the adolescents who retained a diagnosis of ADD, 48% developed conduct disorders as compared with 13% of the adolescents whose ADD remitted and 8% of the control group. They noted that in turn, 59% of adolescents with conduct disorder went on to develop alcohol or substance abuse disorders. As noted by Weiss et al. (1985), the persistence of symptoms of ADD rather than successful treatment with stimulants appears most relevant to adolescent outcome. These studies clearly indicate the need for more thorough assessment of adolescents with conduct disorder for ADD and more treatments directed at the unique needs of the adolescent with ADD.

Neurological Dysfunction

Central nervous system dysfunction has been widely investigated in adolescents with conduct disorder. Studies have focused on identification of active neurological disease, particularly seizure disorder, on signs of "soft" or minimal neurological dysfunction, and on more subtle deficits identifiable by neuropsychological and educational testing. These studies have confirmed a widely held impression that central nervous system dysfunction is common in adolescents with conduct disorder, but they differ substantially in their estimation of the nature of the dysfunction.

The studies by Lewis (Lewis, 1976; Lewis & Shanok, 1978) have focused on the presence of gross neurological dysfunction delinquent adolescents. Lewis found that about 13% of a group of seriously delinquent adolescents had localizing neurological signs on examination and another 30% had abnormal electroencephalograms (EEGs). Lewis postulated that many delinquent adolescents, particularly those with patterns of violent behavior, have undiagnosed seizure disorders, mostly of the psychomotor type.

Later research, however, (Hsu, Wisner, Richey, & Goldstein, 1985;

McManus, Brickman, Alessi, & Grapentine, 1985) has not fully supported these results. Hsu et al. (1985) found that a group of delinquent adolescents hospitalized for evaluation was no more likely than a group of nondelinquent hospitalized adolescents to have abnormal EEGs, and the rate of diagnosable seizure disorders was low in both groups. In a group of violent delinquents, McManus et al. (1985) found that only 4% of adolescents had localizing neurological findings, a rate consistent with hospitalized nondelinquent adolescents and that 1% had active symptoms of seizure disorder. It would appear that gross neurological dysfunction is less common than previously supposed.

There is widespread agreement among a number of researchers that minimal or soft neurological signs are common among conduct disordered and delinquent adolescents. These signs (which are of uncertain prognostic significance) include a variety of findings, such as gross motor clumsiness, failures in lateralization, minor choreiform movements, and so on, indicative of deficits in cortical integration. They have pointed out and other researchers have documented (Tarter, Hegedus, Winston, & Alterman, 1984; McManus et al., 1984a; McManus, Brickman, Alessi, & Grapentine, 1984b) that conduct disordered adolescents are likely to have experienced physical abuse, which may be one source of this type of dysfunction.

Studies differ as to the relationship between soft signs and the symptoms of conduct disorder. Lewis and Shanok (1978) found a significant relationship between soft signs and violent behavior, a relationship not supported by Wolff, Waber, Bauermeister, Cohen, and Ferber (1982) or McManus et al. (1985). McManus et al. found that soft signs were likely to occur in adolescents with undersocialized types of conduct disorder, and Wolff et al. found a relationship between soft signs and age of first arrest in a group of delinquent adolescents. In general, the research suggests that soft signs are associated with an increased risk for antisocial behavior, although the effect may be difficult to specify.

Wolff et al. (1982) demonstrated that an association between soft signs and language deficits is unique to delinquent adolescents, suggesting that a relationship between minor neurological dysfunction and language functioning may be central to the genesis of conduct disorder in some adolescents. A substantial body of research supports impairment of language-based skills as an important accessory symptom in conduct disorder (Brickman, McManus, Grapentine, & Alessi, 1984; Rutter et al., 1981). Reading and other types of learning disability influence conduct disordered behavior by reducing motivation for academic achievement as well as by impairing the social learning necessary for normative behavior. The findings of a number of studies suggest that minimal neurological dysfunction and neuropsychological deficits, particularly in language and reading, increase the risk for undersocialization and conduct disordered behavior in adolescence.

Affective Disorder

Beginning with Aichorn (1965), it was hypothesized that depressive affect leads to delinquent acting out. The later theories about masked depression (Chwast, 1974) postulated that delinquent behavior is a "depressive equivalent" in many adolescents. More recently, empirical research lent some support to the idea that in at least some children and adolescents, conduct disordered behavior follows the onset of a depressed mood or a syndromal depression. Kandel and Davies (1982), in a large scale epidemiological study, found that depressed mood often preceded minor delinquent acts, and the adolescents who reported depressive symptoms were more likely to report minor delinquencies. Puig-Antich (1982) reported that in children with a diagnosis of major depressive disorder, symptoms of conduct disorder waxed and waned depending on the status of their depression. Puig-Antich suggests that for some children conduct disorder may arise as a behavioral component of a major depressive disorder. Alessi, McManus, Grapentine, and Brickman (1983) found that in delinquent adolescents with major depressive disorders, it was common for the predominant mood associated with the depression to be anger and irritability and for features of agitation to be present. Given the tendency for children and adolescents to view affective states as arising from interpersonal or external sources, it is possible to see how the onset of a major depressive episode could lead to conduct disordered behavior. To what extent this pathway is a common one in the genesis of conduct disorder is unknown at present.

There are several studies that have attempted to identify depression in delinquent adolescents. Chiles, Miller, and Cox (1980), Kashani et al. (1980), and McManus et al. (1984a) all have examined incarcerated delinquent populations. All three studies found similar rates of occurrence of major depressive disorder (18% versus 23% versus 15%). In the study of McManus et al. (1984a), dysthymic disorder was diagnosed in 15% of subjects, and an additional 8% were found to have had a major depressive episode in the year prior to evaluation. Kashani et al. (1980) examined a nondelinquent nonincarcerated group of adolescents as a control and found a prevalence of 4%, suggesting as do the other studies that depression occurs with increased frequency in delinquent and conduct disordered adolescents.

In the study of McManus et al. (1984a), it was found that standard clinician and self rating scales (Hamilton and Carroll) could be used reliably in assessing delinquent populations, with a high degree of correlation between clinician and self ratings of depression. Despite theories that depression may lead to delinquent behavior, the majority of adolescents in the McManus et al. study had secondary depressions, meaning that they had a preexisting diagnosis of substance abuse, alcoholism, or conduct disorder. It appears likely that many adolescents with conduct disorder are likely to have "depressive spectrum" rather than "pure familial" types of depression, in which alcoholism and sociopathy as well as depression are common in family members. This distinction may have significance for future studies which attempt to study clinical course, drug response, and biological markers. It is noteworthy that in all three of the studies just mentioned, no relationship was found between the presence of depressive symptoms and severity of delinquency or particular types of delinquent acts.

Borderline personality disorder (BPD), a diagnosis that can be made reliably in adolescence (McManus, Lerner, Robbins, & Barbour, 1984), is common among delinquent adolescents. In their psychodynamic study of hospitalized delinquents, Offer, Marohn, and Ostrov (1979) developed a personality topology to describe their adolescent population. Two of the four types of personality they classified involved borderline psychopathology. McManus et al. (1984c) found that nearly 40% of a group of seriously delinquent adolescents met DSM-III criteria for BPD. The symptoms that were most sensitive and specific for the diagnosis of BPD were affective lability and self-injury. In addition, it was found that a strong association existed between the presence of a diagnosis of BPD and predictors of adult antisocial outcome. Delinquents with BPD were much more likely to meet criteria for antisocial personality disorder than were their nonborderline counterparts, and they were more likely to be assigned a diagnosis of an aggressive conduct disorder. Furthermore, they were significantly more likely to have been adjudicated for a violent felony than the remaining delinquents. While these findings are of interest, further studies are needed to determine if identification of borderline psychopathology in delinquent adolescents segregates a unique population in terms of etiology, treatment, or prognosis.

PSYCHODYNAMIC AND BEHAVIORAL APPROACHES

Unlike the early days of psychoanalysis and the social welfare movement when it was widely believed that conduct disorder could be successfully treated if the appropriate psychotherapeutic and psychosocial interventions were applied, there now is widespread pessimism regarding the potential for successful treatment of conduct disorder by either psychodynamic or behavioral means. While descriptive literature on conduct disorder and delinquency has continued to grow, literature on the treatment of conduct disorder has not. Although successful intervention programs with delinquent adolescents are reported, these most often seem to be the result of fortuitous circumstances involving highly committed professionals combined with a brief period of enlightened funding. Shamsie (1981), in his excellent article, reviewed the many follow-up studies that have examined the effect of a variety of treatments on recidivism. He found that case work, group therapy, behavior modification, family therapy, training school placement, therapeutic community, and psychotherapy all showed no obvious advantage over no treatment.

There are numerous reasons why treatment of conduct disorder has been so unsuccessful. The first and most obvious is that most adolescents with conduct disorder and many of their families are not motivated to change and often are forced to participate in treatment rather than seeking it voluntarily. In addition, faddism is very prevalent, particularly in programs designed to treat delinquents. Programs often are designed in response to legislative and social pressures and then rapidly altered or dropped as the pressures change. A final difficulty is that programs providing the type of treatment likely to be successful with conduct disordered adolescents are also extremely expensive. As Offer et al. (1979) have shown, long term, multidisciplinary, hospital-based treatment of delinquent adolescents has the potential to be successful. However, few public agencies have been willing or able (given the current climate of shrinking funding for social programs) to design such programs. The need is for programs that will allow longitudinal growth of social skills and social awareness coupled with state-of-the-art intervention into the multiple psychiatric, educational, and neuropsychological deficits characteristic of adolescents with conduct disorder.

Despite such a pessimistic state of affairs, clinicians working with children and adolescents with conduct disorders have not been uniformly unsuccessful in their attempts at treatment, and general guidelines can be drawn from the literature. First, it seems clear that treatment of conduct disorder must utilize multiple modalities depending on the vulnerabilities of the adolescent in question. The clinician who ignores symptoms of reading disorder or who attempts to treat ADD while ignoring family conflict, and so on is likely to be unsuccessful. Second, the clinician must determine the setting in which the treatment(s) will take place. One of the unexamined factors in many of the treatment studies in conduct disorder is that treatments that are unable to break the cycle of conduct disordered behavior have little likelihood of success. This statement is particularly true when substance abuse is a concomitant of conduct disorder and requires concurrent treatment. A final general guideline is that adolescents with conduct disorder often are able to respond to clearly defined negative contingencies for their behavior. Thus behavioral treatment programs need to incorporate clear and appropriate negative as well as positive contingencies.

PSYCHOPHARMACOLOGICAL APPROACHES

General Issues

While psychopharmacology has revolutionized the treatment of many psychiatric disorders, this was not the case with conduct disorder.

Psychotropic medications are rarely considered a first choice treatment with behaviorally disturbed adolescents; they most often are utilized when one or more other types of treatment have failed. As is true in much of adolescent psychiatry, few empirical studies have been done that clearly support the use of drug therapy. For that reason, it is difficult at present to know if psychopharmacological interventions are underutilized or overutilized in the treatment of conduct disorder. Much of clinical practice in drug treatment of adolescents with conduct disorder is based on the assumption that those with demonstrated efficacy in adults are likely to be equally effective in adolescents. This assumption has rarely been tested, however. The one conclusion that can be firmly drawn after a review of the literature is that more and better studies are needed before the role of drug therapy in the treatment of conduct disorder can be fully evaluated (Leventhal, 1984).

Many factors complicate research and clinical practice in the drug treatment of adolescents with conduct disorder. Foremost of these is the fact that conduct disorder is one of the broadest and least specific of the diagnoses that can be made in adolescence. For this reason, it is often clinically difficult to determine which adolescents should be selected for medication trials and which adolescents are unlikely to respond to psychotropic agents. Attempts have been made to improve on the specificity of drug treatments by focusing on the treatment of specific symptoms associated with conduct disorder (such as aggression) or by treating disorders like depression or attention deficit disorder (that may coexist with conduct disorder).

In addition to the lack of specificity in the diagnosis of conduct disorder, which makes drug treatment difficult, there is a widespread and valid perception that conduct disorder has significant environmental and interpersonal determinants that must be addressed. Nonmedical professionals and the public at large have attitudes regarding the treatment of biologic or "intrinsic" factors in conduct disorder with medication ranging from mild skepticism to outright hostility. For adolescents whose behavior brings them into contact with the juvenile court, for example, such treatment may be seen as a coercive attempt to control behavior that is unacceptable to society. Similarly, for adolescents who are receiving concurrent treatment for substance abuse, treatment of symptoms of conduct disorder with psychotropic medication may appear to be in direct conflict with maintaining sobriety and solving problems in living without the use of drugs. Given clinical issues of this nature and the conduct disordered adolescent's poor compliance with treatment, the prospect of successful treatment of symptoms of conduct disorder with psychotropic medications is in most instances poor.

Treatment of Associated Psychopathology

One of the main approaches to the treatment of conduct disorder has been the identification and treatment of psychiatric illnesses found in association with conduct disorder, with the assumption that improvement in the symptoms of the coexisting disorder (e.g., attention deficit disorder) will have a beneficial effect on the clinical course of the conduct disorder. In an early study, Eisenberg et al. (1963) found that adolescents in a delinquent training school population frequently had ongoing symptoms of ADD, which when treated with d-amphetamine produced an improvement in symptoms of conduct disorder, including lying, disobedience, and leading others into trouble. Maletzky's (1974) double-blind, placebo-controlled study using d-amphetamine in delinquent adolescents found significant improvement in drug treated versus placebo treated adolescents. Current and past symptoms of ADD were the factors most strongly predictive of a positive drug response.

Several studies, including those of Amery, Minichiello, and Brown (1984) and Conners (1969), have demonstrated a positive effect of psychostimulants on aggressive behavior that occurs as a part of the clinical picture of ADD. Other investigators, such as Allen, Safer, and Covi (1975), have claimed that amphetamine effects on aggression in ADD are independent of their impact on motoric overactivity, a finding supported by a large body of animal literature. These studies indicate that adolescents with combined diagnoses of conduct disorder and ADD may have amelioration of symptoms of both attention deficit disorder and conduct disorder, particularly aggression, when treated with stimulants.

Studies to date, however, have not been able to demonstrate the efficacy of stimulant treatment for adolescents with conduct disorder without ADD. These studies (see Klein, Gittelman, Quitkin, & Rifkin, 1980) indicate that at present there is no role for the treatment of children with conduct disorder with stimulants in the absence of symptoms of ADD. As sophistication in the diagnosis and treatment of ADD in adolescence increases, it is likely that more adolescents with both conduct disorder and ADD will receive treatment.

An area in which there may be potential benefit but where little if any research exists is in the treatment of affective disorders that coexist with conduct disorder. As studies have shown (McManus et al., 1985; Chiles et al., 1980; Kashani et al., 1980), depression can be reliably diagnosed even in severely delinquent adolescents. Research also has shown that dysthymic disorder and borderline personality disorder frequently can be diagnosed in association with conduct disorder (McManus et al., 1984a; Alessi et al., 1983). Both these illnesses have been shown to be related to an increased risk for the development of a major affective disorder and may be amenable to psychopharmacological intervention.

In Puig-Antich's (1982) longitudinal study of prepubescent children with major depressive disorder plus conduct disorder, symptoms of conduct disorder were activated or worsened during depressive episodes and remitted following successful tricyclic antidepressant treatment.

Alessi et al. (1983) also found primary depressives among a group of serious delinquents, but they noted that many had conduct disorders antedating the onset of depressive illnesses. In adolescents with conduct disorder who have affective symptomatology, the distinction between primary versus secondary affective disorder may be important (as has been the case with adults) in understanding clinical course, the importance of biological factors, and response to antidepressants. Because progress of research in the drug treatment of depression in adolescence has been slow, the clinician is presently unable to make treatment decisions based on a firm empirical base. Despite this fact, it is likely that in clinical practice a wide variety of medications, including tricyclic antidepressants, lithium, monamine oxidase (MAO) inhibitors, and carbamazepine, are utilized in adolescents with combined diagnoses of conduct and affective disorder.

Lithium and Neuroleptics

Of the numerous medications suggested as being effective in conduct disorder, lithium and neuroleptics have been the most widely studied and are in the widest clinical use. There is an extensive literature on the antiaggressive effects of lithium and neuroleptics in both adolescents and adults (Campbell, Cohen, & Small, 1982; Lena, 1979; Sheard, Marini, Bridges, & Wagner, 1976). The recent study of Campbell et al. (1984) is the best designed, best controlled study, examining the efficacy of lithium and haloperidol versus placebo in the treatment of aggressive conduct disorder. Although the subjects were mostly prepubertal (age range 5 to 13), the results are equally pertinent to the treatment of adolescents.

In their study, 61 hospitalized children were randomly assigned to placebo, lithium, or haloperidol. Optimal doses of the medications ranged from 1 to 6 mg/day in the case of haloperidol and 500 to 2000 mg/day in the case of lithium. Both lithium and haloperidol were found to diminish hyperactivity, aggression, hostility, and unresponsiveness to a significantly greater degree than placebo, according to child psychiatrists blind to assignment of medications. The global ratings of the hospital staff at the end of the study supported the efficacy of both medications, and the two active drug groups were both considered to be moderately improved. Drug side effects were significant, particularly in the haloperidol group, where 50% of the children had acute dystonic reactions and 80% experienced periods of excessive sedation. Lithium side effects were somewhat less onerous, although from one-third to one-half of subjects reported stomachache, headache, and/or tremor.

These findings are consistent with those of Lena (1979), Werry, Aman, and Lampen (1975), Naruse et al. (1982), and DeLong (1978) in demonstrating that neuroleptics and lithium have a mildly to moderately beneficial impact on symptoms associated with conduct disorder. Because biological markers have not been investigated much in conduct disorder, there has been little research directed using these to predict drug response. In a companion study to the one by Campbell et al. (1984), Bennett, Korein, Kalmijn, Grega, and Campbell (1983) found that drug response to both lithium and haloperidol could be retrospectively predicted by the appearance of EEG abnormalities after the drug was instituted. While this finding may not have direct clinical utility, it does suggest that future research oriented toward classifying the minor EEG abnormalities common in conduct disorder may provide a means for identifying drug responsive groups.

The use of these agents has been questioned on several grounds. The first relates to the impact of these medications on cognitive functioning and learning. As indicated by the findings of Platt, Campbell, Green, and Grega (1984), these effects appear to be much more significant with neuroleptics than with lithium. Decrements in attention, concentration, and visual-motor performance have been documented, and long-term use of neuroleptics may impair academic performance even in the context of improved behavioral control. The most problematic area, of course, is the potential for long-term side effects with neuroleptics. Studies reporting on the prevalence of tardive dyskinesia in retarded children and adolescents treated with neuroleptics found that about one-fourth to one-third developed tardive dyskinesia (Perry et al., 1985; Gualtieri, Quade, Hicks, Mayo, & Schroeder, 1984). Because these findings are consistent with the adult literature on tardive dyskinesia, it is reasonable to assume that if large numbers of adolescents with conduct disorder (a chronic illness) were to be treated with neuroleptics, many would develop tardive dyskinesia. This risk would seem to be unacceptable both from a clinical and possibly a medico-legal perspective. Lithium, however, appears to have a legitimate role in the treatment of conduct disorder, particularly when aggressive symptomatology is predominant.

In summary, lithium has been demonstrated to be an effective treatment for conduct disorder. Neuroleptics, while clinically effective, present the potential for unacceptable side effects and should be reserved for adolescents with frank psychotic symptomatology. Adolescents with conduct disorder who have concurrent ADD or an affective disorder may benefit from drug therapy, with secondary improvement in symptoms of conduct disorder as well.

Propranolol has been shown by Williams, Mehl, Yudofsky, Adams, and Roseman (1982) to be an effective treatment in children and adolescents with episodic outbursts of aggression and rage. All the subjects studied had ongoing neurological impairment, although symptoms in a number consisted of minor neurological dysfunction as seen in ADD. Nearly 80% of subjects met criteria for conduct disorder, with slightly more than half of subjects with conduct disorder also meeting criteria for ADD. Doses of propranolol ranged between 60 to 1600 mg/day, with a median dose of 161 mg/day. Only 6/30 patients failed to show some degree of improvement on propranolol, with nearly 50% of subjects showing moderate improvement. For the most part, side effects were minor, with sedation and hypotension most common. Depression, a frequent side effect in adults treated with propranolol, occurred in one subject. Because of the open design of the study and the fact that the majority of subjects were receiving other medications, including stimulants, neuroleptics, and anticonvulsants, the results must be viewed with some caution.

In brief, psychopharmacological intervention with adolescent conduct disorder has not been widely researched. The clinician can approach treatment of conduct disorder with two basic strategies: treatment of associated psychopathology, such as ADD and depression, which may provide secondary benefits as regards symptoms of conduct disorder; and direct treatment of conduct disorder, in which case lithium would at present be considered the drug of choice.

SUMMARY

Conduct disordered behavior represents a final common pathway in which a multitude of interpersonal, environmental, educational, and biological factors converge. The clinical presentations of adolescents with conduct disorder are varied and produce a wide array of clinical outcomes. Despite the heterogeneity of adolescents included within this diagnosis and the debate about the validity and utility of conduct disorder as a diagnosis, the clinical symptoms associated with conduct disorder have well-documented significance for clinical course, prognosis, and treatment outcome.

At present, a large body of information has been accumulated about conduct disorder, but it has not had a significant impact on actual treatment. Because of widespread discouragement regarding the treatment of conduct disorder, there is a pressing need for this new knowledge to be incorporated into more sophisticated and effective treatment modalities for such adolescents.

REFERENCES

Aichorn, A. (1985). *Wayward youth.* New York: Viking.

Alessi, N. E., McManus, M., Grapentine, W. L., & Brickman, A. (1983). The characterization of depressive disorders in serious juvenile offenders. *Journal of Affective Disorders, 6,* 9–17.

Allen, R. P., Safer, D., & Covi, L. (1975). Effects of psychostimulants on aggression. *Journal of Nervous and Mental Disease, 160,* 138–145.

American Psychiatric Association (1987). *Diagnostic and statistical manual of mental disorders* (3d ed., revised). (DSM-III-R). Washington, DC: Author.

American Psychiatric Association (1980). *Diagnostic and statistical manual of mental disorders* (3d ed.). (DSM-III). Washington, DC: Author.

Amery, B., Minichiello, M. D., & Brown, G. L. (1984). Aggression in hyperactive boys: response to d-amphetamine. *Journal of the American Academy of Child Psychiatry, 23,* 291–292.

Bennett, N. G., Korein, J., Kalmijn, M., Grega, D. M., & Campbell, M. (1983). Electroencephalogram and treatment of hospitalized aggressive children with haloperidol and lithium. *Biological Psychiatry, 18,* 1427–1440.

Bohman, M., Cloninger, R., Sigvardsson, S., & von Knorring, A. (1982). Predisposition to petty criminality in Swedish adoptees: I. Genetic and environmental heterogeneity. *Archives of General Psychiatry, 39,* 1233–1241.

Brickman, A., McManus, M., Grapentine, W. L., & Alessi, N. (1984). Neuropsychological assessment of seriously delinquent adolescents. *Journal of the American Academy of Child Psychiatry, 23,* 453–457.

Campbell, M., Cohen, I. L., & Small, A. M. (1982). Drugs in aggressive behavior. *Journal of the American Academy of Child Psychiatry, 21,* 107–117.

Campbell, M., Small, A. M., Green, W. H., Jennings, S. J., Perry, R., Bennett, W. G., & Anderson, L. (1984). Behavioral efficacy of haloperidol and lithium carbonate: A comparison in hospitalized aggressive children with conduct disorder. *Archives of General Psychiatry, 41,* 650–656.

Cantwell, D. P. (1972). Psychiatric illness in families of hyperactive children. *Archives of General Psychiatry, 27,* 414–417.

Cantwell, D. P. (1978). Hyperactivity and antisocial behavior. *Journal of the American Academy of Child Psychiatry, 17,* 252–262.

Chiles, J. A., Miller, M. L., & Cox, G. B. (1980). Depression in an adolescent delinquent population. *Archives of General Psychiatry, 37,* 1179–1184.

Chwast, J. (1974). Delinquency and criminal behavior as depressive equivalents adolescents. In S. Lesse (Ed.), *Masked depression.* New York: Jason Aronson.

Cloninger, C. R., Sigvardsson, S., Bohman, M., & von Knorring, A. (1982). Predisposition to petty criminality in Swedish adoptees II: Cross fostering analysis of gene-environment interaction. *Archives of General Psychiatry, 39,* 1242–1257.

Conners, C. K. (1969). A teacher rating scale for use in drug studies. *American Journal of Psychiatry, 126,* 884–886.

DeLong, G. R. (1978). Lithium carbonate treatment of select behavior disturbances in children suggesting manic-depressive illness. *Journal of Pediatrics, 93,* 689–694.

Eisenberg, L., Lachman, R., Molling, P. A., Lockner, A., Mizelle, J. D., & Conners, C. K. (1963). A psychopharmacologic experiment in a training school for delinquent boys: methods, problems, findings. *American Journal of Orthopsychiatry, 3,* 431–443.

Gittelman, R., Mannuzza, S., Shenker, R., & Bonagura, N. (1985). Hyperactive boys almost grown up: I. Psychiatric status. *Archives of General Psychiatry, 42,* 937–947.

Glueck, S., & Glueck, E. T. (1962). *Family environment and delinquency.* Boston: Houghton-Mifflin.

Goodwin, D. W., Schilsinger, F., Knop, J., Mednick, S., & Guze, S. B. (1977). Psychopathology in adopted and non-adopted daughters of alcoholics. *Archives of General Psychiatry, 34,* 1005–1009.

Gordon, A. L. (1973). Patterns of delinquency in drug addiction. *British Journal of Psychiatry, 122,* 205–210.

Gualtieri, C. T., Quade, D., Hicks, R. E., Mayo, J. P., & Schroeder, S. R. (1984). Tardive dyskinesia and other clinical consequences of neuroleptic treatment in children and adolescents. *American Journal of Psychiatry, 141,* 20–23.

Hechtman, L., Weiss, G., & Perlman, T. (1984). Young adult outcome of hyperactive children who received long-term stimulant treatment. *Journal of the American Academy of Child Psychiatry, 23,* 261–269.

Hechtman, L., & Weiss, G. (1985). Controlled prospective 15 year follow-up of hyperactives as adults: Non-medical drug and alcohol use and antisocial behavior. *Journal of the American Academy of Child Psychiatry, 24,* 211–220.

Henn, F., Bardwell, R., & Jenkins, R. L. (1980). Juvenile delinquents revisited. *Archives of General Psychiatry, 37,* 1160–1165.

Hsu, L. K. G., Wisner, K., Richey, E. T., & Goldstein, C. (1985). Is juvenile delinquency related to an abnormal EEG? A study of EEG abnormalities in juvenile delinquents and adolescent psychiatric patients. *Journal of the American Academy of Child Psychiatry, 24,* 310–315.

Kandel, D. B. (1982). Epidemiological and psychosocial perspectives on drug use. *Journal of the American Academy of Child Psychiatry, 21,* 238–247.

Kandel, D. B., & Davies, M. (1982). Epidemiology of depressive mood in adolescents. *Archives of General Psychiatry, 39,* 1205–1212.

Kashani, J. H., Manning, G. W., McKnew, D. H., Cytryn, L., Simonds, J. F., & Wooderson, P. C. (1980). Depression among incarcerated delinquents. *Psychiatry Research, 3,* 185–191.

Klein, D. F., Gittelman, R., Quitkin, F., & Rifkin, A. (1980). *Diagnosis and drug treatment of psychiatric disorders: Adults and children.* Baltimore: Williams & Wilkins.

Kraus, J. (1981). Juvenile drug abuse and delinquency: some differential associations. *British Journal of Psychiatry, 139,* 422–430.

Kreuz, L. E., & Rose, R. M. (1972). Assessment of aggressive behavior and plasma testosterone in a young criminal population. *Psychomatic Medicine, 34,* 321–332.

Lena, B. (1979). Lithium in child and adolescent psychiatry. *Archives of General Psychiatry, 36,* 854–855.

Leventhal, B. (1984). The neuropharmacology of violent and aggressive behavior in children and adolescents. In C. Keith (Ed.), *The aggressive adolescent: Clinical perspectives.* New York: Free Press.

Lewis, D. O. (1976). Delinquency, psychomotor epileptic symptoms and paranoid ideation. *American Journal of Psychiatry, 133,* 1395–1398.

Lewis, D. O., & Shanok, S. S. (1978). Delinquency and the schizophrenic spectrum of disorders. *Journal of the American Academy of Child Psychiatry, 17,* 263–276.

Loney, J., Kramer, J., & Milich, R. S. (1981). The hyperactive child grows up: Predictors of symptoms, delinquency and achievement at follow-up. In K. D. Gadow & J. Loney (Eds.), *Psychosocial aspects of drug treatment for hyperactivity* (pp. 381–415). Boulder, CO: Westview.

Maletzky, B. M. (1974). D-amphetamine and delinquency: Hyperkinesis persisting? *Diseases of the Nervous System, 35,* 543–547.

Mannuzza, S., & Gittelman, R. (1984). The adolescent outcome of hyperactive girls. *Psychiatry Research, 13,* 19–29.

McCord, W., & McCord, J. (1959). *Origins of crime.* New York: Columbia University Press.

McGee, R., Williams, S., & Silva, P. A. (1984). Behavioral and developmental characteristics of aggressive, hyperactive and aggressive-hyperactive boys. *Journal of the American Academy of Child Psychiatry, 23,* 270–279.

McManus, M. E., Alessi, N. E., Grapentine, W. L., & Brickman, A. (1984a). Psychiatric disturbance in serious delinquents. *Journal of the American Academy of Child Psychiatry, 23,* 602–615.

McManus, M. E., Brickman, A., Alessi, N. E., & Grapentine, W. L. (1984b). Borderline personality in serious delinquents. *Comprehensive Psychiatry, 25,* 446–454.

McManus, M. E., Brickman, A., Alessi, N. E., & Grapentine, W. L. (1985). Neurological dysfunction in serious delinquents. *Journal of the American Academy of Child Psychiatry, 24,* 481–486.

McManus, M. E., Lerner, H., Robbins, D., & Barbour, C. (1984). Assessment of borderline symptomatology in hospitalized adolescents. *Journal of the American Academy of Child Psychiatry, 23,* 685–694.

Mednick, S. A., Gabrielli, W. F., Jr., & Hutchings, B. (1984). Genetic influences in criminal convictions: evidence from an adoption cohort. *Science, 224,* 891–894.

Naruse, H., Nagahata, M., Nakane, Y., Shirahoshi, K., Takesada, M., Yamazaki, K. (1982). A multicenter double-blind trial of pimozide, haloperidol and placebo in children with behavioral disorders, using crossover design. *Acta Paedopsychiatria, 48,* 173–184.

Offer, D., Marohn, R. C., & Ostrov, E. (1979). *The psychological world of the juvenile delinquent.* New York: Basic Books.

Patterson, G. R. (1974). Interventions for boys with conduct problems: multiple settings, treatments and criteria. *Journal of Consulting Clinical Psychology, 17,* 471–481.

Patterson, G. R., Reid, J. B., Jones, R. R., & Conger, R. (1975). *A social learning approach to family intervention Vol. I: Families with aggressive Children.* Eugene OR: Castalia.

Perry, R., Campbell, M., Green, W. H., Small, A. M., Die Trill, M. L., Meisslas, K., Golden, R. R., & Deutsch, S. I. (1985). Neuroleptic-related dyskinesias in autistic children: A prospective study. *Psychopharmacology Bulletin, 21,* 118–128.

Platt, J. E., Campbell, M., Green, W. H., & Grega, D. M. (1984). Cognitive effects of lithium carbonate and haloperidol in treatment resistant aggressive children. *Archives of General Psychiatry, 41,* 657–662.

Puig-Antich, J. (1982). Major depression and conduct disorder in prepuberty. *Journal of the American Academy of Child Psychiatry, 21,* 118–128.

Robins, L. N. (1966). *Delinquent children grown up: A sociological and psychiatric perspective.* Baltimore: Williams & Wilkins.

Robins, L. N. (1978). Sturdy predictors of adult antisocial behavior: Replications from longitudinal studies. *Psychological Medicine, 8,* 611–622.

Robins, L. N. (1983). Continuities and discontinuities in childhood behavior disorders. In D. E. Mechanic (Ed.), *Handbook of health and health services* (pp. 195–219). New York: Free Press.

Rutter, M., Graham, P., Chadwick, O. F. D., & Yule, W. (1976). Adolescent turmoil: Fact or fiction? *Journal of Child Psychology and Psychiatry and Allied Disciplines, 17,* 35–56.

Rutter, M., Tizard, J., & Whitemore, K. (1981). *Education, health and behavior.* Huntington, NY: Krieger.

Satterfield, J. H., Hoppe, C. M., & Schell, A. M. (1982). A prospective study of delinquency in 110 boys with attention deficit disorder and 88 normal boys. *American Journal of Psychiatry, 139,* 795–798.

Shamsie, S. J. (1981). Antisocial adolescents: Our treatments do not work—where do we go from here? *Canadian Journal of Psychiatry, 26,* 357–364.

Shapiro, S. K., & Garfinkel, B. D. (1986). The occurrence of behavior disorders in children: The interdependence of attention deficit disorder and conduct disorder. *Journal of the American Academy of Child Psychiatry, 25,* 809–819.

Sheard, M. H., Marini, J. L., Bridges, C. I., & Wagner, E. (1976). The effect of lithium on impulsive, aggressive behavior in man. *American Journal of Psychiatry, 133,* 1409–1433.

Sigvardsson, S., Cloninger, C. R., Bohman, N., & von Knorring, A. (1982). Predisposition to petty criminality in Swedish adoptees: III. Sex differences and validation of the male typology. *Archives of General Psychiatry, 39,* 1248–1253.

Simonds, J. F., & Kashani, J. (1979). Drug abuse and criminal behavior in boys committed to a training school. *American Journal of Psychiatry, 136,* 1444–1448.

Stewart, M. A., Cummings, C., Singer, S., & deBlois, C. S. (1981). The overlap between hyperactive and unsocialized aggressive children. *Journal of Child Psychology and Psychiatry, 22,* 35–48.

Stewart, M. A., deBlois, C. S., & Cummings (1980a). Psychiatric disorder in the parents of hyperactive boys and those with conduct disorders. *Journal of Child Psychology and Psychiatry, 21,* 283–292.

Stewart, M. A., deBlois, C., Meardon, J., & Cummings, C. (1980b). Aggressive conduct disorder of children: The clinical picture. *Journal of Nervous and Mental Disease, 168,* 604–610.

Tarter, R. A., Hegedus, A. M., Winston, N. E., & Alterman, A. (1984). Neuropsychological, personality and familial characteristics of physically abused delinquents. *Journal of the American Academy of Child Psychiatry, 23,* 668–674.

Weiss, G., Hechtman, L., Milroy, T., & Perlman, T. (1985). Psychiatric status of hyperactives as young adults: A controlled prospective 15 year follow-up of 63 hyperactive children. *Journal of the American Academy of Child Psychiatry, 24,* 211–220.

Werry, J. S., Aman, M. G., & Lampen, E. (1975). Haloperidol and methylphenidate in children. *Acta Paedopsychiatria, 42,* 26–40.

Williams, D. T., Mehl, R., Yudofsky, S., Adams, D., & Roseman, B. (1982). The effect of propanolol on uncontrolled rage outbursts in children and adolescents with organic brain dysfunction. *Journal of the American Academy of Child Psychiatry, 21,* 129–135.

Wolff, P. H., Waber, D., Bauermeister, M., Cohen, C., & Ferber, R. (1982). The neuropsychological status of adolescent delinquent boys. *Journal of Child Psychology and Psychiatry, 23,* 267–279.

CHAPTER THIRTEEN

Schizophrenia and Schizophreniform Disorder

S. Charles Schulz
Miriam M. Koller

A 14-year-old boy was the subject of Morel's description of a syndrome he labeled demence procose in the middle of the nineteenth century. According to Morel's report, the patient had been highly functioning, socially likable, and intellectually bright. His psychotic illness was devastating and unremitting, leading to the classification of a premature dementia. The term dementia praecox was used by Krapelin as he also observed the early onset of a psychotic illness that was characteristically unrelenting in its course. Therefore, since the modern conceptualization of schizophrenia, the disorder has been inexorably intertwined with adolescence.

Schizophrenia is considered the most severe of psychiatric illnesses and is unfortunately not rare. The seriousness of schizophrenia is attested to by a number of factors. First, schizophrenia is the most prevalent diagnosis in long-term care wards of the state mental hospitals. Many patients are referenced to admissions sections of such hospitals, but patients with schizophrenia are those who are more frequently unable to go home and are transferred to longer-term care units. It is not unusual to find hundreds of patients with schizophrenia who have been in such institutions for 10 to 15 years. Furthermore, for those patients who are able to leave the hospital (clearly the majority in recent times), very few are able to function at a level that would be considered career. In addition, a very large percentage of patients who suffer from schizophrenia require rehospitalization a number of times during the course of their illness.

Another factor, which has been assumed for some time but has been quantified recently, is the number of homeless people who have schizophrenia either as a result of deinstitutionalization or patients who drift out of the mainstream mental health system (Davies, Munetz, Schulz, & Bromet, in press; Baxter & Hopper, 1984). Some of the homeless mentally ill are those referred to as the young adult chronic patient. The serious nature of schizophrenia is further underscored by recent follow-up data by Grinker and associates (1981), who noted that as many as 17% of schizophrenic patients had ended their own lives within the first 5 years of their admission to a research ward. In addition to all of these factors that demonstrate the staggering impact of schizophrenia on the patient, it is now well documented by empirical studies and by the emergence of family advocacy groups that the lives of the relatives of a patient with schizophrenia are severely altered emotionally and financially (Hatfield, 1984, Schulz et al., 1982).

There are no epidemiological studies of the prevalence of schizophrenia in teenage years; however, the prevalence of schizophrenia in adolescents can be estimated to be approximately 50,000 at any time. It is known that the mean age of onset of schizophrenia is approximately 19, indicating that many patients have developed symptoms of the disorder some years earlier. The empirical incidence rate of schizophrenia is 1 in 1000 per year, and the new cases are predominantly in the adolescent age range.

These introductory comments are intended to convey the authors' concern about the serious nature of schizophrenia. The thematic thread that will run through this chapter is the connection between schizophrenia in teenagers and adults and the importance of appropriate management during the early years of the illness.

DIAGNOSTIC ISSUES

A problem for the field of psychiatry and psychology in past years was the inability to communicate accurately about diagnosis. This was particularly a problem for clinicians and researchers interested in schizophrenia. Although the field of psychiatry tried to convey the seriousness of the illness, the public had trouble taking it seriously because they felt psychiatrists were unable to agree on who had the disorder. Furthermore, there was such variance in diagnostic practices that patients who were transferred to different loci of care would have their diagnosis changed based on nonobjective criteria. With the development of the Feighner criteria (1972) and the subsequent development of the Research Diagnostic Criteria (RDC) (Spitzer, Endicott, & Robins, 1977), both of which culminated in the DSM-III (APA, 1980), the diagnosis of schizophrenia became much less mysterious and more reliable (Carpenter, Strauss, & Bartko, 1974). The diagnosis was further refined in the recent DSM-III-R (APA, 1987).

The diagnosis of schizophrenia can be made when the DSM-III-R criteria are fulfilled. To be so classified, the patient must have reported the symptoms listed in the manual; obviously, not every psychotic teenager is to be classified as schizophrenic. The types of symptoms needed for the diagnosis include disturbances in the content and form of thought, perceptions, motor behavior, affect, and relation to the world (autism). These disturbances may take the form of bizarre delusions (meaning that the belief is impossible). A patient with the symptom of bizarre delusions reported to the authors that his mother had been created in a space station circling Jupiter and was then sent to Earth. The Schneiderian symptoms, also known as passive delusions, are part of this category and include such statements as "I feel that a malignant force is controlling me by messages relayed through the toaster." Other characteristic symptoms include auditory hallucinations in which a voice keeps a running commentary on the patient's behavior or two or more voices converse with one another, and thought disorder, usually noted as marked loosening of associations or incoherence. These characteristic symptoms must interfere in the patient's life as evidenced by diminution in function at work or school.

In our opinion, the fourth criterion for the diagnosis of schizophrenia in teenagers, related to the length of time ill, is especially important. Because the psychiatrist interviewing the teenage patient frequently may be the first professional to see the patient, the nature of the prodromal symptoms is more important than in adults, who often have been manifestly ill for years. Such symptoms should be sought in the evaluation of a teenager with psychosis. They include phenomena such as social isolation, recent odd or eccentric behavior, or blunted affect.

When DSM-III-R criteria are fulfilled, the classification of schizophrenia may be made. It is appropriate at this point to note the obvious: The presentation of one teenager with schizophrenia may be quite different from that of another, using the polythetical approach to diagnosis. This has led the field to the frequently discussed topic of heterogeneity of schizophrenia. The heterogeneity concept, which is very important for investigators of schizophrenia, is also important for clinicians. That is, their statements (which are global generalizations about schizophrenia) probably lead to trouble if they are believed as such. Clearly, not all patients have the same symptom profile; for example, some have more positive than negative symptoms, and not all patients have the same course or response to medication.

Although it is rarely mentioned in these times of objective criteria, the mechanism of eliciting diagnostic criteria is as important, and some feel it is inexorably linked to the final classification. This may be especially true for the teenager with schizophrenia. Although a structured interview like the Diagnostic Interview Schedule (DIS) (Robins, Helzer, Croughan, & Ratcliff, 1981) is an instrument which allows for uniform assessment, there are some data (Pulver & Carpenter, 1983) to indicate that when delivered just once, it may under assess for schizophrenia. We feel this may be especially true for teenagers who often feel that they are being criticized or judged for the symptoms they experience. We have noted that such young patients may respond to questions about psychotic symptoms by saying they have them but that it does not make them "bad" or "different." The need for a sympathetic interviewer cannot be stressed enough. This means a clinician who will use data gathered over a period of time to make the best estimate of the diagnostic evaluation.

When the diagnosis of schizophrenia is made in the teenager at the outset of a psychotic illness, this does not mean the clinician's thoughts about diagnosis are over. Certain physical causes of psychosis may declare themselves later in the illness, or a more affective course may unfold. Use of drugs which mimic schizophrenia and may not clear immediately after admission—such as PCP or extended amphetamine use—are to be strongly considered. The laboratory may be especially helpful in this regard because even if a cooperative teenager reports no serious drug use, PCP can be put in other preparations such as marijuana. Medical causes of psychosis need to be carefully investigated in teenagers. Now that noninvasive imaging can be performed, this tool should be strongly considered in any patient's evaluation. In addition, an electroencephalogram (EEG) can be helpful if there is any suspicion of an epileptic disorder. We are not recommending a routine request for these studies at each admission to an inpatient unit, but we want to stress the importance of them in the early stages of the illness. Other psychiatric disorders to be kept in mind include bipolar disorder (see Chapter 10), borderline/schizotypal disorder, brief reactive psychosis, and paranoid disorders. It is clear that the psychiatric differential is of great importance because of the different treatment strategies indicated.

DEVELOPMENTAL ISSUES

Developmental issues have played a large role in the conceptualization of schizophrenia for the majority of the twentieth century. Various psychoenvironmental issues were at the center of theories about the etiology and treatment of schizophrenia. Most of these centered around the interaction of the parents with the patient during his or her early years. Such theories as the "double-bind" hypothesis and the "schizophrenogenic mother" were espoused. However, none of these theories has a strong empirical base, and none has been convincing in the etiology of schizophrenia. It is short-sighted to say that a relationship between environment and illness will never be found or that certain psychoenvironmental issues play a large role for some patients, but future research will answer that question.

In thinking of developmental issues as of this writing, we will focus mainly on the issue of the impact of schizophrenia on the developing teenager. For example, evidence about the subtle difficulties that a person who develops schizophrenia may have had to deal with all his or her life are important to remember. Fish and Hagin (1972) demonstrated neurological abnormalities in infants born to schizophrenic women. In high-risk studies, Erlenmeyer-Kimling and Cornblatt (1978) have shown attentional as well as school difficulties in their sample well before the onset of any symptoms referable to schizophrenia. Persons with such difficulties present throughout early life will have significant difficulty negotiating usual developmental tasks. Furthermore, their difficulties may reverberate within the family, setting up a situation in which emotions are heightened and criticism increased.

In his book, *Clinical Aspects of Child Development,* Melvin Lewis (1982) discusses several phases of adolescence. Using Lewis' rubric, we will consider how these phases may be modified by schizophrenia. It is during middle adolescence, age 15 to 17, that adolescents turn toward peers for external certainties. Schizophrenic children in middle adolescence have enormous difficulty turning toward peers because they often feel ostracized by them. Here, the negative symptoms of schizophrenia (withdrawal, flattened affect, and asocial behavior) interfere dramatically with appropriate development during the middle adolescent years. Important peer group support is rarely available to schizophrenically impaired youngsters. We have found group therapy on an adolescent inpatient unit is often extremely valuable in helping schizophrenic adolescents recognize that they can be valued by peers. We have found that such groups function best when there is a heterogenous group of patients so that the higher functioning patients can help those more seriously impaired. It is in such a situation that schizophrenic adolescents may first experience themselves as members of a group.

It is in the late stage of adolescence that normal individuals become more self-sufficient in their commitments to others and to work. As we have mentioned earlier, it is rare that schizophrenic adolescents are able to develop a genuine career. Schizophrenic youngsters are seriously impaired when it comes to focusing on the tasks needed to be successful at a complicated job. Here, more frustration sets in as the youngsters realize that, again, they are going to function in a different way than their peers. Often the illness has interfered with schooling and these youngsters are behind the other teenagers their age. It is commonly difficult for these youngsters to organize and present themselves in an integrated enough fashion to be accepted by the college of their first choice and to remain in college if accepted. Once again, they fall behind those around them, and this fact usually leads to a sense of alienation and failure.

Thus it is during adolescence when schizophrenia first begins, that many youngsters become severely depressed as they are forced to face the reality of their decreased functioning in virtually every developmental phase. These youngsters require tremendous support from adults around them and positive reinforcement when they are able to succeed either in school, socially, or in the work place. What would be considered routine achievement for normal children may, in fact, be monumental achievements for schizophrenic children. Therefore, a passing grade, a part time job successfully completed, the development of an enduring friendship, and a successful date should be considered as significant achievements for schizophrenic or schizophreniform youngsters.

In addition to the impact of the illness on social and vocational issues, it is during adolescence that cognitive development is characterized by a broadened scope of intellectual activity and a capacity for insight. Piaget termed this stage one of formal operations (Inhalder and Piaget, 1958). It is during this cognitive stage that children can grasp abstract concepts and reason from hypothesis. Schizophrenic youngsters, however, may not be able to think abstractly. Furthermore, the positive signs of their development (hallucinations, delusions, illusions) may interfere with their ability to think clearly even on a concrete level.

Egocentricity was viewed by Piaget (1962) as a normal manifestation of adolescent development. Schizophrenic youngsters may carry this egocentricity to an extreme, and their paranoia may heighten as to what others are thinking or saying about them, as well as being grandiose at times. Normal adolescents may feel scrutinized by others, self-critical, and self-admiring. Schizophrenic youngsters are in need of a supportive and mature adult who can continually put these in perspective for them.

In summary, normal adolescents are faced with issues of self-identity, cognitive development, separation from parents, development of love relationships, and final career goals. Schizophrenic youngsters face all of these normal developmental stressors, and each stress is often exacerbated by their inadequacy to rise up to the developmental task. Thus schizophrenic adolescents need considerable support and guidance from mature adults who can steer them in the correct direction while allowing them to develop as much autonomy as possible.

Another developmental issue in patients with schizophrenia is the age of onset of symptoms. It has been our experience that when a severe psychosis begins in early adolescence, that behavior during the illness seems dramatically immature and childlike. This may appear self-evident, but it may be important for the treatment team to remember so they can help such teenagers rather than criticize them or interpret their behavior as acting out. In a recent study using the experimental antipsychotic medication clozapine, it has been noted that a patient in her midtwenties who had been psychotic since early teenage years had a dramatic remission of symptoms. Interestingly, though now 26, her behavior resembled that of a normal 13- or 14-year-old, including crushes on the male staff, playing pranks on the unit, and dressing as an early teenager (personal communication, Robert Conley, M.D.). These observations are intended to illustrate the impact of schizophrenia on the young patient's development. At this time, we do not know whether these observations are specific for schizophrenia or nonspecific in the sense they may occur following any major chronic illness.

CLINICAL PROBLEMS

It is our concern that the major clinical problem in the treatment of adolescents with schizophrenia is the lack of recognition of schizophrenia as part of the continuum of adult schizophrenia. Although not universal, the case summaries of patients transferred to our care indicate a reticence to diagnose schizophrenia and to use antipsychotic medications. In addition, schizophrenia in teenagers is essentially ignored in the major textbooks of general psychiatry. This lack of recognition may be understandable as a concern of stigma of the diagnosis or a wish to remain hopeful and not assign a serious diagnosis to such young patients. However, the consequences of such a delay in treatment also may have serious consequences.

There have been recent studies by us and others that provide biological data indicating that for some teenagers the parameters of the disorder seen in many adult seriously ill schizophrenic patients are already present at the outset of the illness. Weinberger and colleagues (1979) reported enlargement of the lateral ventricles of the brain in schizophrenic patients as compared to controls. They also reported that the size of the ventricles was not related to age. We assessed ventricular size (expressed as ventricular brain ratio [VBR] in a group of inpatient teenagers with schizophrenia or schizophreniform disorder. It was noted that the teenagers with schizophrenia had significantly enlarged ventricles compared to controls and to borderline personality disordered inpatients (Fig. 13.1) (Schulz et al., 1983a). Compared to other studies, such as Weinberger's, the teenagers in this study had VBRs of nearly equal size, and as large a percentage were outside the control range. Interestingly, some of the patients with the larger ventricles were in the group who had experienced symptoms for less than 6 months.

To extend our findings in parallel to those in adult schizophrenic patients, we then investigated the relationship of the ventricular size to treatment with neuroleptics. Earlier, Weinberger and colleagues (1980) had shown that schizophrenics with increased VBRs had no change as a group to

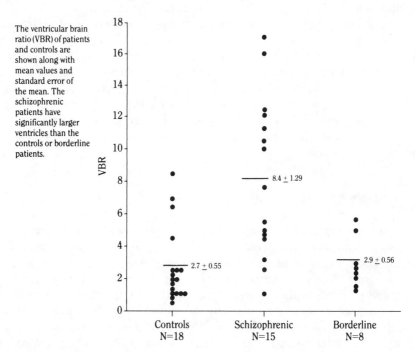

Figure 13.1. Ventricular brain ratio (VBR) measurements in teenage patients and controls.

neuroleptic treatment, while schizophrenic patients with normal-sized ventricles had a significant response. In another group of teenagers (Schulz et al., 1983b), we showed the same relationship; that is, that the patients with enlarged ventricles had poor response to treatment as a group (see Figure 13.2). Thus we posit that for some if not most patients, the factors contributing to poor response to neuroleptics are present at the onset of the disorder and are not a result of the illness.

In our third experiment in this series designed to investigate the relationship of findings in adult schizophrenic patients to teenagers with the syndrome, we explored the relationship between ventricular size and metabolites of the neurotransmitters dopamine and serotonin (Jennings, Schulz, Narasimhachari, Hamer, and Friedel, 1985). Other research groups had found that those patients with larger ventricles had lower levels of the monoamine metabolites homovanillic acid (HVA) and 5-hydroxyindoleacetic acid (5-HIAA), and they hypothesized that this reflected diminished neuronal number or function (Potkin, Weinberger, Linnoila, & Wyatt, 1983; van Kammen et al., 1983; Nyback, Berggren, Hindmarsh, Sedvall, & Wiesel, 1983). However, all the studies on older schizophrenic patients were confounded by previous neuroleptic treatment. Therefore, we examined a group of adolescents with psychotic disorders—schizophrenia, manic-depressive illness, and psychotic depression—and compared the relationship of cerebrospinal fluid (CSF) metabolites to VBR in psychiatric inpatient teenagers without a psychotic illness. The results of this experiment were consistent with the two earlier studies, in that the teenagers with psychotic illness had the same inverse relationship of HVA and 5-HIAA to VBR. The teenagers without psychotic illness did not have a significant relationship of monoamine metabolites and VBR.

These studies are significant because they support the idea that a group of teenagers with schizophrenia already has parameters of adult seriously ill schizophrenic patients. The implication is that for a group of the schizophrenic teenagers, methods which have been found useful for adult patients (such as the early and judicious use of neuroleptics and attention to structured psychosocial interventions) are important. Recently, some empirical evidence has emerged from England (DeLisi, Crow, & Hirsch, 1986). It was noted that May, Tuma, Yale, Potepan, and Dixon (1976) showed that the schizophrenic patients who were assigned to psychotherapy alone spent nearly twice as many days in the hospital as those who had received medication during the 6 months of the experiment. Based on this follow-up study, Crow and colleagues examined the relationship of the duration of symptoms prior to treatment with outcome. As reported by DeLisi et al., (1986) they found that the patients who had been psychotic for a longer period of time prior to initiation of neuroleptic treatment fared worse, as measured by relapse, than the first break patients who

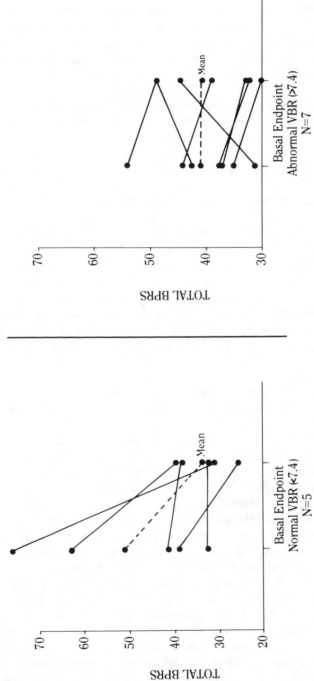

In this figure the amount of improvement as assessed by the Brief Psychiatric Rating Scale (BPRS) during neuroleptic treatment is illustrated. As a group, those patients with ventricular enlargement did not improve with neuroleptics.

Figure 13.2. The relationship between ventricular size and neuroleptic treatment response.

received treatment close to their onset of symptoms. Although this is not a prospective study and the patients who had a long period of time to treatment may have had a slow and insidious onset of illness consistent with a chronic course, such data point to the importance of the early recognition of symptoms of psychosis and prompt treatment.

The concern that seriously disturbed adolescents may be underrecognized is underscored by studies done in Chicago by Offer, Ostrov, and Howard (1981). In their work, it was noted that mental health professionals significantly overestimated the turmoil of adolescence when compared to the perception of normal teenagers. In our view, if clinicians view serious disturbance as part of normal development, they will be less likely to treat serious mental illness or have the appropriate index of suspicion for the consequences of the prodrome of psychosis in teenagers.

In summary, the treatment of the adolescent who becomes psychotic is clearly a complex and difficult issue, as will be described in the next sections of the chapter focusing on treatment. However, present understanding of mental illness in the field of psychiatry provides sufficient data to recognize the significance of psychosis in teenagers and to not delay empirically proven treatments.

PHARMACOLOGICAL APPROACHES

Once there has been agreement on the diagnosis of schizophrenia in the adolescent patient, the pharmacological treatment rests on the dopamine receptor blocking antipsychotic agents. To date, there is no other form of treatment of schizophrenia that has been demonstrated to be efficacious in reducing symptoms of psychosis in these patients. Furthermore, the antipsychotic medications not only reduce hallucinations and paranoia, but they also improve concentration and attention so that patients are able to participate in psychosocial treatments and school or work. Significant improvement can be expected in approximately 70% of patients according to the results of the classic National Institute of Mental Health (NIMH) collaborative studies (Cole, Goldberg, & Klerman, 1964). However, knowledge of the efficacy of the medication is only part of the treatment approach to the psychotic patient, as there are special concerns for the teenager. To optimally treat schizophrenia, the clinician must be able to select a specific medication, decide on a dosing strategy, know how to recognize and manage side effects, how to shift to maintenance treatment, and what to consider if minimal response is seen (for a review of these strategies, see Jennings & Schulz, 1986).

In selecting an antipsychotic medication, the clinician needs to remember that all of the approved medications work through the same mechanism of action, that is, through the blockade of dopamine receptors.

Therefore, there is no "correct" drug. Furthermore, no evidence exists that there is a "correct" drug for specific situations. For example, the idea that an agitated patient needs a sedating neuroleptic in an emergent situation is not borne out by controlled studies. The selection of an antipsychotic medication has been recommended to rest on factors concerning side effects, past response, and familiarity of the clinician with the drug. There is no evidence that changing the class of antipsychotic drug will enhance response, although anecdotal reports are known.

Dosing strategies have changed in recent years from the idea of rapid neuroleptization to a more conservative approach. Recent studies have demonstrated that haloperidol at 10 mg/d has the same effect on a group of schizophrenic patients at the same rate of improvement as much higher doses (Donlon et al., 1980; Nebrosky, Janowsky, Perel, Munson, & Dupry, 1984). Most clinicians treating teenagers probably have used lower doses over the years, so they are accustomed to this approach. It should be remembered also that there is widely replicated evidence that if dosage is below approximately 300–500 chlorpromazine equivalents-cpze/day, a patient has not had an adequate trial of medication. Also, recent biochemical evidence from the NIMH has indicated that the full effect of antipsychotic medications does not occur until 4 or 5 weeks (Pickar et al., 1984).

Our approach to the schizophrenic teenager, based on these studies, is to begin with a relatively low dose of antipsychotic medication (approximately 300 CPZ-E/d in divided doses). We do not change dose before 1 week because the patient will not have reached steady state blood level. We try to make sure that each patient has had a fair neuroleptic trial, so if response is not seen at 300 CPZ/d, we try 500–800 CPZ/d. We do not see a place for so-called megadose strategies consistent with findings of Magliozzi et al., (1980). Preliminary results from medication level studies indicate that for some patients the concentration of the medication in their blood is too low or too high for response even though they are on appropriate doses (Schulz, 1987; Schulz, Butterfield, Garicano, Narasimachari, & Friedel, 1984; van Putten, 1987). In cases of poor response, an assessment of blood level may be helpful.

Perhaps because of the medication-naive nature of schizophrenic patients who are beginning neuroleptic treatment, extrapyramidal side effects are common. Again, in our experience, we have found that if this issue is ignored, some patients never want to take antipsychotic medications again. Some investigators have recommended using prophylactic anticholinergic medication for adolescent patients beginning antipsychotic treatment to avoid painful dystonic reactions. Others recommend closely watching patients so that rapid intervention for dystonia can be made—such as with the use of intramuscular diphenhydramine (Benadryl). Another medication side effect which has received increased attention in recent years is akathesia (van Putten, May, & Marder, 1984). This side effect is very uncomfortable and can lead to increased agitation in patients or discontinuation of medication. As is well known, anticholinergic medication is not very helpful for this condition, but recent controlled trials have shown propranolol to be efficacious (Lipinski, Zubenko, Cohen, & Barriera, 1984; Zubenko, Lipinski, Cohen, & Barriera, 1984; Adler et al., 1986).

Tardive dyskinesia (TD) can no longer be ignored by psychiatrists treating teenagers simply because it is usually seen after some years of treatment. The authors have seen cases arise as early as 9 months after beginning neuroleptics, and large scale epidemiological studies indicate that after 7 years of treatment approximately 25% of patients will have developed TD (Kane et al., 1984). We feel that the APA Task Force on TD guidelines are appropriate for patients of all ages. These guidelines include a candid discussion of the problem and recommend using the lowest dose of neuroleptic possible and frequent examination. Although there is not a treatment for TD, recent studies have demonstrated that by using the lowest dose possible to control symptoms, TD does not progress in most patients and may diminish slightly (Munetz & Toenniessen, 1984).

Maintenance treatment follows the acute phase of neuroleptic administration. No evidence exists that schizophrenic teenagers do not need maintenance treatment, and there is every reason to think that the relapse rate of those not treated will be about 80% in the first year. However, some of the distasteful aspects of maintenance treatment have been addressed by recent research showing that lower doses of maintenance medication can prevent relapse (at least during the first year) and improve the quality of life of the patient by decreasing sedation and a motivational syndrome (Marder et al., 1984). In addition, the use of intermittent neuroleptic medication during maintenance may work for some patients and may even decrease the risk for TD (Herz, 1987).

Last, it is well known that not all patients with schizophrenia respond fully to neuroleptic treatment. The next steps with such patients have never been clear. However, clinical trials have been completed that indicate some hopefulness for the use of nonneuroleptic agents used as augmenters of neuroleptics. In our work with neuroleptic nonresponsive schizophrenic patients, both lithium carbonate and carbamazepine have been shown to reduce psychotic symptoms in some poorly responsive schizophrenic patients (Schulz, Conley, & Benjamin, 1987). Pickar and colleagues (1987) have shown the usefulness of adding the benzodiazepine alprazolam to neuroleptics in reducing both positive and negative symptoms of schizophrenia. To our knowledge, these types of augmentation have not been tried in teenagers in controlled clinical trials. Thus in our opinion, they should be used carefully.

In conclusion, there has been a significant amount of work in the use of neuroleptic medication, management of side effects, and augmentation in the last few years. Consistent with our view of the continuity of schizophrenia in teenagers with the adult disorder, we feel that those clinicians treating teenagers should be aware of these advances and that their patients should have the opportunity to benefit from them.

PSYCHOSOCIAL APPROACHES

A number of movements in psychiatry during the last decade have changed the psychosocial approach to patients with schizophrenia, including teenagers. Shortened hospital stays, the desire of the family group to know more about the illness, the recognized need for structure in the early stage of the illness, and the influence of family emotional environment on the course of the illness have all led to significant changes in adolescent inpatient units and programs.

Perhaps the most important of these developments has been the increasing recognition of the need for structure in the early stage of the illness and the impact of heightened emotionality in the home and the treatment setting. Adolescent units have been in the forefront of a structured environment for their inpatient units because of their recognition of the need for a planned day for young people. Most wards we have visited or worked on have a full day's schedule of school, vocational, and social activities. It is our impression that this spirit be extended to the manner of talking therapy. For the acutely ill patient, straightforward communications about content issues are most helpful. Recognition during the first few weeks of hospitalization of any patients who are becoming overwhelmed by the stimulating environment is needed in order to diminish agitation that can be a response to overwhelming input.

Some schizophrenia programs have begun explicit teaching programs about mental illness and its treatment during or near the end of inpatient stays. Such programs have included a classroom format in which printed handouts of booklets are made available. Slides about the treatment modalities, medications, and their side effects are frequently shown. Some clinicians doing this type of work stress the importance of performing it in groups so discussion can occur among the patient's peers. Hearing that a side effect was successfully managed from another patient, especially with teenagers, can be a meaningful interaction.

Because most teenage patients come to the hospital from a family and most return to a family, the family is more involved in the treatment of schizophrenic teenagers than in most schizophrenic patients. We feel that there are several goals in helping the family of teenagers who have been diagnosed as schizophrenic. These include: (1) a candid and factual discussion of the problem and the conclusions of the evaluation team, (2) an empathetic discussion of the impact of the illness on the family, (3) and a discussion (in a nonpejorative fashion) of the ways to diminish emotionality in the home.

In our experience, the clinicians treating psychiatric patients have been reluctant to discuss diagnostic issues or the evidence for the diagnostic impression with the patients and their families in much the same way that serious medical illnesses were not openly discussed in the 1950s. Now it is clear that families want and deserve to know what the problem is, what the prognosis is, and how the diagnosis was made. This needs to be done in a fashion that allows for extended discussion and, of course, should not be done before the diagnosis is clarified. Also at this time, the clinician should make it clear that he or she is aware of the impact of the illness on the family. These issues are usually discussed with the family in individual sessions during the patient's hospital treatment.

Near the end of an inpatient stay or shortly after discharge, we feel that most families can benefit from participation in groups designed for them (Schulz, House, & Andrews, 1986). Such groups have initial sessions devoted to what are termed psychoeducational issues, and one of the psychiatrists from the treatment program usually joins the other staff to describe what is known about schizophrenia and its treatment. In these initial sessions, adequate time is needed to accommodate questions and discussions. This is followed by a series of group sessions for the discussion of concerns the family has about the illness, sharing their feelings with others who have had similar experiences, and developing coping strategies with other families. We have utilized a short-term group strategy to accomplish this and have found it to be well received. Many of the family members who have participated in the groups go on to join local chapters of the National Alliance for the Mentally Ill (NAMI). Other centers have recommended a more extended group experience for families, which is designed to diminish the isolation of family members with a schizophrenic patient and to bolster them for the adjustment to dealing with the long-term problem of schizophrenia (McFarlane, 1982).

Recently, several groups of researchers (Goldstein, Rodnick, Evans, May, & Steinberg, 1978; Leff, Kuipers, Berkowitz, Eberlein-Freis, & Sturgeon, 1982; Falloon et al., 1982; Hogarty et al., 1986) have found a psychoeducational family therapy approach to be effective in lowering the short-term relapse rate in adult schizophrenic patients maintained on neuroleptics. While the details of each study differed, all emphasized educating the families about schizophrenia and its treatment and improving the families' problem-solving skills, particularly in relation to coping with the schizophrenic illness. It must be emphasized that the rationale of this treatment need not depend on the more controversial concept of expressed emotion (EE) in families. Since most adolescent patients live with their family, the effectiveness of such a treatment deserves to be studied intensively.

The major portion of a section on psychosocial treatment in past years would have concentrated on techniques of talking therapy for the adolescent patient. At this time, the evidence for the efficacy of a psychoanalytically oriented psychotherapy for teenagers with schizophrenia or for adult patients with schizophrenia is not present. In our opinion, the use of regressive techniques and interpretations of thinking and behavior rather than clarifications may slow the progress of a schizophrenic teenager. Nonspecific techniques of interviewing skills (such as empathy, positive regard, hopeful outlook, and the establishment of a therapeutic alliance) are clearly needed, but they are needed in the context of clear, mostly content-oriented communications. Gunderson and Carrol (1983) have described the use of the initial hospitalization as a time for the evaluation of those people early in the course of schizophrenia who may benefit from more intensive talking therapy. This strategy appears to be a good one for identifying the patients best suited to the treatment, and the treatment is begun after the acute phase of the illness resolving.

SUMMARY

We have set out to draw parallels of adult schizophrenia to schizophrenia in adolescents because numbers of advances have been made that can be successfully applied to teenagers. We have described the diagnostic considerations, including our concern for a high index of suspicion for prodromal symptoms and our concern for underrecognition of the disturbed adolescent. Next, we extensively discussed the results of studies that demonstrate a biological continuity with adult schizophrenia. Following this section, we described pharmacological strategies for adolescent schizophrenia, citing a number of recent experiments in adults. The new studies on psychosocial approaches to schizophrenia have not been applied widely to schizophrenic adolescents; however, we propose that their use may be quite helpful, especially as they fit the tradition of the educational and structured nature of adolescent units.

Finally, social skills training, which seems to decrease the short-term relapse rate in adult patients (Hogarty et al., 1986), may benefit these adolescents. A more individualized program tailored to meet the particular adolescent's needs may be more appropriate than a packaged program.

REFERENCES

Adler, L., Angrist, B., Peselow, E., Corwin, J., Maslansky, R., & Rotrosen, J. (1986). A controlled assessment of propranolol in the treatment of neuroleptic-induced akathisia. *British Journal of Psychiatry, 149,* 42–45.

American Psychiatric Association (1987). *Diagnostic and statistical manual of mental disorders* (3rd ed., revised). (DSM-III-R). Washington, DC: Author.

American Psychiatric Association (1980). *Diagnostic and statistical manual of mental disorders,* (3rd ed.). (DSM-III). Washington, DC: Author.

Baxter, E., & Hopper, K. (1984). Troubled on the streets: The mentally disabled homeless poor. In: J. A. Talbott (Ed.), *The chronic mental patient: Five years later* (pp. 49–62). Orlando, Fl: Grune & Stratton, Inc.

Carpenter, W. T., Jr., Strauss, J. S., & Bartko, J. J. (1974). Use of signs and symptoms for the identification of schizophrenic patients. *Schizophrenia Bulletin,* Winters, 37–49.

Cole, J. O., Goldberg, S. C., & Klerman, G. L. (1964). Phenothiazine treatment in acute schizophrenia. *Archives of General Psychiatry, 10,* 246–261.

Conley, R. M. Personal ccommunication, 1987.

Davies, M. A., Munetz, M. R., Schulz, S. C., & Bromet, E. J. (In press). Assessing mental illness in SRO shelter residents: Preventing a "catastrophe." *Hospital and Community Psychiatry.*

DeLisi, L. E., Crow, T. J., & Hirsch, S. R. (1986, January 26–31). The third biannual winter workshop on schizophrenia, Schladming, Austria. (Published erratum appears in 1987 Jan:44(1):76) *Archives of General Psychiatry, 43,* 706–711.

Donlon, P. T., Hopkin, J. T., Tupin, J. P., Wicks, J. J., Wahba, M., & Meadow A. (1980). Haloperidol for acute schizophrenic patients: An evaluation of three oral regimens. *Archives of General Psychiatry, 37,* 691–695.

Erlenmeyer-Kimling, L., & Cornblatt, B. (1978). Attentional measures in a study of children at high risk for schizophrenia. In L. C. Wynne, R. Crombell, & S. Matthysse (Eds.), *Nature of schizophrenia: New approaches to research and treatment* (pp. 359–365). New York: Wiley.

Falloon, I. R. H., Boyd, J. L., McGill, C. W., Razani, J., Moss, H. B., & Gilderman, A. M. (1982). Family management in the prevention of exacerbations of schizophrenia. *New England Journal of Medicine, 306* 1437–1440.

Feighner, J., Robins, E., Guze, S., Woodruff, R., Winokur, G., & Munoz, R. (1972). Diagnostic criteria for use in psychiatric research. *Archives of General Psychiatry, 26,* 57–63.

Fish, B., & Hagin, R. (1972). Visual-motor disorder in infants at risk for schizophrenia. *Archives of General Psychiatry, 27,* 594–596.

Goldstein, M. J., Rodnick, E. H., Evans, J. R., May, P. R. A., & Steinberg, M. R. (1978). Drug and family therapy in the aftercare treatment of acute schizophrenics. *Archives of General Psychiatry, 35,* 1169–1177.

Grinker, R. R., Sr., Harrow, M., Westermeyer, M. A., Silverstein, M., Cohler, B., & Jacobs, B. (1981, May 9–15). Outpatient treatment of schizophrenia: The posthospital course of schizophrenia. Presented at the 134th Annual Meeting of Tomorrow's Psychiatrists at American Psychiatric Association, New Orleans, LA.

Gunderson, J. G., & Carrol, A. (1983). Clinical considerations from Empiric research. *Psychosocial Interventions for Schizophrenia* (pp. 126–142). In H. Sterlin (Ed.). New York: Springer-Verlag.

Hatfield, A. B. (1984). The family. In J. A. Talbott (Ed.), *The Chronic Mental Patient: Five Years Later* (pp. 307–323). Orlando, Florida: Grune & Stratton.

Herz, M. I. (1987, March 28–April 1). Prodromal symptoms and prevention of relapse. Presented at the International Congress on Schizophrenia Research symposium, Clearwater, FL.

Hogarty, G. E., Anderson, C. M., Reiss, D. J., Kornblith, S. J., Greenwald, D. P., Javna, C. D., Madonia, M. J., & EPICS Schizophrenia Research Group (1986). Family psychoeducation, social skills training and maintenance chemotherapy in the aftercare treatment of schizophrenia. *Archives of General Psychiatry, 43,* 633–642.

Inholder, B., & Piaget, J. (1958). The growth of logical thinking from childhood to adolesence. New York: Basic Books.

Jennings, W. S., & Schulz, S. C. (1986). Psychopharmacologic treatment of schizophrenia: Developing a dosing strategy. *Hospital Formulary, 21,* 332–346.

Jennings, W. S., Schulz, S. C., Narasimhachari, N., Hamer, R. M. & Friedel, R. O. (1985). Brain ventricular size and CSF monoamine metabolites in an adolescent inpatient population. *Psychiatry Research,* 87–94.

Kane, J. M., Woerner, M., Weinhold, P., Wegner, J., Kinon, B., & Borenstein, M. (1984). Incidence of tardive dyskinesia: Five-year data from a prospective study. *Psychopharmacology Bulletin, 20,* 39–40.

Leff, J., Kuipers, L., Berkowitz, R., Eberlein-Freis, R., & Sturgeon, D. (1982). A controlled trial of intervention in the families of schizophrenic patients. *British Journal of Psychiatry, 141,* 121–134.

Lewis, M. (1982) Clinical aspects of child development. Philadelphia: Lea & Fabiger, p. 263–300.

Lipinski, J. F., Zubenko, G. S., Cohen, B. M., & Barriera, P. J. (1984). Propranolol in the treatment of neuroleptic-induced akathisia. *American Journal of Psychiatry, 141,* 412–415.

Magliozzi, J. R., Hollister, L. E., Arnold, K. V., & Earle, G. M., (1980). Relationship of serum haloperidol levels to clinical response in schizophrenic patients. *American Journal of Psychiatry, 138,* 365–367.

Marder, S. R., van Putten, T., Mintz, J., McKenzie, J., Labell, M., Faltico, G., & May, P. R. A. (1984). Costs and benefits of two doses of fluphenazine. *Archives of General Psychiatry, 41,* 1025–1029.

May, P. R. A., Tuma, A. H., Yale, C., Potepan, P., & Dixon, W. J. (1976). Schizophrenia—A follow-up study of results of treatment: II. Hospital stay over two to five years. *Archives of General Psychiatry, 33,* 481–506.

McFarlane, W. R. (1982). Multiple family therapy in the psychiatric hospital, in H. T. Harbin (Ed.), *The Psychiatric Hospital and the Family* (pp. 103–129). New York: Spectrum Publications.

Munetz, M. R., & Toenniessen, L. M. (1984, May 2–6). Tardive dyskinesia does not progress over three years despite continued neuroleptics. Presented at the Thirty-Ninth Annual Convention & Scientific Program of the Society of Biological Psychiatry, Los Angeles, CA.

Nebrosky, R. J., Janowsky, D. S., Perel, J. M., Munson, E., & Depry, D. (1984). Plasma/RBS haloperidol ratios and improvement in acute psychotic symptoms. *Journal of Clinical Psychiatry, 45,* 10–13.

Nyback, H., Berggren, B. M., Hindmarsh, T., Sedvall, G., & Wiesel, F. A. (1983). Cerebroventricular size and cerebrospinal fluid monoamine metabolites in schizophrenic patients and healthy volunteers. *Psychiatry Research, 9,* 301.

Offer, D., Ostrov, E., & Howard, K. I. (1981). The mental health professional's concept of the normal adolescent. *Archives of General Psychiatry, 38,* 149–152.

Piaget, J. (1962) Comments on V. Y. Gotsky's "Critical remarks concerning the language and thought of the child." Cambridge, MA: MIT Press, pp. 473–490.

Pickar, D., Labarca, R., Linnoila, M., Roy, A., Hommer, D., Everett, D., & Paul, S. M. (1984). Neuroleptic-induced increase in plasma homovanillic acid and antipsychotic activity in schizophrenic patients. *Science, 225,* 954–957.

Pickar, D., Wolkowitz, O. M., Breier, A. F., Kelsoe, J., & Doran, A. R., (1987, May 9–14). Plasma HVA and models of drug response. Presented at the 140th Annual Meeting of the American Psychiatric Association, Chicago, IL.

Potkin, S. G., Weinberger, D. R., Linnoila, M., & Wyatt, R. J. (1983). Low CSF 5-hydroxyindoleacetic acid in Schizophrenics with enlarged ventricles. *American Journal of Psychiatry, 140,* 21.

Pulver, A. E., & Carpenter, W. T., Jr. (1983). Lifetime psychotic symptoms assessed with the DIS. *Schizophrenia Bulletin, 9,* 377–382.

Robins, L. N., Helzer, J. E., Croughan, J., & Ratcliff, K. S. (1981). National Institute of Mental Health Diagnostic interview schedule: Its history, characteristics and validity. *Archives of General Psychiatry, 38,* 381–389.

Schulz, S. C. (1987). Treatment resistant schizophrenics: A distinct subtype. Presented at the International Congress on Schizophrenia Research symposium, Clearwater, FL.

Schulz, S. C., Conley, R. R., & Benjamin, L. (1987). Progress in the treatment of nonresponders. Presented at the 140th Annual Meeting of the American Psychiatric Association, Chicago, IL.

Schulz, S. C., House, J., & Andrews, M. B. (1986). Helping families in a schizophrenia program. In M.Z. Goldstein (Ed.), *Clinical Insights: Family involvement in the treatment of schizophrenia* (pp. 19–32). Washington DC: American Psychiatric Press.

Schulz, P. M., Schulz, S. C., Dibble, E., Targum, S. D., van Kammen, D. P., & Gershon, E. S. (1982). Patient and family attitudes about schizophrenia: Implications for genetic counseling. *Psychopharmacology Bulletin, 8,* 504–513.

Schulz, S. C., Sinicrope, P., Kishore, P., & Friedel, R. O., (1983b). Treatment response and ventricular brain ratio in young schizophrenic patients. *Psychopharmacology Bulletin, 19,* 510–512.

Schulz, S. C., Koller, M. M., Kishore, P. R., Hamer, R. M., Gehl, J. J., & Friedel, R. O. (1983a). Ventricular enlargement in teenage patients with schizophrenia spectrum disorder. *American Journal of Psychiatry, 140,* 1592–1595.

Schulz, S. C., Butterfield, L., Garicano, M., Narasimhachari, N., & Friedel, R. O. (1984). Beyond the therapeutic window: A case presentation. *Journal of Clinical Psychiatry, 45,* (5)223–225.

Spitzer, R. L., Endicott, J., & Robins, E. (1977). *Research Diagnostic Criteria (RDC) for a Selected Group of Functional Disorders* (3rd ed.). New York: Biometrics Research.

van Kammen, D. P., Mann, L. S., Sternberg, D. E., Scheinin, M., Ninan, P. T., Marder, S. R., van Kammen, W. B., Rieder, R. O., & Linnoila, M. (1983). Dopamine-B-hydroxylase activity and homovanillic acid in spinal fluid of schizophrenics with brain atrophy. *Science, 220,* 974.

van Putten, T. (March 28–April 1) (1987). A controlled dose comparison of haloperidol in newly admitted schizophrenia patients. Presented at the International Congress on Schizophrenia Research symposium, Clearwater, FL.

van Putten, T., May, P. R. A., & Marder, S. R. (1984). Akathisia with haloperidol and thiothixene. *Archives of General Psychiatry, 41,* 1036–1039.

Weinberger, D. R., Torrey, E. F., Neophytides, A., & Wyatt, R. J. (1979). Lateral cerebral ventricular enlargement in chronic schizophrenia. *Archives of General Psychiatry, 36,* 735–739.

Weinberger, D. R., Bigelow, L. B., Kleinman, J. E., Klein, S. T., Rosenblatt, J. E., & Wyatt, R. J. (1980). Cerebral ventricular enlargement in chronic schizophrenia: Association with poor response to treatment. *Archives of General Psychiatry, 37,* 11–14.

Zubenko, G. S., Lipinski, J. F., Cohen, B. M., & Barriera, P. J. (1984). Comparison of metoprolol and propranolol in the treatment of akathisia. *Psychiatry Research, 11,* 143–149.

CHAPTER FOURTEEN

Psychoactive Substance Use Disorders

Geary S. Alford

Chemical substance misuse is one of the most common and significant factors complicating and often disrupting adolescent development. Although abuse of psychoactive chemicals in adolescent and young adult populations has declined slightly and gradually over the past decade, prevalence of substance misuse remains alarmingly high. For example, careful surveys sponsored and reported by the National Institute on Drug Abuse show that in 1984, 48% of high school seniors admitted having used some illicit drug at least once during that school year, and 29% admitted they had used one or more illicit drugs at least once during the immediately preceding 30-day period. While these percentages are slightly lower than those obtained 5 years earlier for 1979, this decline has been partially offset by findings that onset of illicit drug use has tended to occur at younger and younger ages across the past decade.

Alcohol (which was not included in the statistics just cited) and marijuana are by far the most frequently used and abused of the more potent psychoactive substances. Among the 1984 high school seniors, nationwide, 40% admitted having smoked marijuana and 86% admitted having drunk alcohol *at some time* during their senior year. More disturbing still, 5% of those students admitted *daily* use of marijuana, and 4.8% admitted *daily* alcohol consumption. Although prevalence of drug abuse is less for each precedingly lower grade level, clearly a rather significant percentage of the U.S. adolescent population engages in some form of chemical substance abuse. Further, clinical common sense would conclude that many of these adolescents, certainly most of those who engage in daily use, are or are in the process of becoming chemically dependent.

Psychoactive compounds exert a wide variety of effects on sensory, cognitive, affectual, verbal, and motor behaviors. All drugs of abuse when taken frequently, chronically, or in excessive doses disrupt normal neuropsychological functioning, resulting in impaired, maladaptive, and abnormal behaviors. These effects can be seen in such diverse arenas as impaired cognitive and intellectual processes, resulting in diminished academic-scholastic performance and achievement, abnormal affectual and motivational levels, "personality changes" with associated intrapersonal and interpersonal conflicts and problems, and in dysfunctional motor skills. Recent studies indicate that at least 50% of young suicides involve chronic substance abusers (Fowler, Rich, & Young, 1986), while 80 to 90% of vehicular accidents among 16- to 20-year-old drivers involve drinking (Grunby, 1984). Such findings highlight both the diversity and seriousness of catastrophic life events associated with adolescent substance abuse.

THEORETICAL MODELS

Theories of alcoholism and drug dependency abound. In 1980, the National Institute on Drug Abuse published a collection of synopses of 43 different theoretical models (Lettier, Sayers, & Pearson, 1980). Although most of these are multifactorial, their central or basic etiological perspectives can be categorized into one of three general approaches: biopathological-genetic models, psychopathological-personality models, and social-behavioral learning models. While an in-depth examination of each of these approaches is beyond the scope of the present chapter, a brief review of their basic tenets, hypotheses, and theoretical implications will emphasize the range and multiplicity of factors thought to play a role in the etiology of chemical dependency.

Biopathological-Genetic Models

It is necessary to distinguish between biological models of addiction that focus on physiological concomitants and mechanisms of dependency from those biological models that attempt to account for chemical dependency on the basis of genetic and premorbid (indeed, prechemical use) biopathologies. The fundamental etiological assumption of genetic models of addiction is that people who became alcoholic or dependent on any other psychoactive substance are in some significant ways inherently biologically different from people who do not develop a drug dependency. This hypothesized difference has variously been postulated to involve a kind of allergy (a metaphor commonly used by Alcoholics Anonymous [AA] members) and as entailing unusual metabolic products (Schuckit & Rayses, 1979). Appropriately designed and controlled studies have failed to provide consistent and significant evidence of such premorbid differences.

However, evidence from studies of twins and adoptees has strongly implicated genetic predisposition as a contributing factor at least in some alcoholics. Comparative investigations have reported higher concordance rates for alcoholism in identical, monozygotic twins (concordance of approximately 60%), than for fraternal, dizygotic twins (concordance around 30%). Critics have argued that in most twin studies (i.e., except where twins were raised in separate families), it is likely that identical twins are treated even more similarly than are fraternal twins, thus confounding the genetic contribution with environmental influence.

The strongest support to date that genetically transmitted factors play a contributory role in at least some individuals developing alcoholism has come from adoption studies. Goodwin and his colleagues (Goodwin, Schulsinger, Hermansen, Guze, & Winokur, 1973; Goodwin et al., 1974) found that male adoptees who had an alcoholic biological parent were almost four times more likely themselves to become alcoholic than were male adoptees in a matched group without such a parental alcoholic history. Further, when adopted-away sons of alcoholics were compared to biological brothers who had been raised by the alcoholic biological parent, the incidence of subsequent alcoholism in these offspring was equivalent. These and similar adoption studies (Bohman, Sigvardsson, & Cloninger, 1981) do support a genetic influence at least in *some* alcoholics. It is important, however, to note that these very studies also provide evidence that such a genetic predisposition is neither necessary nor sufficient. In Goodwin's studies and also those of Bohman (1978), results did not support such genetic influence (i.e., father to daughter) in females, nor was there evidence for a generalized predisposition toward drug abuse. Further, a significant number of subjects with no apparent genetic predisposition (i.e., no evidence of parental addiction) also developed chemical dependency.

Such findings are consistent with most clinicians' experience that while many chemically dependent patients report one or more biological ancestors as having been alcoholic, many other patients have no such family history. Considering that all drugs of abuse have the psychopharmacological properties of producing very reinforcing sensations or pleasurable psychophysical states and most induce tolerance and withdrawal, it should not be surprising that genetic predisposition is not always a prerequisite for abuse or dependence. Genetic studies, including laboratory studies breeding alcohol-preference strains of rats (e.g., Wister in contrast to Sprague-Dawley rats), do implicate inherited, endogenous factors in at least some alcoholics and possibly in certain other drug dependencies as well. However, the majority of current scientific evidence indicates that a genetic predisposition is neither necessary nor sufficient for development of chemical dependency. Moreover, while biogenetics etiological theories may have some explanatory value, they have not generated useful clinical treatment procedures. Aside from their explanatory functions, such models will likely prove of greater value in *prevention* strategies than in treatment.

Biogenetic *theories* of chemical dependency need to be distinguished from *biological* components or mechanisms or addiction. In contrast to biogenetic theories, which postulate inherited, premorbid biological differences between persons who become chemically dependent and those who do not, biological models of the addiction process make no such assumptions. Instead, their focus is upon physiological changes that *result from* and *accompany* chemical use and abuse. Primary (though not exclusive) among the physiological aspects of the addictive process are, of course, tolerance induction and the appearance of abstinence symptoms upon abrupt cessation of drug use. These do not account for why someone uses or abuses a chemical substance in the first place, but they have much potential for our understanding of increasing dosage and frequency of use and for long-term maintenance of addictive behavior.

Psychopathological and Personality Models

Just as the biogenetic models postulate some underlying physiological predisposition to chemical abuse, psychopathological and personality models argue that certain personality types or personality traits predispose some individuals to chemical abuse and/or to chemical dependency (e.g., Khantzian & Treece, 1977; Spotts & Shontz, 1980). The central element of such theories is the notion that the underlying psychopathology or personality trait generates aversive emotional states that the psychoactive chemical of choice relieves. Chemical abuse is viewed as a form of self-medication and thus is considered only *symptomatic* of the true underlying psychological disorders. It follows, then, that treatment focuses on the presumed underlying disorder and that chemical abuse is expected to cease once the cause of or need for it is removed.

Apparent support for this position rests upon a mass of psychological assessment and testing studies that report significantly increased incidence of various psychological pathologies and deviances among alcoholic and other drug-dependent populations. However, the vast majority of such studies have been conducted *after* emergence of the chemical dependency, and therefore the psychopathologies are at least as likely to be the product of the chemical abuse as its cause. In one of the few studies utilizing extensive data gathered premorbidly (i.e., prior to chemical abuse), McCord and McCord (1960) found no differences in metabolic, glandular, or general physical functioning or in clinically significant levels of abnormal or maladaptive affectual or personality characteristics between teenagers who subsequently became alcoholic teenagers and those who did not later evidence alcoholism. While these researchers found that boys who subsequently became alcoholic were more frequently described as hyperactive and aggressive than boys who did not eventually develop alcoholism, the "prealcoholic" boys also were described as more self-assured. Some studies have reported that such characteristics as antisocial tendencies have been found higher in drug-abusing teenagers *before* as well as *after* a sustained period of chemical abuse (e.g., Cadoret, Troughton, O'Gorman, & Heywood, 1986; Jones, 1968; Loper, Kammeier, & Hoffman, 1973; Monnelly, Harth, & Elderkin, 1983).

That some antecedent personality characteristics are found more frequently among drug abusers than nonabusers may relate more to willingness to experiment with and use drugs than to any special sensitivity to drug effects at some central, "psychic" level. That is, adolescents who, "personality-wise," are more "self-assured," "adventuresome," *and* "sociopathic-antisocial" (i.e., willing if not eager to violate social norms, rules, laws) would be more likely to engage in illicit and illegal drug use than would teenagers less disposed to such violations. This alone could result in a population of teenage drug abusers with a statistical distribution skewed in the direction of such *antecedent,* though not necessarily *causative,* personality characteristics.

Personality characteristics probably do play some interactive role in the etiology of chemical dependency in some people. Like genetic predisposition, however, evidence to date suggests that such characteristics are neither necessary nor sufficient for the development of chemical dependency.

The working assumption that chemical abuse is only symptomatic of some other underlying psychological conflict or disorder has generally led to focusing away from the chemical using behavior and, instead, to addressing such hypothetical causes of drug abuse as "low self-esteem." Such treatment often takes the form of drug substitution. For example, alcoholic patients frequently have a history of benzodiazepine use, if not addiction, having been placed on an anxiolytic in the belief (shared by both patient and physician) that various life stresses were *causing* excessive drinking. Traditional psychotherapy alone or in combination with pharmacotherapy, especially when aimed at psychodynamic, personality, or psychopathology other than chemical dependency itself, has not been demonstrated effective in successfully ameliorating chemical dependency.

Social and Behavioral Models

Sociological and behavioral psychological theories of drug dependency argue that chemical misuse behavior is learned from environmental influences and experiences. According to such theorists, alcohol and drug-abusing behaviors are learned in the same way that language, social customs, and food preferences are learned, primarily by exposure to environmental social models. Such behaviors are then maintained by the various positive and negative reinforcing aspects of the drug-abuse behavior itself. This behavior is considered to be under the control of predominantly external, environmental stimuli. The sociological theories in particular emphasize such environmental conditions as unemployment, poverty, marital discord, job stress, and other environmental pressures as *setting events* for, if not actual *causes* of, drug abuse. Sociological models have a more difficult time formulating persuasive explanations for middle- and upper-class abusers, and they usually invoke presumed intrapsychic conflicts to account for those populations.

Behavioral models conceptualize chemical abuse within the context of classical and operant conditioning and social learning theory (Marlatt & Rose, 1980). While acknowledging the potential roles of "personality characteristics" (Tarter & Edwards, 1986) and biogenetic factors (Nathan, 1986), behavioral theorists view such factors as primarily influencing the reinforcing properties of drug use. The strength of the behavioral models arises from utilization of empirically derived principles of behavior and reliance on carefully designed treatment evaluation studies to determine and document efficacy. The major weakness of most behavioral models of addictive disorders is their tendency to focus too narrowly on the observable, overt stimulus and behavioral events of chemical use, while tending to down-play or even ignore the covert, characterological-personality components. Such personality components include *rationalization, denial,* and *resistance,* which almost all other theoretical approaches view as critical if not central points of focus in treating chemical dependency.

The weaknesses of behavioral models arise not only from the peripheralistic perspective of traditional behaviorism, but they also result in part from the many behavioral studies in which selection criteria require pretreatment subjects to acknowledge "alcoholism" or at least "major problem drinking" (thus automatically excluding alcoholics who are in gross denial). Some other behavioral treatment studies have utilized subjects whose average alcohol intake was far below that seen in most nonbehavioral treatment evaluations. Still, the commitment to an empirical approach eventually results in self-correcting development. This is perhaps the greatest strength of the behavioral approach. For example, most behavioral investigators and clinicians have quietly backed away from endorsing attempts at *controlled drinking training* for the more long-term, chronic "gamma" alcoholics. Indeed, more recently proposed behavioral analyses addressing such problems as relapse prevention show much broader, more comprehensive, more sophisticated formulations of the diverse and complex cognitive, affectual, as well as overt stimulus-response components of chemical dependency (Brownell, Marlatt, Lichtenstein, & Wilson, 1986).

COMMENT

In summary, several factors, ranging from genetics to personality characteristics, have been empirically related to the development of alcoholism. Aside from genetic vulnerability, most intrapersonal-personality characteristics and social psychological factors found as frequent antecedents of alcoholism appear related to other drug dependencies as well. However, such factors are not evidenced in all chemically dependent persons' premorbid (i.e., prechemical abusive) behavior. That is, many chemically dependent patients are not found to have had any identifiable family history of alcoholism or other drug abuse. Also, there may be no evidence of any significantly abnormal levels of common behavioral patterns or personality traits prior to use and misuse of psychoactive chemicals. Further, neither the fact of a biological ancestor having been alcoholic nor the presence of one or more of the behavioral risk factors invariably results in chemical dependency. These genetic and behavioral risk factors, therefore, while often antecedent to chemical abuse in many individuals, do not appear to be either necessary or sufficient to produce drug dependency. In short, there appear to be many avenues of entry into chemical abuse and subsequent dependency, the final common path being the actual behavior of frequent chemical misuse.

One way to organize these various antecedents and avenues of entry and of understanding the development of chemical dependency is to consider the biobehavioral properties of drugs of abuse and the consequences of their misuse. All psychoactive chemical substances with high abuse potential are compounds that can induce very pleasurable sensations and enjoyable perceptual states of well-being. Examples of the psychopharmacological compounds most commonly misused are listed in Table 14.1. These classes of compounds can also significantly reduce unpleasant, painful, aversive sensations and feelings. However, it is not necessary to be in a state of discomfort in order to induce and experience the pleasurable drug effects. This fact is important to bear in mind.

Perplexed parents, for example, frequently ask "Why would anybody want to use a drug anyway?" The unfortunately misleading answer that something must be wrong with the person who would take a drug of abuse perpetuates the myth that preexisting, underlying psychological disorders are always the real problems that cause drug abuse. Such answers

Table 14.1. Psychoactive Drugs Frequently Abused by Adolescents

Drug Class	Common Examples		Approximate percent of High School seniors currently using (*)
Ethyl Alcohol	beer, wine whiskey		70
Cannabis	marijuana, hashish, extracts containing delta-9-tetrahydro-cannabinol (THC)		25
Stimulants	amphetamines, cocaine, methylenedioxyamphet-amine ("Ecstacy")		10-15
Hallucinogens	d-lysergic acid diethyl-amide (LSD),phencyclidine (PCP), psilocybin mushrooms		2.5
Sedative-Anxiolytics	benzodiazepines alprozolam (Xanax) [+] chlorazepate (Tranxene) diazepam (Valium) flurazepam (Dalmane)	barbiturates secobarbital (Seconal) pentobarbital (Nembutal)	2
Narcotic Analgesics	codeine hydromorphone (Dilaudid) [+] meperidine (Demerol) oxycodone (Percodan) pentazocine (Talwin) propoxyphene (Darvon)	less often methadone heroin	.5

*Percentage extrapolated from National Institute on Drug Abuse survey data on 1985 high school seniors admitting the use of particular drugs at least once in the past 30 days.   [+]Trade names are listed for identification purposes only.

correspond to most traditional theories of chemical dependency and also subtly reflect a vestige of the puritan ethic, which views as suspicious if not pathological any behavior engaged in for the shear pleasure of doing so. In contrast, true social drinkers, for example, need not be tense, anxious, depressed, or in any other state of discomfort to enjoy the effects of a cocktail. True social drinking is done to enhance what is already a pleasant occasion and comfortable psychological state. A great deal of adolescent drug use occurs for similar reasons.

Drugs of abuse, then, are compounds which have psychoactive properties of inducing very pleasurable, positively reinforcing effects as well as the property of reducing unpleasant, aversive sensations (i.e., are negatively reinforcing). It is most likely with these two central properties that the predisposing or antecedent risk factors interact. The possibility exists, for example, that some individuals have a genetically transmitted biochemical predisposition to metabolize certain compounds in abnormal ways. Some have suggested that alcoholics tend to produce more reinforcing metabolic by-products (e.g., tetrahydroisoquinolines) than do nonalcoholics (Davis & Walsh, 1970). Although subsequent work has questioned this particular notion (Ellingboe, 1978), such as yet undiscovered metabolic differences are certainly possible. Similarly, individuals who, for whatever reason, suffer more uncomfortable emotional distress would likely experience a correspondingly greater level of negative-reinforcement from drug actions than would individuals free of abnormally frequent or intense aversive feelings. But again, such preexisting biological and psychological factors are not necessary for someone to experience the potent, pleasurable, positively reinforcing effects of drugs.

Just as drugs of abuse produce a range of reinforcing effects, chemical abuse also, of course, results in a wide variety of highly unpleasant, aversive, adverse consequences. Simply examining the various aversive consequences as weighed against the pleasurable ones, it might seem difficult to understand how drug use and abuse ever develop in the first place, especially considering the extremely unpleasant nature of many of the aversive consequences and that most of the pleasurable drug effects can be obtained without drugs. Let us consider the behavioral pharmacology of drug action and briefly examine some of the relationship variables among drug use and its diverse consequences.

BEHAVIORAL PHARMACOLOGY

Latency of Consequences

The time between drug ingestion and onset of its particular desirable effects is generally quite short. Depending on route of administration and the specific pharmacokinetics of a given drug, the latency of onset of many pleasurable effects may range from a few seconds to a couple of hours. Most of the highly aversive consequences, however, do not begin to occur and accrue until after multiple instances of drug use, often months or even years after initiating use. The pleasurable effects tend to be immediate while the most aversive consequences tend to be delayed.

Detectability of Consequences

Not only do most of the pleasurable drug effects tend to come on immediately, but they also tend to produce the peak effect quite rapidly. That is, the user ingests a drug, within a few seconds to minutes he or she begins to feel the desired action, and the full peak "high" is achieved shortly thereafter. There is usually rather rapid change from one psychophysiological state (unintoxicated or "sober") to a markedly different psychophysiological state (intoxicated or "high"). Such relatively rapid and marked changes are easily detectable. Indeed, if the users do not detect such changes, they usually conclude they "made a bad buy;" that is, they were cheated in having been sold weak or fake drugs.

Most of the undesirable, adverse consequences, on the other hand, tend to develop rather gradually. Young users do not start abusing marijuana one day and immediately fail in school the next. Deterioration in intellectual, emotional, social, and physical functioning tends to occur gradually across time. Such gradual changes are far more difficult to detect on a day-to-day basis, particularly for someone whose sensori-perceptual and judgmental capacities may be impaired by the drug action. Frequently, it is only when behaviors are compared across rather long intervals (one semester to the last semester or even one year to the last) that the magnitude of change becomes obvious. Thus the pleasurable effects tend to be easily detectable to the user, while many of the aversive effects tend to be more difficult to detect, at least in the early stages of substance misuse.

Probability of Consequences

Although the psychopharmacological and behavioral-life consequential effects of drugs of abuse are well documented, the *probability* of such effects as *anticipated* and *experienced* by any given individual drug abuser is quite another thing. According to users' own personal experiences, the particular types of pleasurable (positive and negative reinforcing) effects of a given class of drugs occur on every or almost every instance of use. At least in the early phases of abuse, the desirable effects are experienced as having 100% probability. In contrast, since the most aversive effects tend to be delayed, tend to evolve gradually, and are initially relatively more difficult for users to detect, the most significant adverse consequences are experienced and viewed as improbable. In the early stages of chemical abuse, users, supported by their own personal experiences, deny that a drug produces certain adverse consequences or that they as individuals are likely to suffer those consequences.

Attribution of Consequences

The preceding differential relationships between drug abuse and pleasurable versus aversive consequences contribute to one of the most important phenomena in chemical dependency: misattribution as a form of denial. Since the desirable, pleasurable effects of chemical misuse tend to be immediate, tend to reach peak effect rapidly on each occasion of use, and tend to occur with almost 100% probability, they are directly associated cognitively and paired by Pavlovian-classical conditioning with the stimuli of drug usage.

Aversive consequences, on the other hand, tend to be delayed, tend to evolve more gradually and, for so long, *seem* improbable. Therefore, even when and where they do emerge in subjectively detectable magnitude, users often fail to attribute them to the chemical abuse. Instead, many adverse life experiences that are in fact related to chemical misuse are often "safely" misattributed by users to factors ostensibly unrelated to their use pattern. Poor grades in school are attributed to "boring" teachers or subject matter that is not considered "relevant." A late night car accident is blamed on having been sleepy. Unpleasant emotional reactions are blamed on *other* people for hasseling the user, and so forth.

Indeed, in a paradox with much clinical significance, many of the aversive *consequences* of chemical misuse are blamed as *causes* of chemical use. By way of simple example is the husband who, blaming his wife's behavior for his drinking, gets drunk in response to his emotional reaction to a marital argument about his excessive drinking. The differential empirical relationships between drug misuse and the pleasurable versus aversive effects unfortunately provide for the differential conditioning, association, and attribution of those consequences to drug usage. This, then, diminishes the intrinsic punishing (hence response reduction or avoidance) effects that the aversive consequences might otherwise exert on chemical misuse behavior.

Considering these behavioral pharmacologic properties, it can be seen how someone with no specific predisposition and with no clinically significant psychological abnormality could begin chemical misuse for the pleasure of doing so and gradually evolve into a pattern of chemical dependency. This is grasped perhaps more easily when chemicals that induce tolerance and physical addiction are involved. Anyone who uses certain drugs in certain doses on certain schedules will induce addiction. Even in the premorbidly "normal" or "average," nongenetically predisposed individual, once tolerance begins to develop, some aversive withdrawal phenomena will correspondingly begin to occur during falling or abstinent chemical levels. At that point in the use history, such an individual begins to function more like the user who does have noxious preexisting antecedents. Misuse behavior begins to exert significant negative as well as positive reinforcing effects.

Similarly, the role of biological and behavioral antecedents fits well within this abuse model. Any biological or behavioral antecedents that significantly enhance the reinforcing (either positive or negative) properties of chemical substances in given individuals are likely to increase the probability or response strength of abuse behavior. The chemical dependency once developed, whatever factors may have contributed to the misuse behavior in the first place, is almost always functionally autonomous of its roots. That is, by whatever avenue the individual entered the final common pathway of chronic chemical abuse, once this highly reinforced, deeply ingrained pattern develops, it is not reliably modified or ameliorated by addressing the presumed initial contributing factors. Instead, it is its own disorder and will require its own treatment.

Chemically dependent individuals, whether adolescent or adult, rarely come voluntarily into treatment solely out of their own, private concerns about their chemical usage. Instead, potent forces, such as family and often legal pressures, precede their arrival in therapy. Such patients sometimes arrive denying even the use, much less the abuse of drugs. Most initially deny the dependence. In addition to often claiming they "can stop whenever they want" and sometimes accurately noting that they "can go for days (even weeks) without using," chemically dependent adolescents initially deny or minimize many of the adverse drug effects, even those that have occurred in their own lives. Further, even when acknowledging major problems in their lives, the relationship between these and their chemical abuse pattern likewise tends to be initially minimized or rejected outright. In order to generate a valid history, therefore, it is usually necessary to carefully interview parents and often siblings and to obtain records (such as school grade and attendance reports) for periods which may date back several years before the present admission. In examining this history, the clinician should not be so concerned with "which came first" (a specific emotional, social, or scholastic problem or the drug usage), but should be concerned with the pattern of interrelationships that emerges.

Although many of the problems in living traditionally believed to be a *cause* of chemical abuse in fact turn out to be its consequences (e.g., Valliant, 1983), other specific problems that preceded the actual drug usage are often exacerbated by drug use. Such problems thus become partially symptomatic of the drug dependency. That is to say, a chronic pattern of chemical misuse in reaction to unpleasant life events is itself one sign of a substance abuse disorder. Similarly, evidence of coexisting psychiatric disorders is not, in itself, evidence for or against a diagnosis of substance abuse disorder. Not only do most drugs of abuse induce symptoms which closely resemble other disorders (e.g., the stimulant-induced schizophreniform psychosis), but they can actually produce other disorders (e.g., the profound depressions associated with cocaine abstinence). Likewise, chemical dependency can interact with coexisting disorders, as with the case of a young man who was in fact schizophrenic and chemically dependent. He would repeatedly quit taking his Haldol and return to his frequent use of marijuana and occasionally cocaine, much to the chagrin of his psychiatrist. (It took at least three repeated hospitalizations of this patient to convince his primary therapist that the drug abuse was *not* "self-medication," but was itself a coexisting disorder, before this patient was referred to a chemical dependency treatment program!)

Where other psychological disorders coexist with chemical dependency, the rule of thumb regarding treatment alternatives and sequence should be: Cases involving a primary, psychotic disorder, such as schizophrenia or major affective disorder, should be treated first for their thought or affective disorder, then for chemical dependency. Whether the case involves a possible psychotic episode associated with schizophrenia or a schizophreniform psychotic episode of organic, drug-induced origin, treatment may be similar. However, careful evaluation of chemical abuse history should accompany other diagnostic procedures. Considering the prevalence of chemical abuse among the adolescent population and its profound as well as diverse symptomatic sequela, chemical abuse should be considered as one of the possible differential diagnoses in almost every adolescent presenting with psychological symptoms. Where a substance abuse disorder is found coexistent with adjustment disorders, personality disorders, and "neurotic" emotional disorders (e.g., impulse control problems, reactive depression, etc.), the chemical dependency should be treated first. The extensive information accumulated during the diagnostic and evaluative process is useful beyond that stage. It will serve as an integral part of the treatment process.

Chronic chemical abuse impairs and disrupts a broad range of behavioral functions. Particularly in adolescent populations, abuse not only impairs behavioral performance, but it also disrupts critical periods of behavior acquisition, learning, and development. Therefore, termination of drug usage, in itself, does not necessarily result in age appropriate intellectual, cognitive-emotional, or social competencies. Such problems are further compounded in those patients who have histories of significant maladaptive behavior antedating their drug use and in those with coexisting disorders. In addition, many families of drug dependent adolescents are dysfunctional, again, sometimes preceding the drug abuse or often resulting from the family's attempts to respond to and cope with the chemically dependent family member.

It can be seen, therefore, that a multicomponent treatment model is necessary to address these diverse problem areas. The nuclear problem, of course, is the constellation of cognitive, emotional, and overt behavior patterns directly involved in the chemical misuse behavior. Again, however, it should be noted that chemical dependency entails a potently reinforced, highly practiced, and thus deeply ingrained complex behavior pattern. It is, therefore, insufficient to ameliorate or even remove extrinsic factors, be they intrapersonal or environmental, which may have contributed to the initial drug misuse. Rather, in addition to these important targets of intervention, therapy must be primarily focused on the specific cognitive, affectual, and overt behavioral elements of the chemical usage pattern.

Chemical dependency is not substantially modified because patients discover how it was developed; nor is it modified because they intellectually come to understand its multiple and diverse adverse effects. Rather, such patients begin actively to seek, acquire, and practice alternative behaviors when their personal history and anticipatory expectancy of noxious, unpleasant, and aversive consequences become more negatively affectually valenced than the pleasurable effects are positive. Treatment must mitigate the reinforcement history of chemical abuse. This can be partially accomplished by reducing the antecedent conditions, such as aversive feelings states, social affiliations and contacts with active users, and so forth, which frequently have occasioned drug misuse in patients' past. This alone, however, does not directly impact on the reinforcement history. To do so, some variation of aversion training is usually necessary.

Behavioral therapists have addressed this component in the straightforward manner of actually pairing stimuli involved in chemical ingestion with such aversive stimuli as mild faradic shocks, inducing sensations of nausea (see Miller & Hester, 1980), or with use of aversive imagery (Elkins & Murdock, 1977). In a surprisingly similar methodology, AA-oriented counselors have used aversive events from patients' own lives as well as vicarious exposure to aversive events from similar users' lives (which, therefore, carry clear implications regarding additional probable, future aversive consequences) to increase the negative valence of chemical using behavior (a form of vicarious aversive conditioning). Emphasis on these procedures is less often necessary where individuals have, without much external pressure, voluntarily sought treatment because they personally experienced and associated potent aversive effects with their chemical usage* or where misuse of a chemical has been relatively mild and of

---

* AA members refer to this phenomenon as "having hit bottom" and for years believed it was necessary to do so before someone could achieve sobriety. It is now clear that individuals can "hit bottom" in an active treatment program.

relatively short duration. Adolescents, however, most commonly do not come into drug treatment solely on their own volition, and generally they do not have the personal histories of extensive drug-related adverse life experiences typically seen in older patients.

DIAGNOSTIC CONSIDERATIONS

Diagnosing chemical dependency often is a rather complicated process. In spite of the more operationalized format of the current DSM-III-R (APA, 1987), debate continues among clinicians and drug counselors about specific criteria as well as about core concepts in psychoactive substance use disorders. In DSM-III-R, psychoactive substance use disorders are divided, across pharmacologic classes, into two general categories: *dependence* versus *abuse*. DSM-III-R provides a list of psychoactive substance-induced familial, social, academic, occupational, recreational, psychological, and medical-physiological problems, some combination of which is considered indicative of *dependence*. The criteria for *abuse* includes some of the elements cited in the criteria for *dependence*, but the abuse history, pattern, and symptomatic consequences do not meet (and have not previously met) the criteria for *dependence*.

Adaptation of DSM-III-R for adolescent populations is best accomplished by reconsidering the essential features from which the specific criteria are derived, namely, the impact of chemical usage in an individual's daily life. The critical issue in determining whether someone's chemical usage constitutes a clinical problem is whether and to what extent chemical usage contributes to or directly results in significant problems in living. Put another way, chemical dependency can be defined as *a relatively enduring pattern of use of some psychoactive substance which use has contributed to or has directly resulted in severe, aversive, adverse consequences. Moreover, such consequences have not led to reliable and enduring modification of usage pattern of that or similarly acting substances such that no further significant, adverse consequences of use have occurred or have an objectively demonstrable high probability of resulting from such usage.*

This definition does not stipulate any specific quantity, frequency, or particular pattern of chemical usage. Instead, it emphasizes the relationship between chemical usage and consequent adverse life events. In doing so, the definition allows variations in usage practices to be taken into account. For example, someone who drinks only on weekends, but whose drinking is frequently, though not invariably, an antecedent to very offensive, disruptive, or otherwise maladaptive behavior, might be diagnosed chemically dependent on alcohol (assuming, of course, he or she also meets additional criteria). This is the case, even though the actual drinking schedule is only 2 out of every 7 days (i.e., not even close to "daily").

A second feature of this definition is its focus on whether chemical abusive behavior, even if it endured over a significant period of time, ceased or was spontaneously and reliably modified by the individual in a way that does not engender adverse consequences. Thus a circumscribed period of chemical abuse which was terminated by the user would not, in itself, warrant a diagnosis of chemical dependency. By way of example, someone in the midst of a painfully acrimonious divorce might increase his or her alcohol intake to an abusive level and then taper off as emotional and legal conflicts resolve. Similarly, a teenager might go through a period of heavy drug usage ("experimentation") over a summer but self-volitionally cease all chemical misuse at the start of school in the fall. Such spontaneous and reliable cessation of chemical abuse, of course, is to be differentiated from repeated, transient attempts at abstinence or drug substitutions. However, the lines of demarcation are neither clear nor uniformly endorsed.

As discussed earlier, chemical dependency usually does not emerge full-blown suddenly or abruptly. Rather, the initial stage of development of chemical dependency tends to be gradual and unspectacular. In order to make diagnostic determinations, it is necessary to obtain very careful and extensive histories not only from the patient but also from objective records, such as school grades. Cross-sectional data as obtained in current mental status examination and recent drug screens are, of course, valuable, but alone they are grossly insufficient for differential diagnosis. The key elements in the diagnostic algorithm are (1) a relatively long-standing pattern of drug usage, and (2) a history of significant adverse consequences resulting from that chemical usage. This history very often cannot be obtained from the patient alone.

Chemically dependent adolescents, like chemically dependent adults, initially tend to deny or minimize their chemical use, its adverse effects, and the relationships between drug use and various adverse life experiences associated with that use. Once detected, diagnosed, and into treatment, many adolescents then sometimes exaggerate their drug histories. However, during the initial diagnostic process, the clinician must constantly bear in mind that while patients may freely and openly report or admit pain, anxiety, or depression, those who are chemically dependent (and not yet identified as such) are unlikely to offer accurate and valid information about their chemical-abusing behavior. Indeed, some will deny obvious facts such as carefully repeated drug screens that were positive for metabolites of tetrahydrocannabinol (THC) or of other drugs.

Similarly, clinicians must realize that many chemically abusing and dependent adolescents will continue their denial of significant drug use even where they have established an apparently open and trusting relationship with a psychotherapist. Aside from those cases where the therapist learned of chemical abuse but considered it only symptomatic of some other adolescent disorder, I have seen many patients who subsequently admitted that they had never told the truth about their drug history to their private psychotherapists with whom they had been in therapy for months.

TREATMENT

Phase I: Evaluation and Detoxification

Upon inpatient admission, all patients undergo physical examination and mental status examination, and a medical history is taken. In addition to routine laboratory studies (e.g., SMA-18), a complete drug screen is obtained. Many adolescents do not require medical detoxification procedures, particularly those whose primary drug of abuse was marijuana. However, depending upon drug history, medical history, and signs and symptoms evidenced during admission and on the unit, some patients will require a standard detoxification protocol appropriate to the pharmacological class upon which they are physically dependent. During this initial phase, patient's family members are carefully interviewed, school records covering at least 3 to 5 years prior to admission are obtained, and any other recorded information (e.g., arrest and legal records, medical records, etc.) that may be relevant to the patient's presenting problem are gathered and reviewed. Initial psychological testing, including a Minnesota Multiphasic Personality Inventory (MMPI) and Shipley Institute of Living Scale, is administered shortly after completion of detoxification.

Phase II: Individual and Group Therapy, Lectures and Films, and Bibliotherapy

The goals of this phase of treatment are multiple and interactive. First and foremost is to carefully, systematically, and repeatedly examine and elucidate the patient's actual chemical usage pattern and its history. It is also necessary to clarify and make highly salient the relationships among chemical abusing behaviors and the specific adverse consequences that have occurred in the patient's life. While acknowledging that certain kinds of life events (e.g., a family argument) and life experiences (feeling anxious, stressed, depressed) contribute to urges to use, every effort is made to disavow patients of the notion that such factors *cause* or *control* (thus, are responsible for) their continued chemical abuse. Instead, patients are encouraged to recognize that many of their adverse life experiences in fact result from their chemical use. Patients also are encouraged to recognize that those emotional problems or problems in living that antedate or arise independently of chemical abuse are almost invariably exacerbated, not relieved, by chemical use. Each patient's chemical abuse history is repeatedly examined and discussed in individual counseling sessions. Integrally involved in this perspective is the proposition that successful treatment for chemical dependency is necessary to provide a more stable and healthful psychological foundation from which to therapeutically address other acquired ("functional") behavioral disorders. The exceptions to this, as previously noted, are those patients who have carefully differentiated and confirmed major thought or major affective disorders.

A second major goal is to explore and modify cognitive-emotional and overt behavior patterns that contribute to chemical abuse, but that also transcend chemical abuse and result in adverse consequences in other areas of patients' lives as well. Most common among drug-dependent adolescents are: (1) extreme egocentricity, with many self-delusional attitudes and beliefs; and (2) deceptive manipulativeness, anger, and resentment of and conflict with constraints, limits, rules and other symbols of "authority." Underlying these usually are problems of anxiety, insecurity, and depression. Individual psychotherapy, particularly the recently developed cognitive therapies, such as those for depression (Beck, 1976; Beck, Rush, Shaw, & Emery, 1979) and for personality disorders (Alford & Fairbank, 1985), can be employed to address these clinical problems.

These first two treatment goals are the principal targets of individual counseling sessions, which may occur 2 to 5 times a week during the course of hospitalization. Much of this content naturally arises within daily group therapy sessions. Similarly, another of the primary functions of group therapy is to engage each patient in an open and honest self-assessment through interacting with other adolescents who share both common behavior patterns and common consequences. This process not only involves repeated exposure to specific drug-related aversive effects reported by other patients, but it also includes peer feedback regarding stylistic aspects of each patient's current behavior in treatment (e.g., how they "come across," apparent attitude toward treatment, etc.).

A third important goal is educational. Most adolescent patients come into treatment with a kind of streetwise pharmacology, much of which is simply incorrect and even mythical. Along with pseudo-knowledge about psychopharmacology, most patients also hold erroneous stereotypical ideas about what chemical dependency is and is not. Like adult alcoholics, for example, many adolescents believe that if they can go for a day or so, much less a week or more, without using a particular drug, then they cannot be *dependent* on it. Lectures and films, geared to the educational level of patients, are presented daily. Each focuses on a different topic and is addressed in a factual and straightforward style. These topics include: (1) medical and pathophysiological sequels of drug abuse; (2) behavioral pharmacology of drugs of abuse, effects on cognitive, emotive, verbal, and motor behavior; (3) psychological mechanisms of dependence and psychological defenses such as denial and rationalization; (4) a psychological disorder model of chemical dependency; (5) familial, social, educational, and occupational ill effects of chemical abuse; and (6) AA and Narcotics Anonymous (NA) and their 12-steps of recovery, including personal histories presented by young AA/NA members.

The content of each topic area is presented in a straightforward, factual manner. Although presentations are designed to capture attention, and some do entail emotionally evocative issues and information, efforts are made to avoid exaggeration, simplistic "fear tactics," and sensationalism. Film and lecture material tend to evoke questions and discussion in subsequent group therapy sessions. In this way, the material is reviewed, disagreement, debate, and questions are resolved, and the content is related to personal experiences in patients' own lives. Similar personalization and integration of the more factual, more "reality-based" film-lecture content occurs within individual counseling.

Most patients are given reading assignments at the direction of individual counselors. These assignments include selected chapters from *A New Guide to Rational Living* (Ellis & Harper, 1975), *Reality Therapy: A New Approach to Psychiatry* (Glasser, 1965), and *Why Am I Afraid to Tell You Who I Am* (Powell, 1969). Patients are asked to outline the particular assigned chapters and to specifically note associations between the reading material and their own behavior patterns and life experiences. These exercises are then discussed in both individual and group counseling sessions. Patients are not allowed to bring outside reading material (such as novels or magazines) into treatment with the exception of primary religious texts. Reading and study of each patient's own primary religious books is encouraged, as is attendance at their faith's regular religious services. However, no attempt is made to direct any patient toward any particular religion; and reading religious texts and attending religious services is strictly voluntary.

Toward the end of Phase II, patients are reassessed for behavioral disorders and problems which may require additional and specialized treatment. For example, some patients have significant social skill deficits; others have anxiety and phobic reactions; and still others have eating disorders; and so forth. Many chemically dependent adolescents have a history of school and academic problems. Such adolescents are referred to appropriate professionals for remediation, which begins when transferred from the inpatient unit to the half-way house.

Phase III: Half-way House

Almost all adolescents are transferred to a half-way house upon completion of the inpatient phase of treatment. In the half-way house, which is staffed by a house manager ("dorm mother or father") and counselors, patients usually start back to school, or some older adolescents start to work. Patients return each afternoon or evening directly to the half-way house. They attend AA or NA meetings, usually 2 or 3 nights a week, and on alternate evenings they have group therapy sessions in the half-way house. Individual counseling may occur once a week or more as determined by counselors and individual patients. Patients remain in the half-way house from 2 to 6 months before returning to live in their own home environments.

It is during this phase that patients who have additional acquired disorders are then referred to relevant treatment. Most patients will be evaluated and assisted by academic and vocational guidance counselors. For example, those with eating disorders are referred to eating disorder clinics or programs; those with reactive affectual disorders or personality disorders are seen by psychiatrists and psychologists. Those few adolescent patients who have carefully diagnosed major thought or affective disorders and have been on medication throughout inpatient treatment continue to see the psychiatrist who has been following them for that psychotic disorder.

Family Program

Except in unusual circumstances, at least one parent of each adolescent in treatment is required (as a condition of admission) to go through the family program. Meeting 1 or 2 nights a week for several weeks, parents attend the same lecture-film presentations as the patients. In addition, parents meet in their own group therapy sessions. There are two primary foci of these family sessions. The first is to address the parents' own feelings and actions that are associated with their child's chemical abuse. These include parents' feelings of failure and frustration as well as their attempts to cope with their child's behavior and their own contributions to or enabling of their child's chemical abuse. The second primary focus is to develop more effective parenting skills in preparation for their son's or daughter's return to the home. These sessions are conducted by family counselors who have expertise in both chemical dependency treatment and in family therapy.

SUMMARY

Although it has become something of a popular cliché, statistical data in fact document the proposition that chemical abuse has reached epidemic proportions in our society. This is at least as true for adolescent populations as for society as a whole. Advances in psychopharmacological research have not only begun to unravel the complex neurochemistry of drug actions, but they have also more fully elucidated their disruptive impact on normal brain functions and on associated cognitive, affectual, and overt behavioral processes. Similarly, genetic and psychological studies have identified some biological and psychological antecedents that can serve as risk factors for developing chemical dependencies.

While such discoveries are crucial to a comprehensive understanding of substance abuse, the most clinically useful advances have occurred in theoretical conceptualizations and clinical formulations that guide diagnostic and treatment procedures. The most important of these advances are: (1) increasing recognition that a relatively long-standing pattern of chemical abuse as described earlier is *not* a symptom of something else, but is a disorder itself; (2) regardless of biological, environmental, or intrapersonal psychological factors that may have contributed initially to chemical abuse, once the pattern of chemical dependency is well established, it is at that point almost always functionally autonomous of its roots; (3) remediation of the supposed roots alone rarely has a significant or enduring impact on the long-term course of substance abuse disorders; (4) chemical abuse produces as well as contributes to and exacerbates a wide variety of maladaptive, disruptive, problematic behaviors and it is not viewed usually as only symptomatic, but rather other cognitive, affectual, and other behavioral problems are often recognized as symptomatic of substance abuse; and, finally (5) individual psychotherapy alone is not as efficacious in treating chemical dependency as are specialized, multimodal treatment programs. These advances have led informed clinicians to be more alert to signs and symptoms that may be related to chemical substance abuse, to be more aggressive in data gathering and in considering substance abuse and dependency as primary diagnoses, and in placing chemically dependent adolescent patients in appropriate treatment programs.

REFERENCES

Alford, G. S., & Fairbank, J. A. (1985). Personality disorders. In M. Hersen (Ed.), *Practice of inpatient behavior therapy: A clinical guide* (pp. 173–199). Orlando: Grune & Stratton, Inc.

American Psychiatric Association. (1987). *Diagnostic and statistical manual of mental disorders.* (DSM-III-R). Washington, DC: Author.

Beck, A. T. (1976). *Cognitive therapy and the emotional disorders.* New York: International Universities Press.

Beck, A., Rush, A. J., Shaw, B., & Emery, G. (1979). *Cognitive therapy of depression.* New York: Guilford.

Bohman, M. (1978). Some genetic aspects of alcoholism and criminality. *Archives of General Psychiatry, 35,* 269–276.

Bohman, M., Sigvardsson, S., & Cloninger, C. R. (1981). Maternal inheritance of alcohol abuse. *Archives of General Psychiatry, 38,* 965–969.

Brownell, K. D., Marlatt, G. A., Lichtenstein, E., & Wilson, G. T. (1986). Understanding and preventing relapse. *American Psychologist, 41,* 765–782.

Cadoret, R. J., Troughton, E., O'Gorman, T. W., & Heywood, E. (1986). An adoption study of genetic and environmental factors in drug abuse. *Archives of General Psychiatry, 43,* 1131–1136.

Davis, V. E., & Walsh, M. J. (1970). Alcohol, amines and alkaloids: A possible basis for alcohol addiction. *Science, 167,* 1005–1007.

Elkins, R. L., & Murdock, R. P. (1977). The contribution of successful conditioning to abstinence maintenance following covert sensitization (verbal aversion) treatment of alcoholism. *IRCS medical science: Psychology and psychiatry: Social and occupational medicine, 5,* 167.

Ellingboe, J. (1978). Effects of alcohol on neurochemical processes. In M. A. Lipton, A. DiMascio, & K. F. Killam (Eds.), *Psychopharmacology: A generation of progress* (pp. 1653–1664). New York: Raven.

Ellis, A., & Harper, R. A. (1975). *A new guide to rational living.* Hollywood, CA: Wilshire.

Fowler, R. C., Rich, C. L., & Young, D. (1986). San Diego suicide study: Substance abuse in young cases. *Archives of General Psychiatry, 43,* 962–965.

Glasser, W. (1965). *Reality therapy: A new approach to psychiatry.* New York: Harper & Row.

Goodwin, D. W., Schulsinger, F., Hermansen, L., Guze, S., & Winokur, G. (1973). Alcohol problems in adoptees raised apart from alcoholic biological parents. *Archives of General Psychiatry, 28,* 238–243.

Goodwin, D. W., Schulsinger, F., Moller, N., Hermansen, L., Winokur, G., & Guze, S. (1974). Drinking problems in adopted and non-adopted sons of alcoholics. *Archives of General Psychiatry, 31,* 164–169.

Grunby, P. (1984). Deaths decline but drunk driving, other traffic safety hazards remain medical news. *Journal of the American Medical Association, 251,* 1645–1647.

Jones, M. (1968). Personality correlates and antecedents of drinking patterns in adult males. *Journal of Consulting and Clinical Psychology, 32,* 2–12.

Khantzian, E. J., & Treece, C. J. (1977). Psychodynamic aspects of drug dependence: An overview. In J. D. Blaine & D. A. Julius (Eds.), *Psychodynamics of drug dependence.* Research Monograph *No. 12.* Rockville, MD: National Institute on Drug Abuse, 11–25.

Lettier, D. J., Sayers, M., & Pearson, H. W. (Eds.). (1980). *Theories on drug abuse: Selected contemporary perspectives.* NIDA Research Monograph 30. Available from Superintendent of Documents, U.S. Government Printing Office, Washington, DC.

Loper, R., Kammeier, M., & Hoffman, H. (1973). MMPI characteristics of college freshman males who later became alcoholics. *Journal of Abnormal Psychology, 82,* 159–162.

Marlatt, A. G., & Rose, F. (1980). Addictive disorders. In A. E. Kazdin, A. S. Bellack, & M. Hersen (Eds.), *New perspectives in abnormal psychology* (pp. 298–324). New York: Oxford.

McCord, W., & McCord, J. (1960). *Origins of alcoholism.* Stanford, CA: Stanford.

Miller, W. R., & Hester, R. K. (1980). Treating the problem drinker: Modern approaches. In W. R. Miller (Ed.), *The addictive behaviors: Treatment of alcoholism, drug abuse, smoking, and obesity* (pp. 11–141). New York: Pergamon.

Monnelly, E., Harth, E., & Elderkin, R. (1983). Constitutional factors predictive of alcoholism in a follow-up of delinquent boys. *Journal of Studies on Alcohol, 44,* 530–537.

Nathan, P. E. (1986). Some implications of recent biological findings for the behavioral treatment of alcoholism. *The Behavior Therapist, 8,* 159–161.

Powell, J. (1969). *Why am I afraid to tell you who I am.* Allen, TX: Argus.

Schuckit, M. A., & Rayses, V. (1979). Differences in acetaldehyde levels in relatives of alcoholics and controls. *Science, 203,* 54–55.

Spotts, J. V., & Shontz, F. C. (1980). *Cocaine users: A representative case approach.* New York: Free Press.

Tarter, R., & Edwards, K. (1986). Antecedents to alcoholism: Implications for prevention and treatment. *Behavior Therapy, 17,* 346–361.

Vaillant, G. (1983). *The natural history of alcoholism.* Cambridge, MA: Harvard University Press.

CHAPTER FIFTEEN

Psychosexual Disorders

Nathaniel McConaghy

In terms of recognition of psychosexual disorders, the development of adolescent psychiatry remains largely fixated at the latency stage. The Recent texts contain no information concerning sexual dysfunctions or paraphilias (Rutter & Hersov, 1985) or indeed none concerning any aspect of sexual behavior (Weiner, 1982). Meanwhile, health workers in the community are stressing the need for increased awareness and management of the significant problems they are identifying in relation to adolescent sexual behaviors.

One reason that mainstream adolescent psychiatry has ignored these problems could be the marked reluctance of adolescents to reveal their sexual concerns and behaviors to clinicians and investigators. Porteous (1985) commented that when adolescents are surveyed concerning problems, they rarely mention sexual ones. However, a study of the 65 teenagers who committed suicide from 1979 to 1983 in Metro Dade County, Florida, (Copeland, 1985) revealed the following: of the 80% in whom the cause was known, it was a boyfriend/girlfriend problem in 17%; out-of-wedlock pregnancy in 5%; a lover triangle in 5%; and other sexual problems in a further 10%. Sexual problems seem to be of considerable significance to adolescents, though they will not easily reveal them.

This reluctance has proved extremely misleading in regard to theoretical as well as practical developments. Such experienced sex researchers as Ehrhardt, Green, and Money accepted the statements of 110 subjects exposed to increased levels of opposite sex hormones in utero and controls, of whom about half were prepubertal and half adolescent. All but one stated they had not experienced homosexual feelings (McConaghy, 1984). These statements, grossly at variance with evidence that about 50% of adolescents are aware of some homosexual feeling, were attributed major theoretical importance in refuting the theory that such feelings resulted from exposure in utero to increased levels of opposite sex hormones. More recently Money, Schwartz, and Lewis (1984) reported that girls with adrenal hyperplasia when adolescent treated their sexual activity as an unspeakable issue, but as adults they reported a high incidence of homosexual feelings. These workers commented that aging of these subjects brought increased sophistication and the ability to talk about their sexual feelings and behavior.

Knowledge of adolescent sexual problems cannot be based on clinical interview data only. It will require investigation of such behaviors in the community from a variety of perspectives.

DIAGNOSTIC AND DEVELOPMENTAL CONSIDERATIONS

Sexual disorders in the DSM-III-R (APA, 1987) are divided into two groups. The Paraphilias are characterized by arousal to sexual objects or situations that are not part of normative arousal-activity patterns. The Sexual Dysfunctions are characterized by inhibitions in sexual desire or the psychophysiological changes that characterize the sexual response cycle. Other sexual disorders include disorders in sexual functioning that are not classifiable in the two groups. Gender Identity Disorders are characterized by incongruence between assigned sex and gender identity, the sense of knowing to which sex one belongs. Frank, Anderson, and Rubinstein (1978) found that though about half of happily married adults reported by questionnaire that they experienced sexual dysfunctions at times, such dysfunctions correlated less with the subjects' degree of sexual satisfaction than did even more common emotional difficulties in their sexual interactions with their partners. Such difficulties remain largely unclassified in the DSM-III-R.

This tendency of mainstream psychiatry to ignore aspects of adult sexual behavior that produce significant sexual dissatisfaction was considered to contribute to the failure of psychiatry to provide appropriate therapy and to the widely documented explosion of sexual therapies in the 1970s, often provided by minimally qualified or untrained persons (McConaghy, 1987a). There is potential for a similar situation in regard to current developments in the management of problems associated with normal adolescent sexuality, which must inevitably be excluded from disease model classifications such as the DSM-III-R. These developments have been stimulated by factors as diverse as the politics of feminism and the appearance of the AIDS virus. Current developments have led to services for prevention of adolescent pregnancies; for change in sexual activities in relation to sexually transmitted diseases; and for treatment of the victims of sexual abuse, incest and rape, and of sexual discrimination.

Fortunately, the prior development of community psychiatry has meant that many psychiatrists have been prepared to work with health workers from different professional and nonprofessional backgrounds to provide such services. The danger remains that if mainstream adolescent psychiatry ignores these developments, their provision may not be accompanied by adequate critical theoretical analysis and evaluation. At present, the documentation of many such problems of adolescent sexuality and their management is largely through media-reported interviews, with the health workers providing services in schools and walk-in clinics rather than in the adolescent psychiatric literature.

MASTURBATION AND ASSOCIATED GUILT

The sexual activity of adolescents that is most frequently studied in the academic literature is heterosexual intercourse, in particular, age and attitudes at first occurrence. A recent monograph entitled "Adolescent

Sexuality" (Antonovsky, Kav-venaki, Lancet, Modan, & Shoham, 1980) dealt only with these topics, ignoring such behaviors as masturbation, sexual assault, homosexuality, paraphilias, and incest. As masturbation appears to be the most common of adolescents' sexual outlets (certainly in boys) and as the other behaviors provoke marked social disapproval, their incidence and the feelings they provoke also seem worthy of investigation.

No data concerning the incidence or significance of masturbation in representative samples of adolescents appear to have been provided since that of Sorensen (1973). Lo Presto, Sherman, and Sherman (1985) considered that despite the contention of many researchers and clinicians that masturbation is beneficial to self-awareness and sexual behavior, many young people retain societal and religious taboos concerning it. Quoting the strong relationship between masturbatory guilt and low self-esteem widely reported throughout the literature, these workers investigated the effect in reducing such guilt of a single 40-minute masturbation seminar, compared with a discussion of homosexuality of similar duration. Assessment was by the Negative Attitudes Toward Masturbation Inventory. They concluded that the masturbation seminar produced more positive attitudes toward masturbation and reduced sex myths but did not influence guilt feelings. Reduction in negative attitudes was not expressed through increase in self-reported masturbation frequency.

Adolescents continue to be exposed within their families to what must be considered at best ambivalent attitudes toward their masturbation. Gagnon (1985) interviewed a stratified random sample of 1482 parents with 3- to 11-year-old children and found that over 80% of both mothers and fathers believed most preteen children masturbated. About 60% considered this alright, but only about 40% wanted their child to have a positive view of masturbation. Less than 20% of parents discussed the topic with their child; therefore, as Gagnon pointed out, even when parents do approve, their children are unlikely to know about it. About 80% of Sorensen's (1973) sample of adolescents reported their parents had never talked to them about masturbation, suggesting there has been little change in parental behavior in this respect in the last decade. There is thus little data to guide health workers dealing with adolescents concerning the significance or management of the guilt presumably still experienced by most adolescents associated with this common sexual activity.

HETEROSEXUAL INTERCOURSE, SEXUALLY TRANSMITTED DISEASES, AND PREGNANCY IN ADOLESCENCE

In contrast to the situation a decade ago, it is now accepted that there has been a major change in adolescent sexual activity. In 1977, Hopkins discussed the evidence that Americans were then in the midst of a sexual revolution concerning premarital coitus. In 1963, 80% of a representative national sample of adults believed it was always wrong, but in 1975, only 30% believed this (Rodman, Lewis, & Griffith, 1984). Hopkins questioned whether the increase in the social acceptance of premarital coitus was reflected in an increase in its incidence, and he reviewed the studies available, pointing out their methodological weaknesses. In particular, the terminology used could have distorted their findings. Some younger adolescents reported having had "sexual intercourse," considering it meant socializing with the opposite sex, and older adolescents varied considerably as to the meaning they attached to "loss of virginity." As the samples studied were not adequately representative of the total adolescent population, Hopkins was disinclined to accept evidence that a major change had occurred by 1975 in the sexual activity of adolescents under age 20. He accepted the evidence of studies of college-age adolescents in which from the mid-1960s to the mid-1970s premarital coitus incidence figures rose from about 25 to 40% for women and 55 to 60% for men. Hopkins pointed out the strong trend to intergender convergence.

The marked increase in the 1970s in incidence of sexually transmitted disease and of pregnancy in teenagers in the United States has subsequently led to general acceptance that a major change in adolescent sexual activity occurred at least by the end of the 1970s. Most widely quoted are the figures provided by Zelnik, Kantner, and Ford (1981) for the fairly representative sample of unmarried metropolitan teenagers with coital experience: 20% of girls and 35% of boys age 15, and 45% of girls and 56% of boys age 17. In comparison with the data provided over 20 years earlier by Kinsey (Kinsey, Pomeroy, & Martin, 1948; Kinsey, Pomeroy, Martin, & Gebhard, 1953), the figures represent a striking increase in incidence, particularly in girls, demonstrating that marked intergender convergence had occurred. These trends to earlier age of initial coitus and intergender convergence may be restricted to Western cultures. They have been reported from Canada (Barrett, 1980) and Czechoslovakia (Raboch & Bartak, 1980). Studies from West Germany (Clement, Schmidt, & Kruse, 1984) and Sweden (Lewin, 1982) found more girls commenced coitus at earlier ages than boys. However, of unmarried Columbian university students (mean age 22 to 23) studied from 1979 to 1981, 94% of the males reported having experienced coitus, compared with 38% of females (Alzate, 1984). Investigation of Nigerian university students (median age 22) found that 28% of women had experienced coitus by age 16, but only a further 10% by age 21, compared to 7% and 23% of men (Soyinka, 1979). This is suggestive of a different pattern of adolescent sexual development than that in Western countries.

Over the past decade, concern has been expressed in the United States at the rise in incidence of sexually transmitted diseases and pregnancy in teenagers that has accompanied their increased sexual activity (Howard, 1985). From 1960 to 1981, the incidence of gonorrhea rose from 15 to 25/100,000 for boys and 25 to 75/100,000 for girls age 10 to 14 years and from 490 to 1000/100,000 for boys and 350 to 1400/100,000 for girls age 15 to 19. Rates have remained relatively stable since 1975 (Mascola, Albritton, Cates, & Reynolds, 1983). These authors considered that twice as many cases in adolescents remained unreported and pointed out the significance of such future complications in the infected girls as infertility and ectopic pregnancies. They attributed the increased incidence to a change in contraceptive methods less protective against sexually transmitted diseases as well as to increased sexual activity. Though it is generally accepted that adolescents are at high risk for exposure to AIDS and the numbers infected are increasing (Strunin & Hingson, 1987; Rogers & Lifson, 1986), there are no data from representative samples. Burke and colleagues (1987) reported that of 306,001 teenage and young adult applicants for military service 460 (0.15%) carried the virus. Of the 141,900 less than 20 years old, 63 (0.04%) were infected, the male prevalence increasing from 0.02% at 18 to 0.57% at 27 years. A less stable increase was noted in women. For the 3000 teenage applicants from counties in the New York City-Newark area, prevalence was 0.23%.

Luna (1987) pointed out that though the number of cases of AIDS reported in adolescents was small (139 age 13 to 19 years as of March, 1987), the number diagnosed in their 20s (7029, 21% of the total) gave a better indication of those initially infected in their teens, in view of the long incubation period of the disease. Luna considered there were three subpopulations at particularly high risk for AIDS infection: male and female street prostitutes, refugee youth and kept youth, and those youths supported by nonrelative adults. Luna pointed out that street and kept youths generally feared and avoided service agencies, yet to be effective, AIDS prevention programs must reach this population. Furthermore, they should be provided with vocational training and housing.

There has been growing concern in the United States that adolescent pregnancies have reached epidemic proportions (Beck & Davies, 1987), with more than a million 15- to 19-year-olds pregnant (one-tenth of all women in this age group) and 30,000 girls younger than 15 becoming pregnant annually (Rodman et al., 1984). Rodman et al. quoted Zelnik and Kantner's data on metropolitan-area teenagers, showing an increase in premarital pregnancies in women age 15 to 19 from 9% in 1971 to 13% in 1976 and 16% in 1979. This increase was mainly attributable to the larger numbers of adolescents who were sexually active rather than to reduction in their use of effective contraception, as the increase in pregnancies in the sexually active over the same period was much less, from 28 to 30%. That is to say, contraception remained at much the same level of relative inadequacy throughout the decade.

Twenty percent of teenagers who experienced an unwanted pregnancy repeated the experience at least once (Byrne, 1983). Of teenagers who gave birth, one of four was pregnant again within a year (Sugar, 1984). The ratio of first pregnancies in 15- to 19-year-olds terminated by abortion almost doubled from 17% in 1971 to 30% in 1976. However, over 200,000 pregnancies annually resulted in out-of-wedlock births and about 100,000 in hasty unanticipated marriages, disrupting the mothers' educational and vocational plans (Byrne, 1983). Sugar (1984) considered that most unmarried upper- and middle-class girls opted for abortion, but lower- or working-class girls kept their babies in about 95% of cases.

More recently, Flick (1986) also interpreting data from the late 1970s, concluded that 50% of females 15 to 19 years old were sexually active. Thirty-three percent of the 50% became pregnant. Of the 33%, 14% had a miscarriage or stillbirth, 38% an abortion, and 49% delivered a baby, which 90% reared and 10% had adopted out. Hence, 1 in 6 adolescent girls age 15 to 19 years had been pregnant, and 1 in 14 was raising a child premaritally conceived. A recent study by the National Research Council (Hacker, 1987) found that by the mid-1980s, 75% of black and 48% of white teenagers were sexually active before age 18, with 40% of black and 20% of white teenagers becoming pregnant, indicating no increase in effective contraception. The percentages of pregnant black and white teenagers who arranged abortion (35% and 40%, respectively) and who delivered a baby (51 and 46%, respectively) and who subsequently reared the child (99 and 92%, respectively) were fairly similar and showed no meaningful change from the earlier cohort described by Flick. The annual birth rate per 1000 unmarried girls age 15 to 19 was 87 for blacks and 19 for whites.

ADOLESCENT PARENTHOOD

Sugar (1984) reported that of married women giving birth before age 16, nearly one-third lived in poverty, and one-third of the marriages ended in separation or divorce. Of married women first giving birth after age 22, a tenth lived in poverty and a tenth suffered marital breakup. Deliveries in teenagers are associated with a high risk of obstetric complications (Halperin, 1982), and teenage mothers have a high rate of child abuse and a suicide rate 10 times that of the normal population (Byrne, 1983). Two percent of children born to parents younger than 17 die in their first year of life, twice the rate of children in other families (Robinson & Barrett, 1985).

Methodologists continue to plead that in interpreting the results of quasi-experiments (those in which subjects are not randomly allocated to the conditions studied), all other possible explanations should be excluded before casual significance is attributed to correlations found (Cook & Campbell, 1979). Their pleas continue to fall on deaf ears, social scientists appearing in this respect particularly hard of hearing. Motherhood in adolescents almost invariably is held to be responsible for all the negative features associated with it, and a need for preventative programs for such motherhood generally is unquestioned (Flick, 1986).

With the aim of providing information, Flick reviewed the research concerning the four decisions made (or not made) by adolescent mothers: becoming sexually active, failing to use adequate contraception, not obtaining an abortion, and not arranging adoption. Little evidence was available concerning the last decision, but the other three correlated with lower socioeconomic status, lower educational attainment, and membership of large families. Younger age was associated with less adequate contraception but increased likelihood of abortion rather than delivery. The fact that adolescent motherhood is associated with variables existing prior to its occurrence renders more powerful the methodological criticism of the assumption that variables associated with such motherhood were produced by it. At least where black teenagers are concerned, Hacker (1987) considered the fact that most live in neighborhoods that are mainly or all black, increases their demoralization and reduces their confidence they can escape the cycle of poverty.

In light of the current reduction in concern for social welfare characterizing most Western governments, an important finding of Flick was that despite poverty being associated with early sexual activity, less use of contraception, and lower abortion rates, numerous studies have documented that availability of welfare support for single mothers does not encourage either sexual activity or adolescent pregnancy. Hence, though the evidence is not yet available that adolescent motherhood contributes significantly to the cycle of poverty, equally there is no evidence to justify failure to alleviate the poverty with which it is strongly associated. A recent development in attempting its alleviation is by programs aimed at helping teenage fathers to remain more involved with their children and more supportive of the mothers (Robinson & Barrett, 1985). These workers concluded that many teenage fathers go through the same emotional struggle and confusion that young mothers do. They often face unbridled hostility from their girlfriends' families. Those who attempt to provide financial support tend to cease this within a year.

CHANGE IN SEXUAL PRACTICES AND EDUCATION PROGRAMS

Failure to use contraception, though associated with lower socioeconomic and educational status, is common in the sexually active adolescent at all levels. Byrne (1983) found regular use of contraception reported by less than one-third of sexually active unmarried female university students; this frequency of use was not shown to be much superior to that of all sexually active female adolescents, 30% of whom use no, 40% irregular, and 10% ineffective contraception. As abortion is used to terminate many of the pregnancies resulting from failure to use adequate contraception, opposition to contraception might be considered to result only from the activity of religious groups. However, media publicity, given to claimed adverse effects of the contraceptive pill and intrauterine devices, has been considered responsible for a marked decline in their use as a first method from 1976 to 1979 (Kulig, 1985).

As Kulig pointed out, the mortality attributed to pregnancy and childbirth in 15- to 19-year-olds is 12.9 deaths per 100,000 live births, whereas mortality rates attributable to contraception include 0.3 deaths in nonsmokers on the pill, 2.2 deaths in smokers on the pill, and 0.8 deaths in IUD users, per 100,000 users per year. Furthermore, recent studies have found noncontraceptive health benefits with oral contraceptives. Appropriate liaison might ensure that media publicity maintain a pro-contraception perspective. No explanation has been advanced for the failure of the Federal Drug Administration (FDA), and its equivalent in Australia, to approve medroxyprogesterone acetate as a contraceptive despite its being the only effective method for some adolescents, in particular, the retarded, and its excellent safety record with extensive clinical use.

If adolescent and community psychiatrists consider contraception preferable to abortion in preventing unwanted parenthood, it appears necessary that they take a more active role in encouraging effective contraception by teenagers. Psychiatrists may have failed to do so in the past by accepting what Rodman et al. (1984) labeled a clinical myth, the psychoanalytically based theory that many unmarried women become pregnant because they unconsciously desire pregnancy. Rodman et al. argued that before the early 1970s, the most commonly available contraceptive was the condom, which was primarily under the control of men, who were less motivated to use contraception. When effective methods under women's control became available, many women, including teenagers rapidly took advantage of them. In fact, as pointed out earlier, the evidence indicates that contraceptive practices of sexually active teenage girls did not improve in the 1970s.

Rodman et al. warned against the adoption of a new myth of deficient technology, insufficient education, or lack of access to adequate contraception to explain its nonuse by the majority of adolescent girls at risk of an unwanted pregnancy. They considered an important reason was preservation of a "good girl" image; that is, being contraceptively ready implies that one expects to be sexually active. Zelnik et al. (1981) pointed out that the sexual activity of teenagers is irregular, episodic, and unplanned, factors not conducive to efficient contraception.

The 1970s saw the widespread introduction of sex education programs, many of which were directed at adolescents and aimed at prevention of unwanted pregnancies and of sexually transmitted diseases. With the appearance of the AIDS virus, evidence of the efficacy of programs for changing sexual behaviors has a new relevance. Kilmann, Wanlass, Sabalis, and Sullivan (1981) reviewed 33 studies assessing the effectiveness of sex education. Almost all programs evaluated were directed at college or university students, lacked follow-up, and rarely examined behavioral change. Kilmann et al. stressed the need for systematic investigation of programs for younger adolescents.

Howard (1985) commented in a more recent study of exemplary sex education programs in the United States that teenagers experienced knowledge gains but showed little change in behavior. Cvetkovich and Grote (1983) found no difference in sex or contraceptive knowledge between good and poor contraceptive users in their study of white, mainly middle-class high school students age 16 to 18, almost all of whom had attended a health course which included birth control information. Marsiglio and Mott (1986) found no significant association between taking a sex education course and subsequently becoming premaritally pregnant before age 20 in data from the 1984 National Longitudinal Survey of Work Experience of Youth. The conclusion of Rodman et al. (1984) that the presently available positive results are promising enough to warrant developing programs of education in human sexuality seems questionable, although the recommendation to also evaluate them is commendable.

Data supplied by Brown (1983) indicates that the fall in abortion and pregnancy rates in 15- to 19-year-olds in Sweden in 1975 followed the introduction of youth clinics in which school nurses dispensed nonprescription contraceptives, rather than the improved sex education that commenced in 1977. Introduction of services similar to the youth clinics into U. S. high schools also was followed by falls in pregnancy rates (Edwards, Steinman, Arnold, & Hakanson, 1980). Active follow-up of girls appeared essential for high continuation rates (Beck & Davies, 1987).

Gold (1988) reported on a mobile clinic that visited an area frequented mainly by adolescent male prostitutes, that 200 who regularly attended for free condoms and clean needles had remained free of AIDS infection. The condom is still considered the primary contraceptive method for sexually active adolescents (Smith, 1984; Morrison, 1985). Its value in also reducing the risk of sexually transmitted diseases, particularly AIDS, requires that every effort is made to reverse the fall in condom use noted between 1965 and 1975. It would appear this may require not merely education but also the provision of cheap or free condoms to adolescents at risk.

SEXUAL ASSAULT AND PSYCHIATRIC DISTURBANCE

One area of adolescent sexuality that has produced a substantial literature is that of sexual assault. A major stimulus for this literature has been the women's movements, and most of its emphasis has been on the more common situations where women are the victims. Finkelhor (1984) criticized the literature on child sexual abuse as having persistently focused on the question of long-term effects. He considered this to be due to adult ethnocentrism and to the fact that rape was treated as a serious life event whether or not it causes long-term effects. He concluded that research had demonstrated that the negative effects of rape attenuate after 1 or 2 years; however, few would conclude that rape is therefore a less traumatic experience than was previously thought. In fact, the literature on the sexual abuse of adolescents and adults also seems to be biased toward emphasizing its long-term effects in producing psychiatric disturbances rather than on the immediate distress provoked and the evaluation of techniques for managing this.

One of the few studies investigating the effects of sexual assault that attempted to obtain a representative sample was reported in *Sexual Assault among Adolescents* (Ageton, 1983). Sexual assault was defined as all forced sexual behavior involving contact with the sexual parts of the body, the force varying from verbal pressure to physical beatings, in subjects age 11 to 20. Subjects were those in a national probability sample who self-identified as sexual assault victims or offenders. Ageton did not give the data on male victims of homosexual assaults on the questionable grounds that as these were not typical, they could result in misleading conclusions.

From the data, Ageton concluded that in each year from 1978 to 1980, from 5 to 11% of the adolescent female population in the United States, that is, from 700,000 to 1 million teenage females, experienced at least one sexual assault. There were no significant race or social class differences, but urban girls were more vulnerable. The offenders were mainly boyfriends or dates in the same age range as the victim, less than 20% being unknown to her. The most common pressure reported by victims was verbal, but from 27 to 40% experienced some minimal physical force. The majority were successful in deterring the assault. Up to 15% reported physical beating or the presence of a weapon, so that the rate of serious, violent sexual assaults was substantially higher than that in the National Crime Survey, which in turn was over 10 times that of the Uniform Crimes Report. Victims of violent sexual assaults were typically black, lower-class urban adolescents.

Of girls reporting an assault in 1 year, over one-third experienced at least one further assault in the same year and their risk of being assaulted in the next year was three to four times that for all female adolescents. Comparisons between victim and control groups suggested that involvement in delinquent behavior and with delinquent peers might account for the victim's initial and continuing vulnerability. Two years prior to any reported sexual assaults, the victims and controls were substantially different in terms of peer networks, relations with family, and attitudes toward deviance.

Only 5% of the assaults recorded in Ageton's study were reported to the police, mainly those involving unknown or multiple assailants and use of threats or of actual violence. Over half those reported were completed assaults. Ageton suggested that attempted nonviolent assaults by dates or boyfriends may not be defined by the victims as legitimate sexual assaults for purposes of reporting to officials. Over two-thirds of the victims told their friends but not their parents. Personal relationships with husbands or boyfriends were not seriously affected by the assault unless these individuals were the offenders, when the relationships had a high probability of ending. The strongest reactions described within a week of the assault were anger, depression, and embarrassment, but 40% reported some guilt. However, Ageton concluded that the typical assault, a date rape, did not generate many negative reactions that persisted for 6 months. Reactions to the assault were not differentiated by race, age, social class, number of offenders, relationship to the offender, or the amount of force experienced. Only the completion of the assault had a significant influence, being associated with more negative reactions in the following year.

Ageton was able to assess reactions to the assault for up to 3 years in a subsample of victims. After the marked decline noted in the first year, 2 to 3 years later a number of subjects reported depression and fear of men and of being alone. These reactions were not related to features of the assault, and Ageton concluded that factors such as support from significant others, history of traumatic events, and personality traits may be more instrumental in affecting long-term reactions. She also suggested these late reported reactions might have been artifacts of the repeated interview situation. Certainly, if they were not (and many victims of attempted assault by dates or boyfriends experience fear of men and of being alone 2 to 3 years later) these symptoms should be very common in adolescent girls, as this type of assault is sufficiently common that Ageton considered it could be regarded as almost a standard feature of dating.

Koss and Oros (1982) suggested that rape be considered an extreme behavior on a continuum with normal male behavior, a view they supported by the Sexual Experiences Survey responses of 1846 male and 2016 female university students (mean age = 21). Thirty-three percent of women and 23% of men reported having been in situations when the man was so sexually aroused, the woman felt it was useless to stop his having sexual intercourse though she did not want it. The use of physical force to make the woman engage in petting and kissing was reported by 30% of women and 6% of men, and the use of force to successfully make her have intercourse was reported by 8% of women and 2.7% of men. Six percent of women reported having been raped. Men were not asked. Gomez-Schwartz, Horowitz, and Sauzier (1985) compared 14- to 18-year-old victims of sexual abuse that had occurred or been revealed in the preceding 6 months, with adolescents in psychiatric treatment. The Louisville

Behavior Checklist E-3 was used as a measure of emotional distress. On 10 of the 13 scales, sexually abused adolescents showed less pathology than those in treatment. Few exhibited severe pathology on most scales, using the criterion proposed by the author of the checklist.

These studies indicate that sexual abuse of varying degrees of severity, though commonly experienced by female adolescents, does not of itself produce significant long-term psychiatric disturbances. In contrast, other studies (usually with inappropriate or without controls and not using standardized tests) have attributed low self-esteem, promiscuity, homosexuality, prostitution, depression, schizophrenia, suicidal ideation, and murder to earlier sexual assaults (Mrazek & Mrazek, 1981). Psychosexual disorders are the most commonly attributed consequence, though quasi-experimental evidence advanced to support a causal relationship (Tsai, Feldman-Summers, & Edgar, 1979) is certainly open to other interpretations.

Psychosexual disorders also were reported in adolescent males sexually assaulted by women (Sarrel & Masters, 1982) and by men (Groth & Burgess, 1980). Kaufman, Divasto, Jackson, Voorhees, and Christy (1980) reported an increase from 0 to 10% from 1975 to 1978 in percentage of male as compared to female victims of male sexual assault presenting to a Sexual Assault team in New Mexico. Male victims were younger than the female, 5 of the 14 being 13 to 18 years old. They were more likely to have sustained greater physical trauma, more reluctant initially to reveal the genital component of their assault, and more likely to use denial and control their emotions in relation to the assault. The authors speculated that a far smaller proportion of male as compared to female victims report their assault, but they may experience major, hidden trauma.

Emotional disturbances found to follow assault in both males and females may be expressions of preexisting differences. Ageton's evidence indicated that assaulted girls differed from nonassaulted prior to the assault. More follow-up studies similar to that of Ageton appear required, on probability samples of adolescents, comparing the outcome of the assaulted with that of the nonassaulted. If significant differences emerge that bear some meaningful relationship to features of the assault, this would provide the first stage of evidence for a causal relationship.

INCEST

Similar considerations apply to the large number of studies reporting long-term consequences of adolescent incestuous experiences. As with sexual assault, incestuous experiences have been studied mainly in women and have been found to be common. The most widely quoted is Russell's (1983) investigation of 930 women age 18 or older, 50% of a probability sample of residents of San Francisco. Thirty-eight percent reported an experience of sexual abuse before the age of 18, in 31% from a nonrelative, in 16% from a relative. Experiences that were wanted with a relative whose age was within 5 years of that of the subject were not included, though forced kissing was. The incestuous relatives were mainly fathers, 4.5%; uncles, 4.9%; cousins (almost all male), 3%; and brothers, 2.2%. Six percent of the extrafamilial and 2% of the intrafamilial episodes of abuse were reported to the police.

The views of health professionals concerning the effects of incest vary from the belief that "normal development can never be expected from a child who is lover to her father, sexual rival of her mother, and mistress to the household . . ." (Cantwell, 1983), through the finding that the majority of victims are unaffected, to the conclusion that in some cases the experience is emotionally beneficial (Kroth, 1979). There is more agreement that brother-sister incest is relatively innocuous (Steele and Alexander, 1981). In fact, as Henderson (1983) points out in his review "Is Incest Harmful?" the quality of the present research does not enable the effect of incest to be known.

If adolescent psychiatry is to be maintained as an academic as well as a clinical discipline, its practitioners must feel sufficiently confident of their ethical values to disapprove of the sexual exploitation of adolescents without finding it essential to believe such exploitation produces long-term psychiatric disability. Lacking this confidence, they will not require that evidence of such disability be obtained with the methodological rigor expected when issues are investigated that do not evoke the powerful emotional reactions that are inevitable with those of sexual assault and incest.

CLINICAL PROBLEMS

The psychosexual disorders of adolescents differ little from those of adults, according to available accounts of recent developments (McConaghy, 1984). However, adolescents are much less likely to seek treatment for them. Those disorders that come to the attention of psychiatrists because they have led the adolescent into criminal activity tend to be regarded, often incorrectly, as of little significance.

Sexual Dysfunctions

Society appears to have accepted that most adolescents are engaged in sexual activity but has not yet decided whether they should enjoy it. This may explain why though significant numbers of adolescent girls appear to obtain limited pleasure from sexual intercourse, they do not commonly seek advice or treatment concerning this until they are adult and married. There appears to have been no attempt to determine the current validity of Sorensen's (1973) report of the following: 57% of nonvirgin teenage girls rarely or never reached orgasm in heterosexual relations though a third of the 57% considered it very important to do so; and 21% of adolescent males with masturbatory experience reported masturbation without orgasm in the previous month, 12% on five or more occasions. Despite the fact that most adults seeking treatment for sexual dysfunctions report they were established in adolescence, no developments in the study of sexual dysfunctions of adolescents appear to have occurred.

Dysfunction Associated with Adolescent Homosexuality

During the 1980s there has been a growing awareness that gay adolescents may be among those youths at greatest risk for impaired physical, social, and emotional health. Recognizing the problem, the American Academy of Pediatrics issued a Statement of Policy in 1983 encouraging physicians to become involved in the care of homosexual and other young persons struggling with the problem of sexual expression (Remafedi, 1987a, p. 331).

Coincident with the growing awareness of problems associated with adolescent homosexuality, the diagnosis of ego-dystonic homosexuality was dropped from the DSM-III-R. If this has been accompanied by a reduced interest in homosexuality by psychiatrists, it might explain why psychiatrists have not contributed to the recent concern for homosexual adolescents' problems, evidenced by pediatricians and other health workers.

Remafedi (1987b, 1987c) considered his study the first since that of Roesler and Deisher (1972) to understand homosexuality from the adolescent's perspective. He interviewed 29 males age 15 to 19 who were recruited through a gay news publication and radio and a health department clinic. Twenty-three identified themselves as gay and six said they were bisexual. Only six of their mothers and three of their fathers responded or were expected to respond supportively to disclosure of their sexual orientation. Eight were victims of "gay bashings," 2 of sexual assault, and 16 of regular verbal abuse from classmates. Eleven envisioned negative consequences and 11 general uncertainty in regard to the impact of their sexual orientation on their future lives. Six wished to be heterosexual. Thirteen had a history of sexually transmitted diseases, and 17 met DSM-III (APA, 1980) criteria for substance abuse. Approximately half had been arrested or appeared in juvenile court at least once, mainly for substance abuse, truancy, prostitution, or running away from home. Twenty-one had consulted a psychologist or psychiatrist at least once for emotional problems. All but 1 had contemplated and 10 had attempted suicide at least once. Ten reported having a "steady" male partner when interviewed, in only one the relationship being longer than 1 year. The

mean age of the partners was 25 years. The mean number of male partners during 1 year was seven. Fifteen had heterosexual experiences during the previous year with a mean of 5.6 partners. Five admitted
accepting money for sex at least once.

Remafedi considered that it was unlikely the sample was biased by selection toward dysfunctional adolescents, as they were recruited from a wide
variety of settings and none of them were from mental health settings.
Furthermore, their demographic characteristics closely resembled those of
the general adolescent population in the community from which they were
sampled. Remafedi considered that the experience of acquiring a homosexual or bisexual identity at an early age places the individual at risk for
dysfunction, particularly given the stigmata attached to homosexuality in
contemporary American society. Remafedi pointed out that Roesler and
Deisher, in their study of 60 males age 16 to 22 with homosexual experience, reported similar high rates of psychiatric consultation (29/60) and
attempted suicide (19/60).

Adolescents who identify as homosexual or bisexual are only a small
percentage of those who experience some homosexual feeling or who
become involved in homosexual activity, though there appear to have been
no attempts to document the extent of the latter since the study of
Sorensen (1973). Evidence has been reviewed elsewhere (McConaghy,
1984, 1987b) indicating that 30 to 40% of older and 40 to 50% of younger
teenagers are aware of a degree of homosexual feelings. Less than 10%
indicate these are stronger than their heterosexual feelings. Virtually all
adolescents who are aware of a significant but not predominant degree of
homosexual feelings and a percentage of those with predominant homosexual feelings adopt a heterosexual lifestyle and identity in adulthood.
However, some will continue to have occasional or regular clandestine
homosexual experiences (McConaghy, 1978; Brownfain, 1985).

Homosexual experience in adolescence is associated with the greater
likelihood of adoption of a homosexual identity, particularly in males.
In Saghir and Robins' (1973) study, 82% of self-identified homosexual
adult men reported experiencing homosexual activity by age 15 compared
with 23% of heterosexual men. Only 53% of homosexual women had such
experience by age 19. Nevertheless, as Remafedi (1985) commented, to
date no investigator has identified variables that can accurately predict a
young person's ultimate sexual preference, and it would seem appropriate
in counseling adolescents presenting with homosexual feelings or behavior that this be pointed out. The information also is often helpful in aiding
resolution of the intense family discord that commonly accompanies reve-
lation of an adolescent's homosexuality (Remafedi, 1985). While the therapist's first consideration should be to support the adolescent's decision
concerning his or her sexual identity, parents often are able to come to
terms with it and be less rejecting of the adolescent if they accept that the

decision may not be irrevocable. It is important to establish that the parents will not use the information to harass the adolescent into seeking treatment to modify his or her orientation. At the same time, there can be a role for behavioral treatment to help adolescents who for religious or other reasons cannot come to terms with aspects of their homosexuality, which they experience as compulsive. This is more likely to be those who have a significant or predominant heterosexual component and whose homosexual component may become minimal with increasing age.

More attention is being paid to the need for supportive counseling of the overt adolescent male homosexual with obvious effeminate behavior who is commonly treated negatively at school both by staff and other students (Price, 1982; Tartagni, 1978). Martin (1982) pointed out the difficulties adolescents who are aware of a significant homosexual component encounter in their socialization, due to lack of appropriate role models and lack of acceptable situations in which to learn homosexual courting behavior. Paroski (1987) found that of 120 self-identified homosexual adolescents presenting to a New York gay/lesbian community clinic, many had developed a stereotypical view of homosexuality and its associated lifestyle due to their socialization.

With the growing awareness of their significances in relation to the transmission of AIDS, increased attention is being paid to the estimated 300,000 adolescent male prostitutes in the United States, most of whom identify as homosexual (Deisher, Robinson, & Boyer, 1982). The National Institute of Mental Health (NIMH) sponsored study (Luna, 1987) revealed the difficulty the AIDS prevention programs will have in influencing their behavior. Allen's (1980) study indicated the need to do so. The 98 he interviewed had a mean age of 16.6 years. They had commenced homosexual activity at a mean age of 13.6, one-third being initially seduced by an older male. Twenty-five had had sexual intercourse with a female, commencing at a mean age of 12. Nineteen were predominantly heterosexual. Twenty-eight regularly used hard drugs, and 41 were heavy drinkers or alcoholics.

Paraphilias

Paraphilias are commonly established before or during adolescence and are largely restricted to males. Of 45 men who sought treatment for compulsive paraphilias (McConaghy, Armstrong, & Blaszczynski, 1985; McConaghy, Blaszczynski, & Kidson, 1988), 6 were adolescents. A further 21 reported the paraphilic behavior had commenced and was usually fairly regularly repeated in adolescence. This trend was particularly marked in the five fetishists, three of whom showed a marked though apparently not sexual interest in the fetishistic object some years prior to puberty. In the fourth, the fetishistic interest began at age 13. Twelve of 19 exhibitionists, 7 of 11 homosexual pedophiles, and 2 of 3 voyeurs also reported that their behavior commenced in adolescence. Heterosexual pedophiles did not show this trend strongly, only two of seven reporting the behavior in adolescence. Five of the six paraphiliacs seen in adolescence were referred following convictions: two for homosexual and one for heterosexual pedophilia and two for sexual assault. The sixth, a fetishistic transvestite, was brought by his parents, having stolen clothes from schoolmates.

Unlike paraphiliacs seen initially as adults, one-third of whom, mainly pedophiles, sought treatment voluntarily and without prior convictions, adolescents were unlikely to do so. It is noteworthy that none of the subjects who reported regularly exposing in adolescence was charged with this offense until adulthood. Nor were any adolescents referred for treatment of exhibitionism, despite the fact that it is the most common sexual offense in adults and hence at any time must be being regularly carried out by a significant number of adolescents. Presumably, victims do not regard exhibitionism by adolescents as justifying report to the police. Groth, Longo, and McFadin (1982) commented that, unfortunately, sexual offenses by adolescents (in particular, rape and child molestation) are frequently dismissed as sexual curiosity or experimentation, or they are dismissed with the diagnosis of adolescent adjustment reaction. Certainly, in the studies by McConaghy, Blaszczynski, Armstrong, and Kidson (in press-a) the paraphilias of the adolescent subjects showed a trend to be more resistant to treatment than those of adults. Four of the 6 adolescents but only 7 of the 39 adult sex offenders required treatment additional to the initial course.

Rape

The National Crime Survey data indicated that, according to reports of victims, adolescent males were responsible for 15% of forcible rapes in 1978 and 21% in 1979 (Ageton, 1983). As discussed earlier, the rapes recorded in these data are substantially less than those that are unrecorded. How many of the latter are carried out by adolescents who do not differ in personality or degree of emotional disturbance from those who are charged cannot be determined.

If the view is correct that rape is an extreme behavior on a continuum with normal male behavior, the growing acceptance given the view that rape is prompted more by nonsexual needs to dominate than by sexual motives (Groth & Burgess, 1980; Holmstrom & Burgess, 1980) will require questioning. Certainly, nonsexual motives are likely to play a role as they do in nonrape sexual relations (O'Reilly & Aral, 1985). General enjoyment and sexual arousal were average responses of 36 male Canadian undergraduate volunteers to a 12 minute videotape of a motorcycle gang chasing, catching, and raping a young woman (Pfaus, Myronuk, & Jacobs, 1986). Domination would seem to contribute to sexual arousal in a significant percentage of adolescent males. Udry, Billy, Morris, Groff, and Raj (1985) found that free serum testosterone levels in adolescent boys correlated strongly with their levels of sexual interests and behaviors. This indicates that such behaviors were sexually motivated, even though evidence previously reviewed concerning male sexual behavior indicates they often must have been expressed aggressively. Rape may usually be less a result of male pathology than of a lack of social concern to effectively proscribe it. At present, adolescent girls are required to cope with varying degrees of emotional and physical pressure for intercourse from male acquaintances with minimal advice or information from parents or society.

Sexual Asphyxia

Of the 132 cases of fatal sexual asphyxia studied by Hazelwood, Dietz, and Burgess (1983), 37 were teenagers and 5 were female. Hazelwood et al. speculated that it results in 500 to 1000 deaths a year in the United States. It is distinguished from suicide by the characteristic mode of death. The apparatus used to induce strangulation, suffocation, chest compression, or chemical asphyxiation may show signs of regular use or of a fail-safe procedure. There is evidence of autoerotic activity, such as exposure of the genitals and, not infrequently, of cross-dressing, fetishism, bondage, and/or masochistic activity. According to the Hazelwood et al. study, when parents had been aware of their child's involvement in the activity prior to the fatality, they had ignored it.

Gender Identity Disorders

Transvestite behavior is divided in the DSM-III-R classification between the paraphilias and the gender identity disorders. The form presented by adolescents who present for treatment having stolen clothes or having been found using clothes of family members usually approximates the definition of transvestic fetishism, in that they are sexually aroused by the clothes and masturbate while wearing them. Though DSM-III-R states that the disorder has been described only in heterosexual males, one of the author's patients initially stole and used in this way the clothes of boys at his school, to whom he was sexually attracted. Later he switched to using women's clothes (McConaghy et al., in press-a). If questioned about their fantasies during cross-dressing, most say that to some extent they imagine themselves to be girls and may be aroused by the fantasy of the girl they imagine themselves to be. Therefore, they seem to show some degree of gender identity disorder.

There appears to be no literature following up a series of these adolescents. However, men who cross-dress in adulthood with minimal or no sexual arousal and who are classified in DSM-III-R as showing Gender Identity Disorder of Adulthood, Nontranssexual Type (GIDAANT) report transvestic fetishism in adolescence (Buhrich & McConaghy, 1977), indicating that a significant number of adolescents with this condition will develop GIDAANT in adulthood. Transvestic fetishism cannot be regarded as transient in adolescent sexual development. In the author's patient referred to previously, who was followed up until age 22, it was still persisting (McConaghy et al., in press-a). As with the other form of cross-dressing, transsexualism, the majority of youths with transvestic fetishism begin cross-dressing in childhood and almost all the remainder begin in adolescence (Buhrich & McConaghy, 1977). Then, transvestic fetishists are more likely to use only a few items of women's clothes, particularly underclothes, to produce sexual arousal, unlike transsexuals who cross-dress fully and without sexual arousal.

The literature has tended, incorrectly in the author's opinion, to treat gender identity disorder of childhood as a categorical rather than a dimensional condition (McConaghy, 1987a). It would appear to be on a continuum with less extreme opposite sex-linked behaviors. The extent of these behaviors correlates in males with the subsequent balance of their homosexual to heterosexual feelings, even in subjects who are predominantly heterosexual (McConaghy, 1987b).

PHARMACOLOGICAL APPROACHES AND MEDROXYPROGESTERONE THERAPY

Virtually the only pharmacological approach of importance for adolescent psychosexual disorders is medroxyprogesterone therapy for compulsive sexuality. In order to suppress deviant sexual behavior in males, almost all workers have used dosage levels which produced temporary impotence in the patients treated. However, it was shown by McConaghy et al. (1988) that it was not necessary to use such levels to produce what appeared to be an equivalent therapeutic response. If the subject's serum testosterone was lowered to approximately 30% of the pretreatment level, adequate suppression of his deviant or compulsive impulses was obtained. Sexual interest generally was reduced, but he was still aroused by physical stimuli and so maintained previously established acceptable sexual relationships.

The use of medroxyprogesterone in adolescents faces the problem that many have not established acceptable sexual relationships, and reduction of their level of sexual interest would seem likely to weaken their motivation to do so. However, alternative psychological treatment usually requires a significant time commitment within school or working hours. As adolescents are establishing their careers, this can be disruptive, particularly in times of high youth unemployment. Medroxyprogesterone as used in the study by McConaghy and colleagues required a total of eight 150 mg i.m. injections over 6 months, following which almost all adult patients treated were able to control the sexual urges they had experienced as compulsive prior to treatment. Adolescents were likely to require a further course (McConaghy et al., in press-a). Persistence of reduction in the strength of urges following termination of medroxyprogesterone was attributed to a weakening over the period of treatment of the associated behavior completion mechanisms (discussed in the following section). Side effects were minimal. Though Udry, Talbert, and Morris (1986) have reported that androgen levels are significantly related to sexual motivation and masturbation but not coital experience in adolescent girls, the author's experience is that medroxyprogesterone does not weaken compulsive sexual behaviors in women.

The study by Money et al. (1984) referred to in the introduction to this chapter found that significantly more women who were fetally androgenized (due to congenital virilizing adrenal hyperplasia) identified in adulthood as bisexual or homosexual than controls did. However, they had not been willing to reveal such feelings in adolescence. It supports the conclusion by McConaghy (1984) that reports by adolescents concerning their balance of heterosexual/homosexual feeling lack validity. This study by Money et al. must lead to questioning not only of the earlier conclusion of Ehrhardt, Epstein, and Money (1968) that the tomboyism of adrenogenital girls did not include implications of future homosexuality, but also of the similar conclusion reached concerning the tomboyism due to prenatal exposure to androgenizing progestogens (Money & Matthews, 1982). Evidence that prenatal exposure to exogenous hormones in boys affects their subsequent sex-dimorphic behaviors is much less convincing (Ehrhardt, Meyer-Bahlburg, Feldman, & Ince, 1984).

Neuroleptic drugs, the standard treatment for schizophrenia, have been reported to cause decreased libido, erectile impotence, inhibition of ejaculation, and interference with orgasm in males (Nestoros, Lehmann, & Ban, 1981). Evidence of deleterious effects on women's sexual behavior seems less definite (Friedman & Harrison, 1984). Nestoros et al. (1981) pointed out that the reproductive rates of both male and female schizophrenics have increased since introduction of the neuroleptics in the 1950s, and they concluded that the beneficial effects of the drugs on the illness and hence on society's attitude toward the patients outweigh the possible suppression of their sexual behavior. Such suppression needs to be kept in mind when counseling adolescent schizophrenics. The effects of recreational drugs on adolescent sexual behavior appear to have been less explored.

PSYCHODYNAMIC AND BEHAVIORAL APPROACHES

Advances in psychodynamic theories are usually identifiable only retrospectively because they are rarely established by research studies. Instead, they are established by the reception that respected factions give new interpretations and plausible arguments. In addition, psychodynamic theorists traditionally have shown little interest in actual sexual behaviors as opposed to those occurring in fantasy, following Freud's attribution of his patients' memories of childhood incest experiences as being fantasy. The astonishing increase in the accepted incidence of such experiences in the last 20 years from one to two cases to at least several thousand per million of the population (Lester, 1972; Henderson, 1983) inevitably led to questioning of Freud's attribution. The resulting interaction of polemics and personalities was considered of sufficient interest to the New York literati to justify its extensive reporting in the *New Yorker* (Malcolm, 1983). The publicity given by more down-market media to the reported high incidence of incest has led to widespread acceptance of the poorly research-based but emotionally satisfying conclusion that such experiences, unless intensively treated, will result in long-term psychiatric disability.

Together with the publicity given physical child abuse, this publicity has stimulated the rise of a multimillion-dollar social welfare industry (Nelson, 1986). Even though many services in this industry have not been established to be of value, its development is, of course, highly commendable in a society affluent enough to afford it without reducing other welfare commitments. In Australia, this has not proved possible. Provision of such services has been at the expense of housing for runaway homeless adolescents, increasing the number roaming the streets of Sydney at night (Williams, 1986). That homeless youths are considered a high risk group for sexually transmitted disease was pointed out earlier. Hence, there are more than methodological grounds for evaluating the cost-effectiveness of programs for the treatment of sexually abused adolescents and their families, with the same rigor as is applied to the investigation of less emotionally provocative issues.

Sexual Abuse Treatment Programs

The program that has received most publicity and wide acceptance as a model is the Child Sexual Abuse Treatment Program (CSATP) developed by Giarretto (1978, 1981) from a humanistic psychology approach. He considered that to acquire the required compassionate attitude, it was necessary to go into deep exploration of his unconscious for his own incestuous impulses. In turn, patients in his program are coached into self-awareness, so that in the course of treatment the father must acknowledge to the mother and daughter that he was totally responsible for the incestuous behavior; the mother must acknowledge that her poor parenting contributed to it; and in time, the daughter confides she was not entirely a helpless victim. It would seem possible that with less sensitive therapists the treatment could result in a somewhat indulgent wallow in an orgy of guilt. The author's experience is that guilt often results in a weakening of control, as subjects feel that they are so bad it does not matter what more they do. He attempts to decrease the subjects' guilt while encouraging their sense of self-esteem and of responsibility.

Giarretto decided that conjoint family therapy was inappropriate for incestuous families in the early throes of the crisis and that individual counseling was initially required particularly for the daughter, mother, and father. This was usually followed by mother-daughter counseling, then marital counseling, father-daughter counseling, and finally group counseling. The cost of the procedure is not given in most reports nor how it is met, but the average length of treatment for a family is 9 months. Giarretto reported that an independent review conducted by Kroth found an overall recidivism rate of 0.6% compared to an average of 2% reported by other studies, but that Kroth considered a more important statistic to be the increasing rate at which victims, offenders, and families came into the program. No comparison was given with the rate of increase of applicants for treatment to other programs. In evaluating recidivism rates, it is not possible to determine how comparable are the groups treated in various programs. Incestuous families treated in the CSATP would appear to be unrepresentative of the total. Kroth (1979) reported the mean age of the victims to be 12 to 13. This is well above the mean age of victims in population samples (Russell, 1983).

Giarretto, Giarretto, and Sgroi (1978) consider the authority of the criminal justice system absolutely essential in treating incest. Reporting is mandatory in all 50 U.S. states. Sgroi (1975) stated that it was unconscionable that any member of the helping professions would violate the law and withhold potential help from the victim by failure to report suspected child abuse. Despite the pressure such statements put on therapists, Finkelhor (1983) quoted evidence that close to 50% of cases of sexual abuse known to professionals were not officially reported, suggesting that many do not consider this advantageous. He also pointed out that criminal action was taken five times more often in cases of reported sexual than of physical abuse, and foster care placement occurred in 17% of sexual as compared to 12% of physical abuse. When the victims were adolescent, 31% were placed in foster or shelter care. He considered this an excessive response to the emotional outrage sexual abuse provokes.

Wald (1982) and Smith and Meyer (1984) have argued against mandatory reporting of incest on the basis that it can discourage some abusers from seeking voluntary treatment or revealing such abuse in individual or group therapy. A significant percentage of reports made on suspicion of abuse are subsequently not proven, which may have harmful consequences. Given the emphasis placed by Giarretto on the low recidivism rate of the CSATP, a disconcerting finding of Kroth's (1979) evaluation was that the number of perpetrators and spouses who considered that if a future molest occurred they might keep it a secret increased from 18%

at intake to 41% at termination. Kroth considered that this might reflect their unhappiness with the criminal justice system rather than with the treatment program.

Moore, Zusman, and Root (1985) concluded from a survey of Florida mental health facilities that the majority of sex offenders, of whom 41% were incest offenders, were treated in local outpatient services. They considered that this reduced stigmatization and allowed the breadwinner to maintain the family system. Many were under supervision of the court, but 21% of the total were self-referred, and 47%, the majority of whom were incest offenders, had not been convicted of any sex offense. The typical treatment of incest offenders was given in 1 to 1 1/2 hour weekly sessions for 10 months. Only 6 of the 48 facilities treating sex offenders provided special programs for them, 3 of which were limited to incest offenders and victims. The authors pointed out that research and policy discussion of sex offender treatment in Florida has always centered on two residential programs that served only a small proportion of treated offenders. They commented that four basic approaches are used in treatment of sexual aggressors—behavioral, social skills training, psychodynamic, and organic—but did not provide data on those used in the facilities surveyed.

Behavioral Treatment of Sex Offenders: Behavior Completion Hypothesis

The author has developed a treatment approach for sex offenders based on a behavior completion model of compulsive behaviors (McConaghy, 1980, 1983). Utilizing New-Pavlovian concepts of Sokolov and Anokhin, it was hypothesized that as a subject established an habitual behavior, a matching behavior completion mechanism was built up in his nervous system. Then the subject could be stimulated to complete the behavior, for example, by being in a situation where he had carried it out in the past. If he attempted not to complete it, his arousal system would be activated so that he experienced maintained tension and excitement that was sufficiently aversive to cause him to complete the behavior against his will. From this model, it was argued that if the subject were trained to relax and then to repeatedly visualize not carrying out the behavior while remaining relaxed, this would allow him to control the behavior in reality.

The treatment, termed imaginal desensitization, proved significantly more effective than covert sensitization in 15 subjects with compulsive sexuality, 2 of whom were adolescents (McConaghy, Armstrong, & Blaszczynski, 1985). Subsequently, imaginal desensitization was compared with and proved approximately equivalent to medroxyprogesterone alone or to the two treatments combined in the treatment of 30 sex offenders, of whom 4 were adolescents (McConaghy et al., 1988). Imaginal desensitization was administered in 14 sessions over a week's inpatient admission. As discussed earlier, the adolescent subjects in the two sexuality treatment studies were more likely than the adults to relapse following the initial course of the treatment. They did show good response to additional treatment, the use of which should be considered as a routine (McConaghy et al., in press-a). The higher rate of initial relapse could be explained by adolescents' sexual behavior being under greater hormonal control, so that the habitual component associated with behavior completion was not as established as in adults. This is consistent with the strong correlations between sexual behaviors and serum testosterone levels in adolescent (Udry et al., 1985) but not in adult males (McConaghy, 1984).

Both imaginal desensitization and medroxyprogesterone were able to be provided at no cost to the patients and interfered minimally with their education or work commitments. Where indicated, that is, where patients are aware of compulsive deviant sexual urges, either treatment would seem to justify comparison with more intensive and presumably expensive therapies. Smith and Meyer (1984) pointed out the need for low-cost therapy as 80 to 90% of cases of abuse known to the National Study of Child Abuse were in families with annual incomes under $15,000.

Sexual offenders who do not experience their paraphiliac urges as compulsive may be able to control these with counseling and supervision. This approach is less likely to be effective in those who give a history indicative of marked personality disorder. Behavior therapists (Hersen, 1981; McConaghy, 1988) are currently emphasizing the need for assessment and treatment of such disorders now commonly referred to in the behavior therapy literature as organismic factors. The use of appropriate behavioral methods to treat reduced self-esteem, social skills, or sexual responsiveness in victims of sexual assault has not yet been adequately documented.

Periodically, negative reviews of the results of sex conversion operations for transsexualism encourage the alternatives of psychotherapy (Lothstein & Levine, 1981; Morgan, 1978) or behavior therapy (Barlow, Abel, & Blanchard, 1979). Meyer and Reter (1979) found no improvement in social rehabilitation of subjects who received the operation, compared to those who did not because they failed to complete the qualifying period of living and working in the opposite sex role for 1 year. The finding was influential in termination of the surgical program at Johns Hopkins (Lothstein, 1982). Lindemalm, Korlin, and Uddenberg's (1986) finding of poor surgical outcome and little change in sexual and psychosocial adjustment following the operation in male-to-female transsexuals in their and other long-term follow-up studies will presumably further encourage alternative therapies. The lack in follow-up studies of uniform selection and outcome criteria and of adequate controls is not likely to be corrected in the near future. The possibility will remain that positive responses of transsexuals to therapies other than sex conversion are as fortuitous as the reversal in sexual identity reported to occur over a few hours in an adolescent transsexual in response to exorcism (Barlow, Abel, & Blanchard, 1977).

The failure to provide data on the adolescent adjustment of the youngest recipient of sex conversion, a 21-month-old boy, has increased recent questioning of the previously widely accepted psychodynamically based theory advanced by Ellis (1945) that sexual identity was determined by sex of rearing in early childhood. The theory was supported by quasi-experimental evidence that subjects with ambiguous genitals assumed in adolescence a sexual orientation and role consistent with early rearing, rather than their chromosomal sex. On the basis of the theory, the boy who had suffered ablation of the penis at 7 months was reassigned to the female sex at 17 months, later given female steroids, and at about 9 years was reported to have accepted reassignment well though having many tomboyish traits (Money, 1975). The only subsequent data provided was in a British Broadcasting Corporation (BBC) television report, indicating the child's adjustment at puberty was markedly disturbed (Diamond, 1982).

Other evidence questioning the theory had been provided by Peterson, Imperato-McGinley, Gautier, and Sturla (1977). They reported on 33 males with the genetic condition of 5alpha-reductase deficiency, which resulted in their having female-appearing genitals at birth and being raised as girls. With the change to male-appearing genitals and physique consequent on increased testosterone levels as they approached puberty, all but two (roughly the proportion who could be expected to be almost exclusively homosexual of a random sample of 33 males) accepted in adolescence a male sexual role and identity.

The psychodynamic concept that normal males and females have a strong unified sense of sexual identity has recently been questioned (McConaghy & Armstrong, 1983). It was suggested that the concept was largely supported from the study of transsexuals. Assessing sexual identity dimensionally rather than categorically, evidence was advanced that adolescents with a homosexual component have a more consistent sense of being like the opposite sex, while those who were exclusively heterosexual had a less consistent sense of belonging to their own sex.

Orthodox U.S. psychiatric scholarship impressively continues to adhere to psychodynamic theory concerning sexuality (Meyer, 1985; Stoller, 1985), despite the failure of research of the last decade to provide empirical evidence supporting the etiological significance of childhood experiences. The ability to ignore this failure presumably reflects the lack of interest of U.S. psychiatrists in the study of sexual behavior in reality as opposed to fantasy.

SUMMARY

Adolescents commonly fail to reveal sexual problems or disorders, but they admit them subsequently when they are adults. Most experience guilt about the common sexual activity of masturbation, which few parents discuss with them. First occurrence of sexual intercourse is considered an important event in the psychological development of adolescents. The age of first occurrence has significantly reduced in most Western countries in the 1970s, particularly in girls. Associated with this has been a rise in the incidence of sexually transmitted diseases, pregnancy, and abortion in teenagers in the United States. Adolescent mothers as compared with adult mothers are more likely to live in poverty, abuse the child, and commit suicide. If they marry, their marriages are more likely to end in separation or divorce. Research has not yet demonstrated that adolescent motherhood produces these difficulties with which it is associated. Contraceptive use has not improved through the 1970s or 1980s, despite introduction of sex education programs. Clinics that provide contraceptives for adolescents appear to improve effective utilization, both for prevention of unwanted pregnancies and of sexually transmitted diseases.

Sexual assaults of adolescents are being more intensively investigated. Possibly only 5% are reported to the police, mainly those involving unknown assailants. Varying degrees of coercion are a standard feature of dating, and it has been suggested that rape is currently on a continuum of normal male sexual behavior. Evidence that sexual assault has long-term consequences is equivocal, psychosexual disorders being the most common finding in both male and female victims reporting assault. Evidence has been advanced that 16% of women experience incestuous abuse before the age of 18. Professionals tend to agree that brother-sister incest is relatively innocuous, but they disagree concerning the long-term psychiatric consequences of other forms.

Adolescents virtually never seek treatment for sexual disorders, although the majority of adolescent girls rarely reach orgasm in heterosexual relations and an unknown percentage of boys have difficulty ejaculating. Adolescent males identifying as homosexual or bisexual are considered to show significant emotional dysfunction, and those with effeminate behaviors are found to be distressed by the response of their peers and teachers. No variables are known to predict with certainty the sexual identification an adolescent will adopt as an adult.

Paraphilias apart from heterosexual pedophilia are commonly established during adolescence, or before in the case of fetishism. However, they rarely lead to treatment before adulthood unless they result in criminal behavior. Exhibitionism by adolescents appears to be ignored, as does sexual asphyxia, the latter with possible fatal consequences. When treated in adolescence, paraphilias appear to be more likely to recur than when treated in adulthood. An unknown percentage of adolescents who cross-dress with marked sexual arousal continue to cross-dress with minimal arousal in adulthood, leading to their reclassification in the DSM-III-R. Gender identity disorder in childhood is dimensional, not categorical, and it is related to degree of homosexuality in adolescence.

Medroxyprogesterone can give male subjects control over compulsive sexual urges while allowing them to continue acceptable sexual relations. It has a role in treating adolescents with paraphilias if school or work commitments prevent them attending for psychological treatment.

The accepted incidence of incest increased in the last two decades from one or two cases to many thousands per million of the population. This led to questioning of Freud's attribution to fantasies of his patients' reports of childhood incestuous experiences. A multimillion-dollar social welfare industry has arisen to investigate and treat the identified cases of incestuous as well as other sexual and physical abuse. Professionals disagree concerning the advantages of the present mandatory reporting of suspected child and adolescent abuse. No attempt has been made to compare available treatment programs in terms of cost-effectiveness, though some may have been introduced at the expense of other welfare services. A brief treatment based on a behavior completion model of compulsive sexual offenses has been reported. Recent evidence indicates that prenatal exposure to differing ratios of same and opposite sex hormones may be more important than childhood experiences in determining adolescents' balance of heterosexual/homosexual feelings and sexual identity.

REFERENCES

Ageton, S. S. (1983). *Sexual assault among adolescents.* Toronto: Lexington Books.

Allen, D. M. (1980). Young male prostitutes: a psychosocial study. *Archives of Sexual Behavior, 9,* 399–426.

Alzate, H. (1984). Sexual behavior of unmarried Colombian university students: A five-year follow-up. *Archives of Sexual Behavior, 13,* 121–132.

American Psychiatric Association (1980). *Diagnostic and statistical manual of mental disorders* (3rd ed.). (DSM-III). Washington, DC: Author.

American Psychiatric Association (1987). *Diagnostic and statistical manual of mental disorders* (3rd ed. Revised). (DSM-III-R). Washington, DC: Author.

Antonovsky, H. F., Kav-venaki, S., Lancet, M., Modan, B., & Shoham, I. (1980). *Adolescent sexuality.* Lexington, MA: Lexington Books.

Barlow, D. H., Abel, G. G., & Blanchard, E. B. (1977). Gender identity change in a transsexual: An exorcism. *Archives of Sexual Behavior, 6,* 387–395.

Barlow, D. H., Abel, G., & Blanchard, E. (1979). Gender identity change in transsexuals. *Archives of General Psychiatry, 36,* 1001–1007.

Barrett, F. M. (1980). Sexual experience, birth control usage, and sex education of unmarried Canadian university students: Changes between 1968 and 1978. *Archives of Sexual Behavior, 9,* 367–390.

Beck, J. G., & Davies, D. K. (1987). Teen contraception: a review of perspectives on compliance. *Archives of Sexual Behavior, 16,* 337–368.

Brown, P. (1983). The Swedish approach to sex education and adolescent pregnancy: Some impressions. *Family Planning Perspectives, 15,* 90–95.

Brownfain, J. J. (1985). A study of the married bisexual male: Paradox and resolution. *Journal of Homosexuality, 11,* 173–188.

Buhrich, N., & McConaghy, N. (1977). The discrete syndromes of transvestism and transsexualism. *Archives of Sexual Behavior, 6,* 483–495.

Burke, D. S., Brundage, J. F., Herbold, J. R., Berner, W., Gardner, L. I., Gunzenhauser, J. D., Voskovitch, J., & Redfield, R. R. (1987). Human immunodeficiency virus infections among civilian applicants for United States military service, October 1985 to March 1986. Demographic factors associated with seropositivity. *New England Journal of Medicine, 317,* 131–136.

Byrne, D. (1983). Sex Without Contraception. In D. Byrne and W. A. Fisher (Eds.), *Adolescents and Contraception* (pp. 1–31). London: Erlbaum.

Cantwell, H. B. (1983). Vaginal inspection as it relates to child sexual abuse in girls under thirteen. *Child Abuse and Neglect, 7,* 171–176.

Clement, U., Schmidt, G., & Kruse, M. (1984). Changes in sex differences in sexual behavior: A replication of a study on West German students (1966–1981). *Archives of Sexual Behavior, 13,* 99–120.

Cook, T. D., & Campbell, D. T. (1979). *Quasi-experimentation design and analysis issues for field settings.* Chicago: Rand McNally College Publishing Company.

Copeland, A. R. (1985). Teenage suicide—the five-year Metro Dade County experience from 1979 until 1983. *Forensic Science International, 28,* 27–33.

Cvetkovich, G., & Grote, B. (1983). Adolescent development and teenage fertility. In D. Byrne & W. A. Fisher (Eds.), *Adolescents, sex and contraception* (pp. 109–123). London: Erlbaum.

Diamond, M. (1982). Sexual identity, monozygotic twins reared in discordant sex roles and a BBC follow-up. *Archives of Sexual Behavior, 11,* 181–186.

Deisher, R., Robinson, G., & Boyer, D. (1982). The adolescent female and male prostitute. *Pediatric Annals, 11,* 819–825.

Edwards, L. E., Steinman, M. E., Arnold, K. A., & Hakanson, E. Y. (1980). Adolescent pregnancy prevention services in high school clinics. *Family Planning Perspectives, 12,* 6–14.

Ehrhardt, A. A., Epstein, R., & Money, J. (1968). Fetal androgens and female gender identity in the early-treated adrenogenital syndrome. *Johns Hopkins Medical Journal, 122,* 160–167.

Ehrhardt, A. A., Meyer-Bahlburg, H. F. L., Feldman, J. F., & Ince, S. E. (1984). Sex-dimorphic behavior in childhood subsequent to prenatal exposure to exogenous progestogens and estrogens. *Archives of Sexual Behavior, 13,* 457–477.

Ellis, A. (1945). The sexual psychology of human hermaphrodites. *Psychosomatic Medicine, 7,* 108–125.

Finkelhor, D. (1983). Removing the child—Prosecuting the offender in cases of sexual abuse: Evidence from the National Reporting System for Child Abuse and Neglect. *Child Abuse and Neglect, 7,* 195–205.

Finkelhor, D. (1984). *Child sexual abuse.* New York: Free Press.

Flick, L. H. (1986). Paths to adolescent parenthood: Implications for prevention. *Public Health Reports, 101,* 132–147.

Frank, E., Anderson, C., & Rubinstein, D. (1978). Frequency of sexual dysfunction in "normal" couples. *New England Journal of Medicine, 299,* 111–115.

Friedman, S., & Harrison, G. (1984). Sexual histories, attitudes, and behavior of schizophrenic and "normal" women. *Archives of Sexual Behavior, 13,* 555–567.

Gagnon, J. H. (1985). Attitudes and responses of parents to pre-adolescent masturbation. *Archives of Sexual Behavior, 14,* 451–466.

Giarretto, H. (1978). Humanistic treatment of father-daughter incest. *Journal of Humanistic Psychology, 18,* 62–76.

Giarretto, H. (1981). A comprehensive child sexual abuse treatment program. In P. B. Mrazek, & C. H. Kempe (Eds.), *Sexually abused children and their families* (pp. 179–197). Oxford: Pergamon.

Giarretto, H., Giarretto, A., & Sgroi, S. M. (1978). Coordinated community treatment of incest. In A. N. Burgess, A. W. Groth, L. L. Holmstrom, & S. M. Sgroi (Eds.), *Sexual assault of children and adolescents* (pp. 231–241). Toronto: Lexington Books.

Gold, J. (1988). Personal communication.

Gomes-Schwartz, B., Horowitz, J., & Sauzier, M. (1985). Severity of emotional distress among sexually abused preschool, school-age, and adolescent children. *Hospital and Community Psychiatry, 36,* 503–508.

Groth, A. N., & Burgess, A. W. (1980). Male rape: Offenders and victims. *American Journal of Psychiatry, 137,* 806–810.

Groth, A. N., Longo, R. E., & McFadin, J. B. (1982). Undetected recidivism among rapists and child molesters. *Crime and Delinquency, 28,* 450–458.

Hacker, A. (1987). American apartheid. *The New York Review of Books, 34(19),* 26–33.

Halperin, M. E. (1982). Teenage pregnancy—myths and facts. In B. N. Barwin & S. Belisle (Eds.), *Adolescent gynecology and sexuality* (pp. 107–111). New York: Masson Publishing USA, Inc.

Hazelwood, R. R., Dietz, P. E., & Burgess, A. W. (1983). *Autoerotic fatalities.* Lexington, MA: Lexington Books.

Henderson, J. (1983). Is incest harmful?. *Canadian Journal of Psychiatry, 28,* 34–40.

Hersen, M. (1981). Complex problems require complex solutions. *Behavior Therapy, 12,* 15–29.

Holmstrom, L. L., & Burgess, A. W. (1980). Sexual behavior of assailants during reported rapes. *Archives of Sexual Behavior, 9,* 427–439.

Hopkins, J. R. (1977). Sexual behavior in adolescence. *Journal of Social Issues, 33,* 67–85.

Howard, M. (1985). Postponing sexual involvement among adolescents. *Journal of Adolescent Health Care, 6,* 271–277.

Kaufman, A., Divasto, P., Jackson, R., Voorhees, D., & Christy, J. (1980). Male rape victims: noninstitutionalized assault. *American Journal of Psychiatry, 137,* 221–223.

Kilmann, P. R., Wanlass, R.L., Sabalis, R. F., & Sullivan, B. (1981). Sex education: A review of its effects. *Archives of Sexual Behavior, 10,* 177–205.

Kinsey, A. C., Pomeroy, W. B., & Martin, C. E. (1948). *Sexual behavior in the human male.* Philadelphia: Saunders.

Kinsey, A. C., Pomeroy, W. B., Martin, C. E., & Gebhard, P. H. (1953). *Sexual behavior in the human female.* Philadelphia: Saunders.

Koss, M. P., & Oros, C. J. (1982). Sexual experiences survey: A research instrument investigating sexual aggression and victimization. *Journal of Consulting and Clinical Psychology, 50,* 455–457.

Kroth, J. A. (1979). Family therapy impact on intrafamilial child sexual abuse. *Child Abuse and Neglect, 3,* 297–302.

Kulig, J. W. (1985). Adolescent contraception: An update. *Pediatrics, 76,* 675–680.

Lester, D. (1972). Incest. *The Journal of Sex Research, 8,* 268–285.

Lewin, B. (1982). The adolescent boy and girl: First and other experiences with intercourse from a representative sample of Swedish School adolescents, *Archives of Sexual Behavior, 11,* 417–428.

Lindemalm, G., Korlin, D., & Uddenberg, N. (1986). Long-term follow-up of "sex change" in 13 male-to-female transsexuals. *Archives of Sexual Behavior, 15,* 187–210.

Lo Presto, C. T., Sherman, M. G., & Sherman, N. C. (1985). The effects of a masturbation seminar on high school males' attitudes, false beliefs, guilt, and behavior. *The Journal of Sex Research, 21,* 142–156.

Lothstein, L. M. (1982). Sex reassignment surgery: Historical, bioethical, and theoretical issues. *American Journal of Psychiatry, 139,* 417–426.

Lothstein, L., & Levine, S. (1981). Expressive psychotherapy with gender dysphoric patients. *Archives of General Psychiatry, 38,* 924–929.

Luna, G. C., (1987). HIV and homeless youth. *Focus, 2,* 3.

Malcolm, J. (1983). Annals of scholarship I and II. *New Yorker, 59,* Dec. 5, 59–152, Dec. 12, 60–119.

Marsiglio, W., & Mott, F. L. (1986). The impact of sex education on sexual activity, contraceptive use and premarital pregnancy among American teenagers. *Family Planning Perspective, 18,* 151–162.

Martin, A. D. (1982). Learning to hide: The socialization of the gay adolescent. *Adolescent Psychiatry, 10,* 52–65.

Mascola, L., Albritton, W. L., Cates, W., & Reynolds, G. H. (1983). Gonorrhea in American teenagers, 1960–1981. *Pediatric Infectious Disease, 2,* 302–303.

McConaghy, N. (1978). Heterosexual experience, marital status, and orientation of homosexual males. *Archives of Sexual Behavior, 7,* 575–581.

McConaghy, N. (1980). Behavior completion mechanisms rather than primary drives maintain behavioral patterns. *Activitis Nervosa Superior (Praha), 22,* 138–151.

McConaghy, N. (1983). Agoraphobia, compulsive behaviors and behavior completion mechanisms. *Australian and New Zealand Journal of Psychiatry, 17,* 170–179.

McConaghy, N. (1984). Psychosexual disorders. In S. M. Turner & M. Hersen (Eds.), *Adult psychopathology and diagnosis* (pp. 370–405). New York: Wiley.

McConaghy, N. (1987a). A learning approach. In J. H. Geer & W. T. O'Donohue (Eds.). *Theories of human sexuality* (pp. 287–333). New York: Plenum.

McConaghy, N. (1987b). Heterosexuality/homosexuality: dichotomy or continuum. *Archives of Sexual Behavior, 16,* 411–424.

McConaghy, N. (1988). Assessment of sexual dysfunction and deviation. In A. S. Bellack & M. Hersen (Eds.), *Behavioral assessment. A practical handbook* (3rd ed.) (pp. 490–541). Pergamon.

McConaghy, N., & Armstrong, M. S. (1983). Sexual orientation and consistency of sexual identity. *Archives of Sexual Behavior, 12,* 317–327.

McConaghy, N., Armstrong, M. S., & Blaszczynski, A. (1985). Expectancy, covert sensitization and imaginal desensitization in compulsive sexuality. *Acta Psychiatrica Scandinavica, 72,* 176–187.

McConaghy, N., Blaszczynski, A., & Kidson, W. (1988). Treatment of sex offenders with imaginal desensitization and/or medroxyprogesterone, *Acta Psychiatrica Scandinavica, 77,* 199–206.

McConaghy, N., Blaszczynski, A., Armstrong, M. S., & Kidson, W. (in press-a). Resistance to treatment of adolescent sex offenders. *Archives of Sexual Behavior.*

Meyer, J. K. (1985). Paraphilias. In H. I. Kaplan & B. J. Sadock (Eds.), *Comprehensive textbook of psychiatry/IV. Vol. 1* (pp. 1065–1077). Baltimore: Williams & Wilkins.

Meyer, J., & Reter, C. (1979). Sex-assignment: Follow-up. *Archives of General Psychiatry, 36,* 1010–1015.

Money, J. (1975). Ablatio penis: Normal male infant sex-reassigned as a girl. *Archives of Sexual Behavior, 4,* 65–71.

Money, J., & Matthews, D. (1982). Prenatal exposure to virilizing progestins: An adult follow-up study of twelve women. *Archives of Sexual Behavior, 11,* 73–83.

Money, J., Schwartz, M., & Lewis, V. G. (1984). Adult erotosexual status and fetal hormonal masculinization and demasculinization: 46,XX congenital virilizing adrenal hyperplasia and 46,XY androgen-insensitivity syndrome compared. *Psychoneuroendocrinology, 9,* 405–414.

Moore, H. A., Zusman, J., & Root, G. C. (1985). Noninstitutional treatment for sex offenders in Florida. *American Journal of Psychiatry, 142,* 964–967.

Morgan, A. (1978). Psychotherapy for transsexual candidates screened out of surgery. *Archives of Sexual Behavior, 7,* 273–283.

Morrison, D. M. (1985). Adolescent contraceptive behavior: a review. *Psychological Bulletin, 98,* 538–568.

Mrazek, P. B., & Mrazek, D. A. (1981). The effects of child sexual abuse: Methodological considerations. In P. B. Mrazek & C. H. Kempe (Eds.), *Sexually abused children and their families* (pp. 235–245). Oxford: Pergamon.

Nelson, B. J. (1986). *Making an issue of child abuse.* Chicago: University of Chicago Press.

Nestoros, J. N., Lehmann, H. E., & Ban, T. A. (1981). Sexual behavior of the male schizophrenic: The impact of illness and medications. *Archives of Sexual Behavior, 10,* 421–442.

O'Reilly, K. R., & Aral, S. O. (1985). Adolescence and sexual behavior. *Journal of Adolescent Health Care, 6,* 262–270.

Paroski, P. A. (1987). Health care delivery and the concerns of gay and lesbian adolescents. *Journal of Adolescent Health Care, 8,* 188–192.

Peterson, R. E., Imperato-McGinley, J., Gautier, T., & Sturla, E. (1977). Male pseudohermaphroditism due to steroid alpha-reductase deficiency. *The American Journal of Medicine, 62,* 170–191.

Pfaus, J. G., Myronuk, L. D. S., & Jacobs, W. J. (1986). Soundtrack contents and depicted sexual violence. *Archives of Sexual Behavior, 15,* 231–237.

Porteous, M. A. (1985). Developmental aspects of adolescent problem disclosure in England and Ireland. *Journal of Child Psychology and Psychiatry, 26,* 465–478.

Price, J. H. (1982). High school students' attitudes toward homosexuality. *The Journal of School Health, 52,* 469–474.

Raboch, J., & Bartak, V. (1980). Changes in the sexual life of Czechoslovak women born between 1911 and 1958. *Archives of Sexual Behavior, 9,* 495–502.

Remafedi, G. J. (1985). Adolescent homosexuality. Clinical *Pediatrics, 24,* 481–485.

Remafedi, G. (1987a). Homosexual youth a challenge to contemporary society. *Journal of the American Medical Association, 258,* 222–225.

Remafedi, G. (1987b). Adolescent homosexuality: psychosocial and medical implications. *Pediatrics, 79,* 331–377.

Remafedi, G. (1987c). Male homosexuality: the adolescent's perspective. *Pediatrics, 79,* 326–329.

Robinson, B. E., & Barret, R. L. (1985). Teenage fathers. *Psychology Today, 19,* 68–70.

Rodman, H., Lewis, S. H., & Griffith, S. B. (1984). *The sexual rights of adolescents.* New York: Columbia University Press.

Roesler, T., & Deisher, R. W. (1972). Youthful male homosexuality. *Journal of the American Medical Association, 219,* 1018–1023.

Rogers, M. F., & Lifson, A. R. (1986). Acquired immunodeficiency syndrome and HTLV-III/LAV infection. *Seminars in Adolescent Medicine, 2,* 163–173.

Russell, D. E. H. (1983). The incidence and prevalence of intrafamilial and extrafamilial sexual abuse of female children. *Child Abuse and Neglect, 7,* 133–146.

Rutter, M., & Hersov, L. (1985). *Child and adolescent psychiatry.* Oxford: Blackwell.

Saghir, M. T., & Robins, E. (1973). *Male and female homosexuality: A comprehensive investigation.* Baltimore: Williams & Wilkins.

Sarrel, P. M., & Masters, W. H. (1982). Sexual molestation of men by women. *Archives of Sexual Behavior, 11,* 117–131.

Sgori, S. M. (1975). Sexual molestation of children. The last frontier in child abuse. *Children Today, 4,* 18–44.

Smith, P. B. (1984). Reproductive health care for teens. In M. Sugar (Ed.), *Adolescent parenthood* (pp. 159–179). New York: MTP Press.

Smith, S. R., & Meyer, R. G. (1984). Child abuse reporting laws and psychotherapy: A time for reconsideration. *International Journal of Law and Psychiatry, 7,* 351–366.

Sorensen, R. C. (1973). *Adolescent sexuality in contemporary America,* New York: World Publishing.

Soyinka, F. (1979). Sexual behavior among university students in Nigeria. *Archives of Sexual Behavior, 8,* 15–26.

Steele, B. F., & Alexander, H. (1981). Long term effects of sexual abuse in childhood. In P. B. Mrazek & C. H. Kempe (Eds.), *Sexually abused children and their families* (pp. 223–236). Oxford: Pergamon.

Stoller, R. J. (1985). Gender identity disorders in children and adults. In H. I. Kaplan & B. J. Sadock (Eds.), *Comprehensive textbook of Psychiatry/IV. Vol. I* (pp. 1034–1041). Baltimore: Williams & Wilkins.

Strunin, L., & Hingson, R. (1987). Acquired immunodeficiency syndrome and adolescents; knowledge, beliefs, attitudes, and behaviors. *Pediatrics, 79,* 825–828.

Sugar, M. (1984), Adolescent decision-making toward motherhood. In M. Sugar (Ed.), *Adolescent parenthood* (pp. 21–33). New York: MTP Press.

Tartagni, D. (1978). Counseling gays in a school setting. *The School Counselor, 26,* 26–32.

Tsai, M., Feldman-Summers, S., & Edgar, M. (1979). Childhood molestation: Variables related to differential impacts on psychosexual functioning in adult women. *Journal of Abnormal Psychology, 88,* 407–417.

Udry, J. R., Billy, J. O. G., Morris, N. M., Groff, T. R., & Raj, M. H. (1985). Serum androgenic hormones motivate sexual behavior in adolescent boys. *Fertility and Sterility, 43,* 90–94.

Udry, J. R., Talbert, L. M., & Morris, N. M. (1986). Biosocial foundations for adolescent female sexuality. *Demography, 23,* 217–227.

Wald, M. S. (1982). State intervention on behalf of endangered children—A proposed legal response. *Child Abuse and Neglect, 6,* 3–45.

Weiner, I. (1982). *Child and adolescent psychopathology.* New York: Wiley.

Williams, G. (1986, September 19). Little aid for runaways, says paper. *The Sydney Morning Herald,* pp. 1.

Zelnik, M., Kantner, J. F., & Ford, K. (1981). *Sex and pregnancy in adolescence.* Beverly Hills: Sage Publications.

CHAPTER SIXTEEN

Mental Retardation

Arthur M. Small

During the past two decades, there has been a slow but steadily increasing interest in the problems of the mentally retarded. This interest has arisen from a new social awareness of the needs of the handicapped and from a concerted effort to establish a health care system appropriate to the needs of this handicapped population. The apathy which traditionally has been shown toward the retarded has been giving way to a new enlightenment rooted in fundamental changes in the law protecting the rights of the retarded. These changes in attitude also recognize the fiscal necessity and the moral and social obligation to help the retarded gain both economic and personal independence.

Because 98% of the mental retardation population lives out of an institution and those within the institution are being slowly domiciled within the community, there has been a newly heightened visibility of the retarded population in our communities. They are appearing in schools and workshops, hospitals, clinics, and group residences. It is therefore mandatory that all health professionals, not only psychiatrists and psychologists, be informed as to the problems of the retarded and be trained in methods to cope with their difficulties.

Although we are making progress to fill the void of services, understanding, and compassion, there is still a large gap in our knowledge of the mentally retarded adolescent, in general, and the mentally retarded adolescent with emotional problems, in particular. This chapter will review the current status of our knowledge in this area and will draw, when appropriate, from the child and young adult studies as well.

Adolescence, as can be seen readily from the other chapters in this book, is difficult under normal conditions. For the mentally retarded youngster, adolescence represents an extremely trying period. Adolescents have to cope with a world that they have difficulty understanding and with bodily changes and feelings that frequently are confusing and sometimes disturbing. The coping mechanisms that normal adolescents have may not be available to the mentally retarded adolescent.

Over the years, it has been well documented that there is a high incidence of emotional problems in the retarded population. Rutter, Graham, & Yule, (1970) found from a large sample of English children that those who were mentally retarded were five to six times more likely to suffer emotional problems than nonretarded children. Penrose (1962) concluded that emotional instability is one of the most frequent contributory factors in the selection of mentally retarded individuals for institutionalization. Chazan (1964) evaluated mentally retarded children in an educational setting and found that the mentally retarded children were twice as likely to exhibit emotional problems as the overall population of children. Foale (1956) concluded that mildly retarded adolescents who were admitted to institutions were placed there because of their emotional instability and not because of their low intelligence. Kirman (1973) reported his findings that mildly retarded individuals with an IQ greater than 50 seldom fail on a job or in social adjustment because of low intelligence. Rather, many mildly retarded individuals fail because of temperamental instability, neurosis, or psychosis. These findings have been confirmed repeatedly by other researchers for both children and adults.

Matson (1985) points out that the literature has typically contended that emotionally disturbed, mentally retarded persons may be one of the most underserved handicapped populations in the country and unfortunately, until recently, research in this area has been slow in coming. He further points out several reasons why there has been a lack of attention in this area. First, he states that until recently, advocates of the mentally retarded feared having mental retardation linked with emotional problems. Historically, mental retardation has been linked with and sometimes considered synonymous with psychosis. Because of this, parents of the mentally retarded were concerned about additional and unfair prejudices against their children. Second, he states that psychiatrists as a group have very little contact with the mentally retarded and tend to attribute deviant behaviors to the mental retardation rather than to view them as coexisting emotional disturbances. Finally, according to Matson, the existing service delivery system is not conducive to providing services to this dual-diagnosed group.

For the purposes of this chapter, the definition of mental retardation will follow the criteria of the American Association of Mental Deficiency (Grossman, 1983) and the DSM-III-R (APA, 1987). To establish the diagnosis of mental retardation the following three diagnostic criteria must be established:

1. Subaverage intellectual functioning, that is, IQ 70 or under
2. Deficits in adaptive functioning
3. Age of onset under 18 years

In addition, the term "mental retardation" encompasses those persons who are mildly retarded on one end of the spectrum to the most severely retarded at the other. When possible, this chapter will refer to each segment of the retarded population that is under discussion.

Chess (1970) proposed a system for classifying mental retardation that takes into account the varying relationships between mental retardation and mental illness. She suggests the following categories:

1. *Mental retardation with no behavior disorder:* In these individuals the deviance is understood only in terms of slow cognition because their behavior is appropriate to their mental age.
2. *Mental retardation with behavior disorder due to cerebral dysfunction:* This category includes such symptoms as hypo- and

hyper-mobility, shortened attention span, distractibility, hypo-
or hyper-irritability, lability or sameness of mood, dependence
or independence, obsessive/compulsive behaviors, stereotype
behaviors, and self-stimulatory behaviors.

3. *Mental retardation with reactive behavior disorder:* Overdependent,
aggressive, fearful, and markedly unorganized activity is noted
herein.

4. *Mental retardation with neurotic behavior disorder:* This pattern reflects the elaboration of a variety of personality defenses against
anxiety.

5. *Mental retardation with psychosis:* The presence of major disorder
of thinking and feeling and the very poor ability to relate to ani-
mate objects typifies these psychoses.

DIAGNOSTIC AND DEVELOPMENTAL CONSIDERATIONS

The mildly to moderately retarded child is highly vulnerable to stresses
from an environment organized primarily for youngsters of average intelligence. Long before retardation has been accurately identified, the child
experiences a host of inappropriate demands for levels of performance,
judgment, and impulse control that are beyond his or her capacity. Even
after the child's defective development has been recognized, he or she
continues to be thrust into situations where functioning in accord with his
or her chronological age is expected (Chess, 1970). Inability to do so
evokes disapproval and ridicule, particularly after the child reaches school
age. As a result of such interpersonal stresses, the retarded child may be
considered at risk for the development of behavioral problems and emotional disorders. The retarded child's ego development from birth is frequently constricted, and responses to stress can be insufficient and/or
inappropriate.

Contributing to the child's difficulties with coping are frequent and concomitant medical problems such as seizures and motor and sensory deficits.
These medical conditions necessitate numerous evaluations, laboratory
testing, and at times hospitalization. These all add to the child's anxiety and
lead to regression, which delays normal emotional development. The motor
and sensory deficits may also impair the development of normal coping
mechanisms and normal responses to changes in the environment by impairing reality testing. This impairment results in the retaining of primitive
modes of thinking past their normal time. Delayed speech/language development results in delayed expression of wishes. Poor development of object
relations, conceptualization, and comprehension and the retaining of fears
are all seen in the mentally retarded child. Thinking becomes concrete and
is less suited for coping with stress.

Almost all mentally retarded adolescents have low self-esteem. They feel they are disappointments to their families and receive very little support from the environment outside the family. They become overly dependent on their families or caretakers. Coping with change, individualization, and separation becomes difficult, especially in the adolescent period. As the child matures chronologically and has limited coping mechanisms for stress, the vulnerability for emotional problems greatly increases (LaVietes, 1978).

Because mentally retarded adolescents have a high incidence of emotional problems, it is important for the clinician to be able to make an assessment of the mental status of the retarded population. Achieving this task is not necessarily an easy one. It is difficult to know what symptoms profoundly retarded adolescents display when they are anxious, depressed, or schizophrenic. Since treatment for mental disorder depends upon an accurate assessment of the mental status, all clinicians need to become familiar with the variety of symptoms that can be presented by a mentally retarded, emotionally handicapped individual.

Mental Status Examination

The method of the mental status examination of the mentally retarded will depend upon the degree of the retardation and psychopathology. In order to make an appropriate diagnosis and institute treatment, the mental status examination has to be performed precisely and accurately. At times it will be difficult to perform a structured, traditional mental status examination because of the patient's inability to understand the examiner or because of poor concentration and distractibility. Several short sessions may be necessary to obtain the appropriate information. For those who are not verbal, it may be necessary to observe the retarded adolescent in his or her own setting to gain information about behavior and peer interaction. Equally important is a careful history from a family member or caretaker. For those retarded people who have verbal ability, direct questions should be kept simple and concrete. Ruedrich and Menolascino (1984) point out that when attempting to accurately diagnose the presence of mental illness in the retarded, the clinician must obviously rely more on signs (i.e., disturbed behavior) and less on symptoms (i.e., verbally reported distress or dysfunction that characterizes the various psychiatric disorders), especially in those individuals at the severe to profound end of the intellectual-social spectrum.

Depression

Depression is one of the most widely prevalent psychiatric disorders. It was estimated that up to 23% of the population will have, at some time in their lives, a major depressive episode of clinical significance. At the present time, it is felt that no age group is exempt and that children as well as the elderly are at risk for this syndrome. Most authors believe that mentally retarded individuals also suffer from depression, probably in the same ratio as do normal individuals. There are no meaningful statistics at the present time to indicate the prevalence of depression in the adolescent mentally retarded population. It is probably safe to assume that they develop depressions at least as frequently as the nonretarded population (Sovner & Hurley, 1983).

The diagnosis of a major depression in the verbal mentally retarded adolescent will depend upon the reported feelings of sadness, hopelessness, helplessness, irritability, restlessness, poor concentration, somatic complaints, and suicidal ideations. The clinical observations by the examiner of a depressed mood, psychomotor retardation, and other vegetative signs are significant elements necessary for making an accurate diagnosis. This does not differ from the manner in which a psychiatric assessment is made with a nonretarded patient.

For those adolescents who are nonverbal or who have difficulty verbalizing their feelings, the examiner must rely on the observations of family members of other significant caretakers. Areas of importance include questions regarding changes in appetite. This is best monitored by periodic weighing. Sleep pattern changes, such as difficulty falling asleep, early wakenings, or increased time sleeping are significant observations. Hyperactivity, hypoactivity, decreased concentration, and loss of interest in activities, as well as self-destructive behavior are all important areas that have to be investigated. The diagnosis of depression, or for that matter, any diagnosis in the mentally retarded, is made more readily if the clinician has been familiar with the patient prior to the onset of any clinical signs.

The introduction of the dexamethasone suppression test may be helpful in making an objective diagnosis of depression in the retarded. Although few studies have been done with retarded adolescent clients, it is hopeful that future research using this test will prove useful in this population as well (Hsu et al., 1983).

Schizophrenia

Not too much is written in the literature on the mentally retarded adolescent who suffers from schizophrenia. However, a review of the literature indicates most authors agree that mentally retarded persons can develop schizophrenia. Corbett (1979) found that 6.5% of mentally retarded adults he reported on either had a current diagnosis of schizophrenia or had a past history of the illness. Several authors agree that it is not possible to make a definitive diagnosis of schizophrenia in the profoundly and severely retarded population. As with depression, a schizophrenic diagnosis depends mainly upon the patient's ability to communicate his or her feelings and ideas to the examiner, and these skills can be impaired in many retarded individuals. With verbal mildly to moderately retarded patients, the traditional clinical signs and symptoms of schizophrenia are used for diagnostic purposes. With clients who are more retarded, a deterioration in their usual behavior and attitude may be helpful in making a diagnosis.

Manic Depressive Psychosis

Recent clinical research has confirmed the existence of bipolar disorders in the adolescent population (Carlson & Strober, 1978). Symptoms can be experienced starting with early puberty. Although bipolar illness has been frequently diagnosed in the adult mentally retarded population, no clinical studies have been reported on the mentally retarded adolescent population. We can assume that adolescent mentally retarded people can suffer from bipolar illness as well. Until specific criteria can be formulated to diagnose the mentally retarded adolescent who suffers from bipolar illness, we must rely on our experience with the nonretarded adolescent. We must keep in mind that the adolescent period is normally characterized as stormy and moody. In addition, many retarded adolescents show signs of immaturity in their emotional development and can manifest labile moods under certain pressures. In the adolescent mentally retarded population, clinicians should look for manic mood swings, hyperactivity, increased rate of speech in those patients who are verbal, increased distractibility, and a positive family history of bipolar illness. Bipolar illness is difficult to diagnose in the mentally retarded adolescent, but it should not be overlooked as it can be successfully treated with psychotropic drug therapy.

Down's Syndrome

Down's Syndrome is the most common chromosomal disorder causing mental retardation, occurring approximately once in every 900 births. Trisomy-21 is the most prevalent form of this disorder. A recent review of the literature by Parsons, May, and Menolascino (1984) reveals that Down's Syndrome patients seem to have less emotional problems than other populations of retarded people. Menolascino (1965) reported a 13% mental illness rate among 86 Down's Syndrome outpatient children. Nevertheless, Down's Syndrome patients can develop significant disturbances in their emotional health. Affective disorder, schizophrenia, anorexia, and other emotional problems can be present in any Down's Syndrome patient.

Fragile X Syndrome

After Down's Syndrome, the most common known inherited cause of mental retardation is the Fragile X Syndrome. This syndrome is identifiable by chromosome analysis and is characterized by the finding of a fragile site on the X chromosome. It is inherited in an X-linked recessive manner. Moderate to severe mental retardation usually has been the associated clinical finding. This syndrome explains the 35% excess of males over females in institutions and classes for the mentally retarded. Boys born with the Fragile X are a little heavy at birth and are taller as youngsters than are normal children, but their growth lags and they are short adults. They have relatively large heads and prominent jaws, foreheads, and ears. As adults they tend to have markedly larger testes than normal. Most boys who have Fragile X Syndrome are moderately to severely retarded. Retardation of a lesser degree is present in about one-third to one-half of the girls who have the Fragile X.

In a study of 37 autistic children, Goldfine et al. (1985) did not find an association between autism and the Fragile X Syndrome. However, Fisch et al. (1986), studying a larger sample of 144 autistic males, did find 18 to have the Fragile X chromosome, supporting other epidemiological findings that the association between Fragile X and autism occurs with relative frequency. Most authors agree that the Fragile X Syndrome should be looked for in any unexplained mental retardation, especially those children showing signs of autism (Turner, Robinson, Laing, & Purvis-Smith, 1986).

Tourette's Syndrome

Tourette's Syndrome (TS), a disorder of the nervous system, is characterized by tics, vocal noise, coprolalia, ritualistic behavior, and, at times, psychosis. It becomes evident during childhood and is frequently diagnosed during the ages of 4 to 12 years. It is important to make an early diagnosis because if left untreated, it can have a significant deleterious effect on the child's emotional growth. The DSM-III-R lists the following criteria for a diagnosis of TS:

1. Both multiple motor and one or more vocal tics, not necessarily at the same time
2. Tics occurring many times a day, nearly every day, or intermittently over more than 1 year
3. Part of the body affected and frequency and intensity of the tics changing over time
4. Age of onset before 21, usually before 14
5. Occurrence not necessarily during psychoactive substance intoxication or known central nervous system disease

The earliest manifestation of TS is usually the recurrence of a single tic, most commonly eye blinking. Other body tics that are seen frequently include tongue protrusion, sniffing, hopping, and snorting. Vocal tics reported are: barking, grunting, throat clearing, and yelping. Coprolalia is frequently present. The disorder is significantly more common in males than in females.

There have been several reports of mentally retarded persons developing TS. Izmeth (1979) and Barr, Lovibond, and Katarus (1981) described adolescents 13 and 16 years old, respectively, who were mildly retarded and had been diagnosed as suffering from TS. In both cases the patient responded well to drug therapy. Golden and Greenhill (1981) reported on 6 mentally retarded children 6 to 12 years old who were suffering from TS. Four of the patients were treated with haloperidol or thioridazine. Of the four, three developed tardive dyskinesia. The authors suggested that the reason for the unusually high percentage of tardive dyskinesia was due to the patients' vulnerability stemming from their central nervous system abnormalities. Tourette's Syndrome usually persists into adulthood, but the lifelong course of the syndrome is not yet known. Most authors believe that a biochemical defect, perhaps on a genetic basis, is a significant factor in the development of this disorder. Drugs, such as haloperidol and clonidine, can produce a marked reduction in TS symptomatology.

Prader-Willi Syndrome

Prader-Willi Syndrome is a relatively rare disorder that is characterized by insatiable appetite, obesity, hypogonadism, hypotonia, and mental retardation. The severe obesity leads to impaired oxygen intake, mild diabetes mellitis, and heart disease, frequently resulting in early death. It is most important to recognize this disease early in life to prevent the complications of overeating (Wett, 1983). Obesity is usually present by early adolescence. The etiology of this disorder is unknown. Treatment is geared toward preventing the weight gain by psychotherapy and a strict behavior modification program.

CLINICAL PROBLEMS

Clinicians frequently are called upon to deal with a variety of problems faced by the mentally retarded/emotionally handicapped adolescent. All the problems seen in nonretarded adolescents are seen in retarded ones as well, but they take on an added dimension due to the dual diagnosis. Parents, teachers, and caretakers concerned with the behavior of adolescents under their care turn to the mental health professional for advice and guidance. Unfortunately, in most cases, the clinician has to proceed on his or her own personal experience rather than on proven clinical methods for assessment and treatment, as these issues are not well documented in the literature.

Adolescent Sexuality

Concerns about a mentally retarded adolescent's psychosexual development is frequently the major concern of parents and caretakers. Issues of masturbation, nudity, touching, sexual activity, and both heterosexual and homosexual behaviors often are feared. It is obvious that mentally retarded adolescents may not have the understanding, and frequently they do not have the judgment to make socially acceptable choices to express their sexual feelings. Within the past several years, sex education programs have been developed in schools and institutions geared to the intelligence level of the adolescent (Robinault, 1978). These programs deal with the issues of anatomy, menstruation, touching, dating, feeling, privacy, hygiene, venereal disease, and pregnancy in concrete and nonjudgmental terms. Those clients who do not have the capacity to participate in these educational programs can be treated with behavioral or psychopharmacological therapies, depending upon the clinical diagnosis and other factors. Placing adolescent females on birth control pills to control pregnancy from either voluntary or nonvoluntary sexual intercourse has to be decided on a case-by-case basis. Similarly, the issues of dating, marriage, and the desire to have children have to be handled on an individual basis as they arise. Genetic counseling should be provided when appropriate.

Aggressive, Assaultive, Self-Mutilatory Behavior

Although aggressive, assaultive, and self-mutilatory behaviors can be seen in any psychiatric patient, they are most difficult to manage in the severely retarded client. A patient who exhibits these behaviors for the first time should be evaluated for a treatable and/or reversible condition. It is well known that severely retarded patients, like children, have only a small repertoire of ways to indicate irritability or frustration. Frequently, these behaviors will result from a physical illness, change in routine, or change in personnel. All correctable environmental measures should be attempted before behavioral or pharmacological methods are tried. Those patients with destructive tendencies toward self or others on a chronic basis could be treated with these measures as needed and for as long as necessary (Campbell, Cohen, & Small, 1982b; Mikkelsen, 1986).

Suicidal Behavior

There are only a few references in the literature concerning suicidal behavior in the retarded. One study by Sternlicht, Pustel, and Deutsch (1970) reported on the incidence of suicidal behavior at a residential state school in New York. They reported an incidence of 1% of suicidal behavior in the population, which they say closely approximated the general population. They concluded that the rate probably would have been higher had the staff not been so watchful. This problem, however, probably will become more intensified with the deinstitutionalization process, whereby patients are placed in a less restrictive and less supervised environment with more social pressures. This is another area that needs further clinical investigation.

Psychological Problems Associated with Community Living

With more community living residences being opened and many more in the planning stage, the adolescent mentally retarded are becoming more highly visible in the towns in which they reside. In many communities, there has been tremendous pressure to prevent these residences from opening; furthermore, when they are opened, the clients are subject to unneighborly behaviors and remarks. Coping with these pressures and other pressures, such as physical stigmata, has direct effects on the developing self-image of the adolescent.

Health Facilities

An enormous problem in the health delivery system is the lack of facilities for medical, dental, and hospital care of the retarded. Most physicians, dentists, and nurses receive no training in the health care of the retarded and have little understanding of the emotional needs of such patients. This lack of training frequently results in substandard care for the mentally retarded adolescent who, at times, only receives emergency-type care. Preventive health issues is another area which needs greater exploration.

Professional Staff

It cannot be overemphasized that there is a great need for psychologists, psychiatrists, family physicians, nurses, child care workers, and other health professionals to acquaint themselves with the needs of the mentally retarded, emotionally handicapped adolescent. All professional training programs also should include didactic teaching as well as clinical experience in this important area (Cytryn, 1970).

Sibling Coping

A recent area of attention has been to focus on the nonretarded siblings of mentally retarded clients. Frequently, nonretarded siblings not only develop their own problems, but by their behaviors and attitudes also have a deleterious effect on the retarded sibling. Their feelings of neglect, guilt, and anger can complicate the overall adjustment of their retarded sibling. Early preventive intervention is necessary to ensure the maximum emotional growth of all family members.

PHARMACOLOGICAL APPROACHES

There have been several recent studies (summarized by Intagliata & Rinck, 1985) documenting the apparent excessive use of psychoactive and/or anticonvulsant medication with mentally retarded persons. Various surveys of public institutions indicate that approximately 40 to 50% of the residents of all ages are on some type of psychoactive medication and that 35 to 45% are receiving anticonvulsant medication as well. These drugs are administered to produce changes in behavior, emotion, or cognition. Surveys of the incidence of drug administration to mentally retarded persons in community residential facilities indicate similar but relatively lower levels of drug usage, with 25 to 30% receiving anticonvulsants. One study, relating to the prevalence of psychotropic administration to mentally retarded clients ages 1 to 18, showed that 18% of the clients living in community residential facilities and 42% of those living in public residential facilities were on major tranquilizers. Twenty-four percent of the community clients and 30% of the public residential clients were on anticonvulsant medication. It seems that the more restrictive the environment, the more prevalence there was for them to be on some sort of medication. The results of these studies and others showed that psychoactive drugs represent a type of treatment being received by vast numbers of mentally retarded persons, including adolescents. Frequently, the psychoactive drug treatment was the only treatment available to these clients.

The type of facility in which the clients reside can influence the likelihood of receiving psychoactive drugs independent of the client's own behavior. This finding, while not surprising, highlights the need to examine environmental factors, such as physician prescribing habits, staff attitudes, levels of stimulation available to clients, and client characteristics, in attempting to understand or influence the way the psychotropic drugs are being used with mentally retarded persons. Although psychoactive drugs have been the focus of much of this attention, it should be noted that mentally retarded persons residing in both public and community residential settings often are being treated with a large variety of other medications as well. These medications include laxatives, analgesics, antibiotics, cold medication, and vitamins. Aman (1984) considers the mentally retarded as one of the most medicated groups in our society.

Intagliata and Rinck (1985) discuss other concerns for the recent attention given to psychoactive drug use in this population. One is the undesirable side effects associated with the use of these drugs even when they are effective in dealing with the problems for which they are prescribed. These undesirable and unwanted side effects include the impaired ability to learn, impaired work production, and a general suppression of certain behaviors that may be adaptive and desirable for the mentally retarded patient. Psychoactive drugs that are used on a long-term basis also can increase the probability of causing tardive dyskinesia. Aman (1983) points out that because of mentally retarded persons' poor ability to communicate, the observed side effects may be mistakenly attributed to their intellectual or neurological condition and not to the offending drug in question.

An additional reason for the new focus on the psychoactive medication is the fact that the medication used among mentally retarded persons can result in law suits concerning the rights of the mentally retarded. This includes their right to refuse psychotropic medication.

Although a number of studies have been conducted to assess the effects of psychotropic medication in mentally retarded persons, there are still significant gaps in our knowledge. However, the majority of these published studies have focused exclusively on institutional populations. In spite of the fact that mentally retarded patients are a highly medicated group, only a few well-designed studies address the efficacy of the medication for these patients. Most striking is the almost complete lack of such studies on the adolescent mentally retarded population with emotional problems. Many of the reported studies are poorly designed, are not well controlled, use heterogeneous populations, and utilize poor methods to assess change or drug effect. Sprague and Werry (1971) indicate six minimal criteria which should be incorporated into any scientifically sound study. These criteria are:

1. The use of placebo controls
2. Random assignment to treatment conditions
3. Line elevation of drug effects to protect against potential observer bias
4. Standardized dosages
5. Standardized evaluation
6. Appropriate statistical tests

In addition, Aman and Singh (1980) state that clinical drug trials should be free of other confounding medications, and they note how often these self-evident criteria have been violated in drug studies with retarded people. Lipman (1986) states, "It is interesting that although the data base of psychotropic studies with the retarded is particularly lacking in scientific merit the quality of scientific review is particularly good." In spite of this lack of documentation, many clinicians prescribe psychotropic medication and other medication at high dosages to treat a variety of behaviors in the mentally retarded adolescent. Many psychiatrists are asked by parents and caretaker staff to prescribe drugs to control hyperactivity, severe aggressiveness, and self-injurious behaviors. These medications are frequently given to poorly selected patients at dosages that are frequently above the optimum and are given for excessive periods of time without follow-up or trials of drug holidays. Moreover, there frequently are no laboratory studies or physical examinations for the side effects of drugs.

Donaldson (1984) and others point out that there are many instances in which drugs have no effect on the mentally retarded population, and a frequent error is to increase the dosage rather than discontinue the medication. He argues that psychotropic medication for nonretarded patients has a beneficial effect on their thinking that permits them to utilize the other psychotherapeutic modalities to effect changes (i.e., to learn self-control). Retarded individuals, especially the severely retarded, however, are not able to benefit in a similar manner and are given psychotropic medication usually as a chemical restraint.

Neuroleptic Medication

There are only a few studies in the psychiatric literature with reference to the efficacy of the psychotropic medication on adolescent psychopathology. There are even fewer studies reporting on mentally retarded adolescents. Most reviewers conclude that given careful diagnosis and until further clinical trials are carried out, mentally retarded people could be treated with drugs using the same careful monitoring as nonretarded people. Until proven otherwise, we extend this to mentally retarded adolescents.

In previously cited surveys of mentally retarded institutions and community residences, thioridazine is the most prevalent medication prescribed in this population, followed by chlorpromazine and haloperidol. Pregelj and Barkauskas (1967) presented the results of a retrospective evaluation of the efficacy of thioridazine in a heterogeneous sample of 304 hospitalized mentally retarded patients. These patients ranged in age from 2 to 68, with a mean of 17 years. They had been receiving medication for at least 4 months prior to the enrollment into this study. The patients' global assessment and specific symptom assessment prior to receiving the drug were compared to their status on optimal dosages of thioridazine. Dosages had been individually regulated and ranged from 10 to 800 mgm per day. Approximately 80% of the patients showed a good to very good response, which was interpreted as being at least a 60% reduction in the severity of symptoms. Hyperactivity, temper tantrums, and aggressiveness were among the most prominent of the specific target symptoms occurring in 40 to 50% of the patient population. The authors did not report any serious side effects due to the medication in this retrospective review.

Singh and Aman (1981) reported on a double-blind placebo-controlled study involving 19 severely retarded, institutionalized patients who were treated with thioridazine. The population included 14 males and 5 females whose mean age was 15.8 years. The patient population's IQ ranged from unmeasureable to 30. In addition, due to a virtual absence of investigations exploring optimal thioridazine dosage in this population or adequate guidelines for dosage regulation, the authors included within their study design a comparison of the efficacy of a "low" standardized thioridazine dose, that is 2.5 mgm per kilogram per day, with dose titrated individually for each patient by ward clinicians.

Prior to enrollment in the study, the patients were receiving thioridazine as their sole psychoactive medication for at least 6 months to control specific target behaviors. These behaviors included stereotypic, self-stimulatory, self-injurious, aggressive, and destructive behaviors in addition to excessive motor activity. The authors concluded that a highly significant reduction of hyperactivity and a modest reduction in the amount of screaming was shown during the active medication condition. Bizarre behavior was also sensitive to drug effect. Clinically significant was the reduction of self-stimulatory behavior while on active drug conditions. This study supports a clinical role for thioridazine in carefully selected patients.

Although thioridazine appears to be effective for the reduction of aggression, hyperactivity, and self-stimulation in some mentally retarded patients, these therapeutic effects may be associated with the reduction of adaptive/habilitative behaviors. Psychotropic medication, specifically thioridazine administered to mentally retarded patients, has been shown to interfere with their ability to perform well on intellectual tests and workshop assignments. In view of these adverse affects on learning, cognition, and workshop performance, the careful selection of patients and regulation of thioridazine dosage are necessary to minimize the occurrence and severity of these adverse affects while achieving desired behavioral control.

Campbell et al. (1978) studied the effects of haloperidol, a behavioral intervention, and the interaction of these two treatments on language acquisition and behavioral symptoms. A sample of 40 autistic children, 32 boys and 8 girls, (ages 2.6 to 7.2 years) was assessed in a placebo-controlled, double-blind study. The results showed that the combination of haloperidol and contingent reinforcement worked synergistically to facilitate acquisition of imitative speech. The authors concluded their discussion with questions regarding the mechanism of haloperidol's action to improve learning. They suggested that improved learning could have resulted from a reduction of behaviors that would interfere with this process or an actual positive effect on attention or other learning mechanisms. In order to address these issues further, the effects of haloperidol on a discrimination task performed in the laboratory and behavioral symptoms were assessed in 33 autistic children, 24 boys and 9 girls, ages 2.3 to 7.9 years (Campbell et al., 1982a). It was concluded that doses not causing sedation may decrease the severity of target symptoms and may improve discrimination learning in a laboratory setting. The improved learning performance did not appear to be due to a reduction of maladaptive behaviors.

Common side effects of major tranquilizers in children and adolescents include drowsiness, weight gain, increased appetite, dry mouth, photosensitivity, enuresis, and neurological symptoms of drooling, rigidity, tremor, akathisia, and dystonia. Thioridazine, with its extreme anticholinergic properties, is beginning to decline as the most popular medication. Chlorpromazine decreases the seizure threshold in epileptic mentally retarded children and adolescents. Although abnormalities in laboratory studies are rare in children and adolescents on phenothiazines, determination of alkaline phosphatase, SGPT, SGOT, CBC, and urinalysis should be performed periodically.

Tardive Dyskinesia (TD)

Tardive and withdrawal dyskinesias can occur in children and adolescents treated with major tranquilizers (Gualtieri, Quade, Hicks, Mayo, & Schroeder, 1984). In retarded and nonretarded children and adolescents, the dyskinesias manifest themselves by buccolingual masticatory movements, facial tics and grimaces, choreoathetoid movements of the extremities, abnormal posturing, generalized motor restlessness, and ataxia. Such tardive dyskinesias can be seen with low dose, short-term treatment as well as high dose, long-term therapy.

There has been very little systematic research on the long-term safety of neuroleptics in the retarded population, especially with respect to the occurrence of tardive dyskinesia, which may occur in 15 to 25% of adult psychiatric patients. Gualtieri, Schroeder, Hicks, and Quade (1986) recently published the results of a systematic neuroleptic withdrawal study in 38 mentally retarded children, adolescents, and young adults. In a well-designed study, they showed that transient side effects were noted in 34% of the subjects and TD in an additional 34%. Withdrawal dyskinesias have been described more frequently in children than in adults. Gualtieri and colleagues conclude that TD is a serious and not infrequent problem in the retarded.

The uncertain and poorly investigated benefits of neuroleptics should be weighed carefully against the risks in this population. Physicians who are called upon to prescribe medication for behavior control and developmentally handicapped individuals should be aware that drug treatment should be instituted for specific purposes and not as a substitute for habilitation. Long-term, high-dose neuroleptic treatment is not always necessary. The lowest effective dose should be prescribed. In a long-term, low-dose study of autistic/retarded children using haloperidol, Perry et al. (1985) found that 22% of the population showed transient dyskinetic symptoms. All symptoms were temporary and spontaneously disappeared. At the present time, there is no known treatment for TD.

Another side effect resulting from treatment with high potency neuroleptics, such as haloperidol and piperazine phenothiazines in therapeutic dosages, is the "neuroleptic malignant syndrome." This syndrome, which is potentially lethal, is characterized by muscular rigidity, hyperthermia, altered consciousness, and autonomic dysfunction. Several cases have been reported as occurring in adolescents (Geller & Greydanus, 1979). Treatment consists of early recognition, immediate discontinuation of psychotropic medication, and the prompt institution of intensive supportive medical and nursing care (Levenson, 1985).

Sedatives-Antianxiety Agents and Anticonvulsants

The role of sedatives, such as chloral hydrate and diphenhydramine, has not been established with the retarded population. Similarly, anticonvulsants (such as carbamazepine, which has been recently used for acting out behavior) have not been demonstrated to date to be effective in the retarded population. Aman (1983), in his review of the literature, concluded that the minor tranquilizers are contraindicated in the retarded.

Antidepressants

The concept of depression in children and adolescents and its treatment with antidepressant medication has been a recent interest of several investigators. However, their investigations have not yet been extended to the retarded population. We only can assume that the antidepressants will have a beneficial effect on the appropriately diagnosed, depressed, retarded adolescent. Aman (1983) states that antidepressant medications have not been adequately tested in well-designed studies in the retarded population.

Lithium

Lithium carbonate therapy has not been documented at the present time as alleviating any symptoms in the mentally retarded child or adolescent. Lithium has been used as an antiaggressive medication in latency children with an efficacy paralleling that of haloperidol (Campbell, et al., 1984). Lithium was less sedating than haloperidol, but it had other side effects which were found to be disturbing to the patient. The assessment of the efficacy of lithium in retarded adolescents awaits further exploration.

Propranolol

In a retrospective study of 30 patients (including 11 children and 15 adolescents), all of whom were diagnosed as having uncontrolled rage outbursts with organic brain syndrome, Williams, Mehl, Yudofsky, Adams, and Roseman (1982) reported that propranolol demonstrated a moderate to marked improvement in control of these rage outbursts and aggressive behavior in 75% of the subjects. Propranolol did not seem to have a positive effect on cognitive dysfunction or psychotic thinking. It may be useful (Deutsch, 1986) for aggressive outbursts refractory to neuroleptics, lithium, and anticonvulsant medication in brain damaged and retarded persons. Although bradycardia and hypotension are the most common side effects, these could be tolerated if initial dosages are low and are raised gradually.

CONCLUDING REMARKS

The psychopharmacological treatment of emotionally disturbed, mentally retarded adolescents remains largely on an empirical basis. Psychotropic medication should not be used for the treatment of mild disturbances of the mentally retarded adolescent. When severe symptomatology presents itself, psychotropic medications should be used only as an adjunct to the total treatment modality for such individuals. Medication should never be the sole treatment. The medication should help patients become more amenable to specific education, rehabilitation, behavior modification, psychotherapy, and other social adaptations in the family, halfway house, or institution. The hazards of drug treatment should always be weighed against the dangers of the nonmedicated adolescent. Physicians should utilize low, divided dosages and short trials whenever possible. The clinician should be aware, for example, that symptom relief by medication may decrease the retarded adolescent's ability to learn in school or work in a workshop. Until better designed studies are carried out, the following are recommended:

1. Careful diagnosis to establish clear reasons and target symptoms for drug intervention
2. Use of drugs with the retarded adolescent as with the nonretarded adolescent
3. Lowest possible dosages to effect target symptom change
4. Polypharmacy to be discouraged
5. Periodic drug holidays to see if the patient can maintain positive effects without the drug and possibly to prevent tardive dyskinesia
6. Drug treatment to be considered only one therapeutic measure of the total treatment plan for the mentally retarded, emotionally handicapped adolescent

PSYCHODYNAMIC APPROACHES

The use of individual psychotherapy for mentally retarded patients has been gaining wider acceptance among many therapists who deal with this population. Previously, it was felt that the mentally retarded lacked the necessary prerequisites to benefit from this form of therapy. It was argued that they had poor verbal skills, lacked the capacity to form therapeutic alliances, were too distractible or easily frustrated, lacked the capacity to view their behavior objectively, or that their personality structure was too rigid for change. Many authors now agree, however, that psychotherapy can be used to treat a wide variety of emotional problems in the mentally retarded client.

The degree of retardation and the severity of the emotional handicap are factors in the selection of the patients but are not necessarily contraindications for therapy. The problems for which the mentally retarded, emotionally handicapped adolescent are treated are not different from their nonretarded peers. However, mentally retarded adolescents may have additional problems stemming from the mental retardation or other handicapping conditions. Their ego development can be limited from infancy. Physiological difficulties necessitating medical evaluations or hospitalizations, which are frequent in the retarded, can result in a higher anxiety level and coping difficulties (LaVietes, 1978). Low self-esteem resulting from their inability to compete with peers and/or from their medical problems is seen frequently in mentally retarded adolescents. Coping with anger, frustration, and impulsivity, school, social, and family pressures can be dealt with in the psychotherapeutic process. Contraindications to treatment include acute psychosis or assaultive behavior.

The goals of treatment, as in therapy with the nonretarded, need an initial diagnostic assessment of the problem followed by the formulation of a realistic treatment plan. The treatment plan should be concrete, well defined, practical, and measurable (Rosen, Clark, & Kivitz, 1977). A contract between the therapist and client is frequently useful to set goals (Monfils & Menolascino, 1984). Specific goals often include better workshop adjustment, better peer interaction, more specific symptom relief, and acceptance of limitations while still feeling good about himself or herself. The ultimate goal is to help the mentally retarded adolescent function to the best of his or her capacity in the least restrictive environment without major behavioral or psychological problems.

The therapist is usually a more active participant in the therapeutic process with the mentally retarded than with a nonretarded patient. The therapist is more directive and concrete, especially when dealing with problems of daily living. The hallmark of a psychotherapy technique with the mentally retarded adolescent is flexibility. The techniques employed must be adapted to the need and ability of the patient, and the therapist must be willing to change techniques as the therapeutic process progresses. Establishing an adequate therapeutic atmosphere is most important to enable the patient to freely express feelings in an acceptable and nonthreatening atmosphere. To decrease poor impulse control in the therapeutic setting, strict limitations have to be set. Because mentally retarded adolescents may have difficulty with verbal expression, other techniques such as play therapy are frequently used. Psychotherapy is never performed in a vacuum with mentally retarded adolescents, and close counseling of parents or caretakers form an integral part of the therapeutic process.

Most authors make a particularly strong point about the qualities needed to be a therapist for the retarded. The therapist must be comfortable taking an active role in the therapy and in using a flexible eclectic approach. The therapist also must be comfortable with frequently settling for modest goals in the patients treated.

Group Therapy

Group therapy often has been used over the years to treat the mentally retarded adolescent. Although it is difficult to measure the efficacy of this technique, it is nevertheless advocated by many authors in the retardation field. There are several good reviews of this area in which the authors recommend this approach for many mentally retarded adolescents who have the ability to relate to a therapist either verbally or nonverbally (Slivan & Bernstein, 1970; Monfils & Menolascino, 1984). Goals of this technique include learning to verbalize feelings instead of acting them out, fostering and gratifying more appropriate identifications, encouraging acceptance of limits, and enhancing daily living problem-solving ability. Many of the techniques used in individual therapy are used in the group therapy process as well. Most authors feel that there are definite benefits in the technique alone or in addition to individual psychotherapy.

BEHAVIORAL APPROACHES

In this model, behaviors that are considered maladaptive, inappropriate, or pathological are considered as learned behaviors, and different behavioral techniques are used to alter behavior in a beneficial manner (Gardner & Cole, 1984). Problems are therefore thought of as resulting from an interaction of the mentally retarded person and his or her physical and social environment. Assessment of the problems is made by direct observation in the setting in which the problems arise. Behavior plans are then formulated and implemented in the client's natural setting. Over the years, behavior modification has gained wide acceptance as a useful tool to decrease maladaptive behavior and to make the client more manageable and better able to adjust to his or her work and/or living environment. The behavioral techniques are commonly used in school, workshop, and residential settings. The behavior modification techniques can help in establishing the basic self-help skills. In addition, behavioral therapy can frequently eliminate the symptoms of emotional disturbances by rewarding the desired behavior. Other areas of behavior for which behavioral programs are used include self-stimulatory and aggressive/assaultive behavior. In addition, still other programs can be useful to increase the patient's language, eye contact, attention span, or self-management. Some authors report that behavioral methods are useful in reducing a variety of sexual deviations.

There are numerous different techniques used in behavior modification, which include desensitization techniques, reciprocal inhibition techniques, reciprocal inhibition, conditions avoidance technique, positive reinforcement, negative reinforcement, aversion therapy, extinction technique, negative practice techniques, overcorrection, and token economy. All of these techniques have been reported as helpful in assisting mentally retarded people to become better adjusted to their environment. The description of each technique is beyond the scope of this paper, and the reader is referred to several sources (Szymanski & Tanguay, 1980; Matson & McCartney, 1981; Hersen, Eisler, & Miller, 1981; Karan & Gardner, 1983). Well-designed, controlled studies for mentally retarded adolescents with emotional problems are lacking in the literature. However, there is enough anecdotal reporting to recommend behavioral techniques in most cases of deviant behavior. Combining drug therapy with behavior technique has been shown to be of value in certain autistic retarded children and could prove to be useful in mentally retarded adolescents as well (Campbell et al., 1984).

SUMMARY

The need to understand the problems of the mentally retarded adolescent is great; however, the literature, at the present time, does not reflect the importance of these problems. Appropriate clinical research is needed to document and assess the problems and to institute and assess therapy: behavior modification, psychotherapy, and psychopharmacology. On the community level, more sheltered workshops, community residences, and specialized schools to cater to these special problems are needed. Last and most important, we need to involve more professionals to take an interest in the mentally retarded and help them adjust to their environment to the best of their abilities (Menolascino & Gutnik, 1984).

REFERENCES

Aman, M. G. (1983). Psychoactive drugs in mental retardation. In J. L. Matson & F. Andrasik (Eds.), *Treatment issues and innovations in mental retardation* (pp. 455–513). New York: Plenum.

Aman, M. G. (1984). Drugs and learning in mentally retarded persons. In G. D. Burrows & J. S. Werry (Eds.), *Advances in human psychopharmacology* (pp. 121–163) Greenwich: JAI.

Aman, M. G., & Singh, N. N. (1980). The usefulness of thioridazine for treating childhood disorders—fact or folklore. *American Journal of Mental Deficiency, 84*, 331–338.

American Psychiatric Association (1987). *Diagnostic and statistical manual of mental disorders* (3rd ed., revised). (DSM-III-R). Washington, DC: Author.

Barr, R. F., Lovibond, S. H., & Katarus, E. (1981). Gilles de la Tourette syndrome in a brain-damaged child. *Medical Journal of Australia, 2*, 372–374.

Campbell, M., Anderson, L. T., Meier, M., Cohen, I. L., Small, A. M., Samit, C., & Sacher, E. J. (1978). A comparison of haloperidol and behavior therapy and their interaction in autistic children. *Journal of the American Academy of Child Psychiatry, 17*, 640–655.

Campbell, M., Anderson, L. T., Small, A. M., Perry, R., Green, W. H., & Caplan, R. (1982a). The effects of haloperidol on learning and behavior in autistic children. *Journal of Autism and Developmental Disorders, 12*, 167–175.

Campbell, M., Cohen, I. L., & Small, A. M. (1982b). Drugs in aggressive behavior. *Journal of The American Academy of Child Psychiatry, 21*, 107–117.

Campbell, M., Small, A. M., Green, W. H., Jennings, S. J., Perry, R., Bennett, W. G., & Anderson, L. (1984). Behavioral efficacy of haloperidol and lithium carbonate. *Archives of General Psychiatry, 41*, 650–656.

Carlson, G. A., & Strober, M. (1978). Manic depressive illness in early adolescence. A study of clinical and diagnostic characteristics in six cases. *Journal of the American Academy of Child Psychiatry, 17*, 138–153.

Chazan, M. (1964). The incidence and nature of maladjustment among children in schools for the educationally subnormal. *British Journal of Educational Psychology, 34*, 292–304.

Chess, S. (1970). Emotional problems in mentally retarded children. In F. Menolascino (Ed.), *Psychiatric approaches to mental retardation* (pp. 55–67). New York: Basic Books.

Corbett, J. A. (1979). Psychiatric morbidity and mental retardation. In F. E. James & R. P. Snaith (Eds.), *Psychiatric illness and mental retardation* (pp. 11–25). London: Gaskell Press.

Cytryn, L. (1970). The training of pediatricians and psychiatrists in mental retardation. In F. Menolascino (Ed.), *Psychiatric approaches to mental retardation* (pp. 651–660). New York: Basic Books.

Deutsch, S. I. (1986). Managing behavior in mentally retarded residential populations. *Hospital and Community Psychiatry, 37*, 221–222.

Donaldson, J. Y. (1984). Specific psychopharmacological approaches and rationale for mentally ill-mentally retarded children. In F. J. Menolascino & J. A. Stark (Eds.), *Handbook of mental illness in the mentally retarded* (pp. 171–187). New York: Plenum.

Fisch, G. S., Cohen, I. L., Wolf, E. G., Brown, W. T., Jenkins, E. C., & Gross, A. (1986). Autism and the fragile X syndrome. *American Journal of Psychiatry, 143*, 71–73.

Foale, M. (1956). The specific difficulties of the high grade mentally defective adolescent. *American Journal of Mental Deficiency, 60,* 867–877.

Gardner, W. I., & Cole, C. L. (1984). Use of behavior therapy with the mentally retarded in community settings. In F. J. Menolascino & J. A. Stark (Eds.), *Handbook of mental illness in the mentally retarded* (pp. 97–153). New York: Plenum.

Geller, B., & Greydanus, B. E. (1979). Haloperidol-induced comatose state with hyperthermia and rigidity in adolescence. Two case reports and a literature review. *Journal of Clinical Psychiatry, 40,* 102–103.

Golden, G. S., & Greenhill, L. (1981). Tourette syndrome in mentally retarded children. *Mental Retardation, 19,* 17–19.

Goldfine, P. E., McPherson, P. M., Heath, G. A., Hardesty, V. A., Beaugregard, L. J., & Gordon, B. (1985). Association of fragile x syndrome with autism. *American Journal of Psychiatry, 142,* 108–110.

Grossman, H. J. (Ed.). (1983). *Classification in mental retardation.* Washington, DC: American Association on Mental Deficiency.

Gualtieri, C. T., Quade, D., Hicks, R. E., Mayo, J. P., & Schroeder, S. R. (1984). Tardive dyskinesia and other clinical consequences of neuroleptic treatment in children and adolescents. *American Journal of Psychiatry, 141,* 20–23.

Gualtieri, C. T., Schroeder, S. R., Hicks, R. E., & Quade, D. (1986). Tardive dyskinesia in young mentally retarded individuals. *Archives of General Psychiatry, 43,* 335–340.

Hersen, M., Eisler, R. M., & Miller, P. M. (Eds.). (1981). *Progress in behavior modification: Vol. 12.* New York: Academic.

Hsu, L. K. G., Molcan, K., Cashman, M. A., Lee, S., Lohr, J., & Hindmarsh, D. (1983). The dexamethasone suppression test in adolescent depression. *Journal of the American Academy of Child Psychiatry, 22,* 470–473.

Intagliata, J., & Rinck, C. (1985). Psychoactive drug use in public and community residential facilities for mentally retarded persons. *Psychopharmacology Bulletin, 21,* 268–278.

Izmeth, A. (1979). Gilles de la Tourette syndrome. *Journal of Mental Deficiency, 23,* 25–27.

Karan, O. C., & Gardner, W. I. (Eds.). (1983). *Habilitation practices with the developmentally disabled who present behavioral and emotional problems.* Madison, WI: Rehabilitation Research and Training Center in Mental Retardation.

Kirman, B. H. (1973). Clinical aspects. In J. Wortis (Ed.), *Mental retardation and developmental disabilities: An annual review: VI* (pp. 1–9). New York: Brunner/Mazel.

LaVietes, R. (1978). Mental retardation. Psychological treatment. In B. B. Wolman, J. Egan, & A. O. Ross (Eds.), *Handbook of treatment of mental disorders in childhood and adolescence* (pp. 202–211). Englewood Cliffs: Prentice Hall.

Levenson, J. L. (1985). Neuroleptic malignant syndrome. *American Journal of Psychiatry, 142,* 1137–1145.

Lipman, R. S. (1986, May). Overview of research in psychopharmacological treatment of the mentally ill/mentally retarded. Paper presented at the annual meeting of the NCDEU, Key Biscayne, FL.

Matson, J. L. (1985). Emotional problems in the mentally retarded: The need for assessment and treatment. *Psychopharmacology Bulletin, 21,* 258–261.

Matson, J. L., & McCartney, J. R. (1981). *Handbook of behavior modification with the mentally retarded.* New York: Plenum.

Menolascino, F. J. (1965). Psychiatric aspects of mongolism. *American Journal of Mental Deficiency, 69,* 653–660.

Menolascino, F. J., & Gutnik, B. (1984). Training mental health personnel in mental retardation. In F. S. Menolascino and J. A. Stark (Eds.), *Handbook of mental illness in the mentally retarded* (pp. 347–368). New York: Plenum.

Mikkelsen, E. J. (1986). Low-dose haloperidol for stereotypic self injurious behavior in the mentally retarded. *The New England Journal of Medicine, 315,* 398–399.

Monfils, M. J., & Menolascino, F. J. (1984). Modified individual and group treatment approaches for the mentally retarded-mentally ill. In F. J. Menolascino & J. A. Stark (Eds.), *Handbook of mental illness in the mentally retarded* (pp. 155–169). New York: Plenum.

Parsons, J. A., May, J. G., & Menolascino, F. J. (1984). The nature and incidence of mental illness in mentally retarded individuals. In F. J. Menolascino & J. A. Stark (Eds.), *Handbook of mental illness in the mentally retarded* (pp. 3–43). New York: Plenum.

Penrose, L. S. (1962). *Biology and mental defect* (rev. ed.). New York: Grune & Stratton, Inc.

Perry, R., Campbell, M., Green, W. H., Small, A. M., Die Trill, M. L., Meiselas, K., Golden, R. R., & Deutsch, S. I. (1985). Neuroleptic-related dyskinesias in autistic children: A prospective study. *Psychopharmacology Bulletin, 21,* 140–143.

Pregelj, S., & Barkauskas, A. (1967). Thioridazine in the treatment of mentally retarded children. *Canadian Psychiatric Association Journal, 12,* 213–215.

Robinault, I. P. (1978). *Sex, society, and the disabled.* New York: Harper & Row.

Rosen, M., Clark, G. R., & Kivitz, M. S. (1977). *Habilitation of the handicapped.* Baltimore: University Park Press.

Ruedrich, S., & Menolascino, F. J. (1984). Dual diagnosis of mental retardation and mental illness: An overview. In F. J. Menolascino & J. A. Stark (Eds.), *Handbook of mental illness in the mentally retarded* (pp. 45–81). New York: Plenum.

Rutter, M., Graham, P., & Yule, W. (1970). A neuropsychiatric study in childhood. *Clinics in Developmental Medicine,* Nos. 35/36. London: Simp/Heinemann.

Singh, N. N., & Aman, M. G. (1981). Effects of thioridazine dosage on the behavior of severely mentally retarded persons. *American Journal of Mental Deficiency, 85,* 580–587.

Slivan, S. E., & Bernstein, N. R. (1970). Group approaches to treating retarded adolescents. In F. Menolascino (Ed.), *Psychiatric approaches to mental retardation* (pp. 435–454). New York: Basic Books.

Sovner, R., & Hurley, A. D. (1983). Do the mentally retarded suffer from affective illness? *Archives of General Psychiatry, 40,* 61–67.

Sprague, R. L., & Werry, J. S. (1971). Methodology of Psychopharmacoligical studies with the retarded. In N. R. Ellis (Ed.), *International review of research in mental illness: Vol. 5.* (pp. 147–219). New York: Academic.

Sternlicht, M., Pustel, G., & Deutsch, M. (1970). Suicidal tendencies among institutionalized retardates. *Journal of Mental Subnormality, 16,* 93–102.

Szymanski, L. S., & Tanguay, P. E. (Eds.). (1980). *Emotional problems of mentally retarded persons.* Baltimore: University Park Press.

Turner, G., Robinson, H., Laing, S., & Purvis-Smith, S. (1986). Preventive screening for the fragile X syndrome. *New England Journal of Medicine, 315,* 607–609.

Wett, R. J. (1983). Prader-Willi syndrome. *Journal of the American Medical Association, 249,* 1836.

Williams, D. T., Mehl, R., Yudofsky, S., Adams, D., & Roseman, B. (1982). The effects of propranolol on uncontrolled rage outbursts in children and adolescents with organic brain dysfunction. *Journal of the American Academy of Child Psychiatry, 21,* 129–135.

CHAPTER SEVENTEEN

Eating Disorders

L.K. George Hsu

The eating disorders of anorexia nervosa and bulimia nervosa are potentially fatal illnesses. The recent increase in the number of eating disordered patients may reflect either a genuine rise in the incidence or simply increased referral. For anorexia nervosa, the evidence from case registers, medical records, and school surveys in Europe and this country strongly favors the former. Kendell, Hall, Hailey, and Babigan (1973) studied psychiatric case registers of Monroe County in New York State (1960–1969), Camberwell in North East London (1965–1971), and the entire region of North East Scotland (1966–1969). The incidence of anorexia nervosa varied from 0.37 per 100,000 per year in Monroe County to 0.66 in Camberwell to 1.6 in North East Scotland. In all three areas, the number of cases reported per year was increasing, and in Camberwell, but not in Monroe County or North East Scotland, there was a significant excess of patients from middle-class backgrounds.

Jones, Fox, Babigan, and Hutton (1980) restudied the psychiatric case registers as well as the medical records of a university affiliated hospital in Monroe County during the period 1960 to 1976. They found an increase in the incidence of anorexia nervosa from 0.35 per 100,000 per year during the period 1960 to 1969 to 0.65 during the years 1970 to 1976. They also found an upper-class preponderance for females age 15 to 44. Szmukler, McCance, McCrone, and Hunter (1986) restudied the Aberdeen psychiatric case register for the incidence of anorexia nervosa in North East Scotland for the period 1965 to 1982. They also found an increase in the total number of cases over time; the average annual incidence for the period 1978 to 1982 was 4.06 per 100,000. The peak incidence rate for females occurred at the age of 18 years at 0.5 per 1,000. Increase in incidence over time was found for females under the age of 34, but not for older females or males. In contrast to the earlier findings of Kendell et al. (1973), there was significant overrepresentation of social class 1 and 2 over the period studied. Theander (1970) used the records of all women admitted to the departments of psychiatry, internal medicine, pediatrics, and gynecology at two university general hospitals in a defined region in Southern Sweden from 1930 to 1960. He found an annual incidence of 0.24 per 100,000 over the 30-year period, and this increased to 0.45 during the last decade of the study. Again, women from a middle-class background were overrepresented. Willi and Grossman (1983) studied the case histories from nearly all medical, pediatric, and psychiatric clinics in the industrialized canton of Zurich, Switzerland, during three randomly selected sampling periods from 1956 to 1975. The incidence of anorexia nervosa increased significantly, from 0.38 per 100,000 for 1956 to 1958 to 0.55 for 1963 to 1965 to 1.12 for 1973 to 1975. Thus the available case registers and hospital record studies all suggested that incidence of anorexia nervosa has been increasing and that the illness predominantly affected those from a middle- to upper-class background.

Crisp, Palmer, and Kalucy (1976) in an attempt to overcome the limitations of case register studies relied on teachers' reports, medical records, and in an unspecified proportion of cases, personal interviews. They found an incidence of one severe case in every 200 school girls in nine school populations in South West London. In those age 16 and over, it amounted to one severe case per 100 pupils. The incidence in the seven private schools studied was four times higher than in the two state comprehensive schools. Pressures to be slim and achievement expectations were additional risk factors in the development of anorexia nervosa. Garner and Garfinkel (1980) found that 7% of a group of professional dance students and modeling students were suffering from anorexia nervosa, while none of the university and music students studied had diagnosable anorexia nervosa. Other studies also have found excessive weight loss, food aversion, and menstrual irregularities to be common in female ballerinas and athletes (Druss & Silverman, 1979; Frisch, Wyshak, & Vincent, 1980).

The incidence of anorexia nervosa in nonwhites has never been properly studied. Several case reports of the disorder in blacks have recently appeared (for review, see Hsu, 1987). Relatively large series of anorexia nervosa (Miyai, Yamamoto, Azukizawa, Ishibashi, & Kumahara, 1975) and bulimia nervosa patients (Nogami & Yabana, 1977) have appeared in Japan. Buhrich (1981) reported that the disorder is rare in Malaysia. It is this author's impression that the disorder may be on the increase in Hong Kong in recent years.

No good epidemiological studies of bulimia nervosa have been reported. Self-report questionnaire studies suggest that between 3 to 19% of high school and college females meet various modified DSM-III (APA, 1980) criteria for bulimia (Halmi, Falk, & Schwartz, 1981; Button & Whitehouse, 1981; Pyle, Mitchell, & Eckert, 1983; Johnson, Lewis, Love, Stuckey, & Lewis, 1983; Pope, Hudson, Yurgelun-Todd, & Hutton, 1984). These studies suffer generally from problems of sample selection and doubtful respondent understanding of the questionnaires. A better designed questionnaire study with relatively high response rate found 2.8% of female and 0% of male Dublin college students to fulfill DSM-III criteria for bulimia (Healey, Conroy, & Walsh, 1985). A two-stage questionnaire and interview survey of English high school girls found 1 in 270 (0.4%) to have bulimia nervosa. Taken together, these findings suggest that the prevalence rate for bulimia nervosa in college women is of the order of 1 to 2% (Szmukler, 1983). Clearly, better designed studies are needed, using at least a two-stage methodology as described by Szmukler.

Thus the eating disorders occur mainly in individuals who are female, age 15 to 45, Caucasian, from an upper social class, and in developed countries. Such characteristics suggest that the disorders are related to social cultural influences. The Ten State Nutrition Study (Garn & Clark, 1975) conducted in the late 1960s in response to concern about starvation in the United States found fatness to be related to being female in both whites and blacks. In the male, fatness was related to higher family income and being white. In the female, a peculiar reversal of fatness occurred at middle adolescence; whites and higher-income females who started out in life being fatter subsequently became thinner than their black and lower-income counterparts. The researchers had no doubt that the fatness reversal occurred as a result of dieting.

Garner and Garfinkel (1980), reviewing the evidence for increasing emphasis on slimness from 1959 to 1978, suggested that such emphasis may have led directly to the increased incidence of the eating disorders. This emphasis is particularly unfortunate in that it is occurring at a time when the younger population on the whole is becoming heavier due presumably to better health care and improved nutrition. Notwithstanding the views of Bruch (1985) and Crisp (1980) that adolescent dieting and onset of an eating disorder are distinctly different events, the available evidence strongly indicates that rigorous dieting is a powerful precipitant for the onset of an eating disorder. Thus it is safe to assume that the number of eating disorder individuals within a population occurs directly in proportion to the number of individuals engaged in dieting to control or lose weight. Since dieting is much more common among young Caucasian females from high-income families in developed countries, it is not surprising that eating disorders occur mainly within this group of individuals.

Obviously, not everyone who goes on a diet will develop an eating disorder. Other risk factors that have been identified include personality characteristics, such as low self-esteem, low interoceptive awareness, and low interpersonal trust on the Eating Disorder Inventory (Garner, Olmsted, Polivy, & Garfinkel, 1984). A family history of alcoholism and affective disorder also increases the risk particularly of the development of the bulimic disorder (Gershon et al., 1984; Rivinus et al., 1984).

To the best of our knowledge, there have not been any twin studies in bulimia nervosa. Our own unpublished series of 8 pairs indicated a concordance rate of 50% among the 4 monozygotic pairs, and 0% among the 4 dizygotic pairs (including one who was adopted). For anorexia nervosa, a collaborative Maudsley and St. George's study (Holland, Hall, Murray, Russell, & Crisp, 1984) found the concordance rate of monozygotic twins to be about eight times that of dizygotic twins. The authors concluded that a genetic predisposition explanation for concordance is more plausible than an equal environment induction explanation.

Adolescence is a period of great stress. Several chapters in this book have discussed the historical development of the concept of adolescence and its relevance to the onset of psychiatric disorders. Suffice it to say here that the most common age of onset for the eating disorders is the teen years (Theander, 1970; Morgan & Russell, 1975; Hsu, Crisp, & Harding, 1979). This is not surprising given that adolescence is a period of rapid physical and sexual development with its social and psychological implications and their attendant conflicts. Although researchers such as Rutter, Graham, Chadwick, and Yule (1976) and Offer (1969) have demonstrated that adolescents' storm and turmoil and severe conflict with parents are not universal even in Western countries, it is nevertheless true that a significant minority (perhaps up to 20%) of teenagers report substantial feelings of misery or depression and self-deprecation (Rutter et al., 1976; Kandel & Davies, 1982). There is also good evidence to suggest that the proportion of teenagers reporting such feelings increases with age (Shepherd, Oppenheim, & Mitchell, 1971; Rutter et al., 1976). Mean levels of self-reported depression were higher in female than in male adolescents from age 14 onward, and the levels of depression were higher among the adolescents than their parents (Kandel & Davies, 1982).

The white female adolescent is particularly prone to develop a poor self-image, greater self-consciousness, lower self-esteem, and less emotional stability (Simmons & Rosenberg, 1975). Furthermore, many researchers have found that self-definition and identity formation, traditional adolescence tasks, may be particularly problematic for the modern female, even for those with high achievements (Marsha & Friedman, 1970; Hoffman, 1974; Orlofsky, 1978). Presumably the role diffusion of the female adolescent increases insecurity and intensifies the striving for perfection and control. Such dilemma that confronts modern females may explain why they are particularly susceptible to the development of eating disorders. Huenemann, Shapiro, Hampton, and Mitchell (1966) found that about 70% of 12th-grade girls classified themselves as obese, whereas only 25% of them were actually overweight. For the boys, the effort was directed mainly at gaining weight or size and strength, whereas for the girls, it was directed mainly toward losing weight and size. Nylander (1971) reported that in a survey of school girls in Sweden in the year of 1970, 10% of 14-year-olds and 40% of 18-year-olds had attempted to diet to control their weight. In a questionnaire survey of 3 separate school districts of North Eastern United States, Hsu, Milliones, Friedman, Holder, and Klepper (1982) reported that 26% of 1102 female high school students were dieting often to control their weight, as compared to 8% of the 1082 high school boys. Forty-two percent of the girls and 17% of the boys in the survey reported often feeling fat.

Crisp (1980) has long suggested that anorexia nervosa represents a psychobiosocial retreat from the maturational and sexual demands of adolescence, and that at the same time, it serves to protect the family from the turmoil that would have occurred if not for the onset of the illness. He has also postulated that anorexia nervosa is a weight phobia (i.e., a morbid fear of normal adult weight). Obviously, anorexia nervosa does serve to express discipline and control, while bulimia nervosa, at least during the times of gorging and purging, expresses impulsivity and rebelliousness.

To the extent that both disorders become the dominant experience of the patients' existence and often that of their parents, it can be argued that both disorders simplify matters of existence (Crisp, 1980). Nevertheless, the same can be said of any adolescent psychiatric disorder, such as an obsessive-compulsive illness or a major depression. If the uniqueness of the developmental nature of anorexia nervosa lies in the fact that it is rooted in the biological regression to a prepubertal body, then the same cannot be said of bulimia nervosa, at least if the patient is at normal weight. Bruch (1985) certainly refused to accept that bulimia is a clinical entity related to anorexia nervosa. In summary, the notion that the eating disorders represent certain maladaptive adolescent developmental processes is plausible; that they are directly the result of disturbances of adolescent development is unproven.

Finally, it may be pertinent at this point to summarize the findings of the Minnesota Study (Keys, Brozek, Henschel, Mickelsen, & Taylor, 1950; see also Schiele & Brozek, 1948; Franklin, Schiele, Brozek, & Keys, 1948), which today could not be carried out for obvious ethical reasons. Briefly, 36 normal male conscientious objectors were subjected to a semistarvation diet of 1500 calories per day divided into two meals for 24 weeks. This diet was begun after a 12-week control period when the subjects on average ate 3100 calories per day, and it was followed by a 12-week restricted rehabilitation period when the subjects were given different diets of rehabilitation. The subjects lived in a nutritional laboratory, but they were encouraged to use the facilities of a nearby college campus and to participate in a wide range of activities both recreational and educational in nature. They were also allowed to go out initially unmonitored, and thus eating outside of the laboratory (i.e., breaking the diet) was possible. It appears that four subjects were most probably violating their diet and were taken out of the study. In the latter part of the study, a buddy system was therefore established to enforce closer monitoring.

After 24 weeks of semistarvation, the subjects lost on average nearly 25% of body weight. Some developed ankle edema. On self-rating measures, they reported an increase in the following: tiredness, appetite, muscle soreness, irritability, apathy, moodiness, depression, and hunger pain. They also reported decreased ambition, concentration, self-discipline, and sexual interest. Intense preoccupation with food, interest in menus and recipes, a possessive attitude toward food, preoccupation with how to prolong the pleasures of the food versus gulping it all at once to curb their hunger, spending up to 2 hours a day at a meal, and increased use of spice and salt were very common. Food substitution such as gum chewing (up to 40 packs a day in several subjects) and drinking large quantities of hot water, tea, and coffee were also widespread. During the semistarvation period, two subjects admitted to binge eating followed by remorse for breaking their diet and vomiting. One ate food from garbage cans. Two

subjects were hospitalized in a psychiatric unit for severe affective disturbances. One subject made two self-mutilative attempts; in the second one he
cut three fingers off his left hand.

These adverse effects were not totally reversed by the end of the 12
weeks of restrictive rehabilitation. Twelve subjects agreed to continue
staying in the laboratory for an additional 8 weeks of unrestrictive rehabilitation, during the weekends of which their eating was unstructured.
Splurges of 8000 to 10,000 calories a day were not uncommon. Despite
these splurges, the subjects still complained of being unsatisfied, and
several had spells of nausea and vomiting. Some of the men then became
concerned about fat accumulation in their abdomen and buttocks.

While it may be argued that the motivation for these men to go on a diet
was very different from that of an eating disorder subject, the consequences of the starvation resemble so closely the symptoms of the eating
disordered patients that we can conclude safely that most of the clinical
features of the eating disorders are due to the self-imposed starvation.

DIAGNOSTIC CONSIDERATIONS

There is relatively little disagreement among researchers on the cardinal
features of the eating disorders. Differences, however, occur as to the
definition of these features. For anorexia nervosa, the DSM-III-R (APA,
1987) retained the first criterion of the DSM-III (i.e., intense fear of becoming obese even when overweight). The disturbance of body image
criterion is changed to disturbance in the way in which one's body
weight, size, or shape is experienced. This is welcome in view of the
debate over the issue of body image disturbance (Hsu, 1982). The third
criterion of refusal to maintain body weight over a minimal weight now
encompasses the previous third and fourth DSM-III criteria, and weight
loss of 15% is now sufficient instead of 25%. A fourth criterion of amenorrhea for three consecutive cycles in the female is now added. For
bulimia nervosa, the DSM-III-R distinguishes the symptomatic behavior
(bulimia) from the disorder (bulimia nervosa). Following a definition of
binge eating similar to DSM-III, the DSM-III-R now lists a lack of control, self-induced vomiting, purging, dieting to counteract the effects
(undefined) of binge eating, and a minimal frequency of two binges
per week. Body weight is not specified, but the last criterion lists a
persistent overconcern with body shape and weight. Whereas the DSM-
III would probably classify a bulimic anorectic as having anorexia nervosa, the DSM-III-R would now probably require that both diagnoses be
given.

There is no consensus of what constitutes a binge. Several self-report
surveys (Mitchell, Hatsukami, Eckert, & Pyle, 1985; Johnson, Stuckey,

Lewis, & Schwartz, 1982; Fairburn & Cooper, 1982) found most patients to have started binge eating at the age of 18 and to begin purging a year later. The foods consumed during a binge mainly consist of sweet foods, and subjects report their preference for snacks and desserts. The typical binge in two laboratory studies (Mitchell & Laine, 1985; Kaye, Gwirtsman, George, Weiss, & Jimerson, 1986) amounted to about 4000 calories and consisted on average of 50% carbohydrates, 40% fat, and 10% protein.

The intriguing question remains: Are the two disorders of anorexia nervosa and bulimia nervosa two ends of a spectrum or distinct from each other? Certainly, some 40% of anorectics in time develop bulimia (Hsu, Crisp, & Harding, 1979), and about the same proportion of bulimics report a history of anorexia nervosa (Hsu & Holder, 1986). The percentage of bulimics without a history of anorexia nervosa who later developed anorexia nervosa is unknown, but clinical experience suggests that it might be rare. Bulimic anorectics are less inhibited than their restricting counterparts (Casper, Eckert, Halmi, Goldberg, & Davis, 1980; Garfinkel, Moldofsky, & Garner, 1980) and perhaps have a poorer outcome (Hsu, 1980). They also seem to resemble more the normal weight bulimics in terms of their personality characteristics (Garner, Garfinkel, & O'Shaughnessy, 1985).

Russell (1985) suggested that the term bulimia nervosa be used for those bulimic patients who previously had an overt or cryptic form of anorexia nervosa. Mickalide and Andersen (1985) proposed that the eating disorders may be represented as four diagnostic subgroups occurring on a spectrum: (1) anorexia nervosa restricting, (2) anorexia nervosa with bulimic complications, (3) normal weight bulimia with history of anorexia nervosa, and (4) normal weight bulimia without a history of anorexia nervosa. However, this still leaves the question of where obese subjects with a bulimic disorder would fit into this scheme. While there is support that the restricting anorectics and bulimic anorectics are relatively distinct (Casper et al., 1980; Garfinkel et al., 1980), it remains unclear if bulimics with or without a history of diagnosable anorexia nervosa are distinct. At least three studies found that such a history was not predictive of short-term outcome (Lacey, 1983; Hsu & Holder, 1986; Hughes, Wells, Cunningham, & Ilstrup, 1986).

The debate continues as to whether the eating disorders are variants of affective disorders (for review, see Swift, Andrews, & Barklage, 1986). The evidence that they are rests on the high percentage of eating disordered patients who are also depressed, the high prevalence of affective illness in the families of eating disordered patients, the similar response to antidepressant treatment, and the finding in some outcome studies that anorectics apparently gave up their anorexia nervosa only to develop an affective illness. The evidence that they are not variants of each other rests on arguments that these findings could have different interpretations. For instance, the high familial prevalence of affective illness may simply predispose a youngster to develop an eating disorder; however, this finding does not therefore necessarily imply that the disorders are variants of each other. The clinical picture of eating disordered patients who are depressed is usually not a primary affective disorder. The biochemical changes in the eating disorders are more likely to be the result of the chaotic eating and weight change rather than being markers of an affective illness. A similar response to a medication carries no implication that the disorders are necessarily related to each other. Outcome studies finding that anorectics gave up their eating disorder and instead developed an affective illness generally suffer from a high failure-to-trace rate (Hsu, 1980) and therefore are methodologically flawed. On balance, the evidence that the eating disorders are *not* variants of affective disorders outweigh those that suggest they are.

The endocrine disturbances in anorexia nervosa have been reviewed extensively elsewhere (Isaacs, 1979; Garfinkel & Garner, 1982; Russell & Beumont, 1987). Many of the changes that occur in anorexia nervosa are probably the direct result of malnutrition and starvation. Since some bulimic patients also suffer from starvation (Pirke, Pahl, Schweiger, & Warnhoff, 1985), they may also show the endocrine changes that occur in anorexia nervosa. In addition, self-induced vomiting, intake of diet pills, diuretics, and emetics, and unusual amounts of foods sometimes eaten (such as cheese and carrots) may produce as yet unknown metabolic and endocrine changes. In general, the search for an etiological factor among the numerous endocrine disturbances of the eating disorders has proven unfruitful, since most of the disturbances quite promptly revert to normal once malnutrition and starvation are corrected. More recently, interest has focused on the neuroendocrine changes in the eating disorders. Of particular interest is the recent preliminary finding that infusion of norepinehrine to the medical hypothalamus of rats increases the animals' eating, while serotonin has the opposite effect (for review, see Leibowitz & Shor-Posner, 1986). There is some indication that the serotonin metabolite, 5-hydroxyindoleaceticacid, is reduced in the cerebral spinal fluid of some bulimic patients (Kaye, Ebert, Gwirtsman, & Weiss, 1984). There also is evidence that serotonergic drugs (e.g., fenfluramine) may decrease the craving of carbohydrates for some obese subjects (for review, see Silverstone & Goodall, 1986; Wurtman & Wurtman, 1986).

A full physical examination should be performed for every patient, along with a carefully taken history of her physical health. Substance abuse, particularly of diuretics, diet pills, or emetics, should be carefully and systematically assessed. If done tactfully, such history taking is probably unlikely to teach the patient new techniques of purging or substance abuse. Positive findings on physical examination in bulimic patients are usually rare, but some may have swollen perotid glands and calluses on the dorsum of the

Table 17.1. Physical Manifestations of the Eating Disorders

System	Anorexia Nervosa	Bulimia Nervosa
Endocrine	Amenorrhea Low LH & FSH Blunted LH response to LHRH Low T_4 & T_3 Variable changes in growth Hormone, Prolactin, Somatomedin and Sometostatin, norepinephrine, TSH, Cortisol, Arginine Vasopressin, and others	Irregular cycles, may show other endocrine disturbances similar to those in AN
Metabolic	Electrolytes usually normal but may show disturbances similar to BN Osteoporosis & retarded bone growth Low cholesterol (from fasting) or high cholesterol (mechanism unclear) Hypercarotenemia Abnormal glucose tolerance Abnormal temperature regulation	Low Potassium Low Sodium Low Chloride High or low Bicarbonate Other metabolic disturbances may occur similar to AN
Cardiovascular	Bradycardia Hypotension Heart failure EKG changes Refeeding edema	Cardiomyopathy Heart failure EKG changes
Pulmonary		Aspiration pneumonia
Gastrointestinal	Constipation Decreased gastric emptying Acute gastric dilatation Increased hepatic enzymes	Constipation Decreased gastric emptying Dental enamel erosion Parotid enlargement Esophagitis Bleeding or rupture of esophagus Acute gastric dilatation Gastric ulcers Increased Amylase
Renal	Low blood urea nitrogen (BUN) (from fasting) Increased BUN (from renal function impairment)	Increased BUN Decreased GFR Nephropathy and renal failure

Table 17.1. *Physical Manifestations of the Eating Disorders* (continued)

System	Anorexia Nervosa	Bulimia Nervosa
Renal	Decreased glomerular filtration rare (GFR) Renal calculi	
Neurological	Epileptic seizures	Epileptic seizures
Hematologic	Anemia Low Erythrocyte Sedimentation Rate	Anemia

dominant hand. For anorectic patients, emaciation is evident and cold extremities and lanugo hair may be present. A full blood count and electrolyte levels should always be taken, as should an electrocardiogram. Other tests may be ordered as indicated. Particular care should be given to the management of a bulimic anorectic who is also taking diuretics or emetics since she may be at risk for serious complications such as cardiac arrest and failure. In our own series, abnormal renal function occurs in 5 to 10% of normal weight bulimics, and it is unclear if this reverts to normal with improvement in the clinical condition. An internist should be consulted if there are abnormal findings.

Patients may present with nonpsychiatric problems such as amenorrhea, recurrent abdominal pain, or rectal bleeding. Epileptic seizures occur in perhaps 10% of bulimic anorectics (Crisp, 1980). Tooth decay may be the first sign of bulimia nervosa. Rarely, a patient may present with an emergency such as esophageal bleeding or rupture. One of the author's first bulimic patients presented as a surgical emergency after she had swallowed the fork she had used to induce a gag reflex. A list of the more common physical manifestations of the eating disorders may be found in Table 17.1.

CLINICAL PROBLEMS

A clinician called upon to treat a patient with an eating disorder has to make a series of decisions. Obviously, the first task is to decide if the patient has an eating disorder. If she presents with an eating or weight problem, the diagnosis is not usually difficult. However, if she presents with other psychiatric symptoms and if the clinician fails to ask systematically for disturbances relating to eating and weight, the disorder may remain undiagnosed. In perhaps 20% of the older patients, there is a concurrent diagnosis of personality disorder and/or substance/alcohol abuse. In this situation (fortunately rare in the adolescent patient) it is often difficult to decide which is the primary diagnosis, and management may have to involve several clinicians, each dealing with a part of the overall problem. Open communication between clinicians and patient is essential since therapist splitting or rivalry may undermine treatment.

Once a diagnosis is made, the clinician has to engage the patient and family as collaborators in treatment. This task is particularly difficult in an adolescent patient unwillingly brought to treatment by her parents. Treatment alliance is probably best achieved by the clinician openly acknowledging the significance and meaning of the patient's striving for thinness and control (Casper, 1982; Strober & Yager, 1985). This may be accompanied by the clinician's acknowledgment of the current cultural emphasis on slimness and the significance attached to weight control. At the same time, the clinician should specifically address the negative and potentially life-threatening nature of the effects of starvation and/or binging or vomiting. The benefits of treatment should then be emphasized, including the assurance that the patient's need to be special will be respected and not destroyed. Before seeing the parents, the issue of confidentiality and right to privacy must be discussed. If consent is given, every effort should then be made to secure the understanding and cooperation of the parents. Several family sessions at this stage in order to address the parents' concerns and also to begin exploring general family dynamics may be particularly helpful.

The next question for the clinician is where to treat the patient. For bulimia nervosa, unless the patient is dangerously ill or suicidal, the initial treatment setting is usually outpatient. However, for the refractory patient, the external structure and control of an inpatient unit may help to break the vicious binge/purge/starve cycle. For anorexia nervosa, inpatient treatment is usually recommended if the patient's body weight is below 70% of normal (Garfinkel & Garner, 1982; Casper, 1982), although a bulimic anorectic at a higher weight may also need inpatient treatment because of the particular dangers of electrolyte imbalance and heart failure. For inpatients, there is no consensus on treatment duration. For anorectics, Crisp (1980) and Russell (1977) usually keep their patients in the hospital for several weeks after they have reached target weight, while Collins, Hodas, and Liebman (1983) discharge their patients after they have reached 50% of what is needed to achieve their target weight. It would appear that the minimum goals of inpatient treatment for anorexia nervosa are a reasonably healthy body weight and healthy eating pattern; for bulimia nervosa minimum goals are a reasonably healthy eating pattern and infrequent bulimic behavior.

Although many clinicians admit eating disorder patients to general adolescent or even adult wards, perhaps more commonly these patients are treated in an eating disorders unit. Strober and Yager (1985) have argued that admission to an adolescent unit exposes the patient to a variety of adolescent behavior and pathology, and the exposure may be beneficial to the withdrawn and rigid patient with a limited behavioral repertoire. This author has treated eating disorder patients both on an adolescent unit and an eating disorder unit, and it is his experience that the latter is preferable to the staff, the patient, and the family. The issue cannot be settled without further research.

The issue of target weight for the eating disorders is not resolved. For anorexia nervosa perhaps most clinicians aim at a low normal weight (Garfinkel & Garner, 1982), an age-appropriate weight (Casper, 1982), or a matched population mean weight at the onset of illness (Crisp, 1980). For bulimia nervosa, the issue has not been directly addressed, although Garner, Rockert, Olmsted, Johnson, and Coscina (1985) seem to indicate that some weight gain may be beneficial even in normal weight bulimics who were premorbidly obese.

For anorexia nervosa, the treatment of choice to achieve target weight is unclear. Some clinicians leave it to the patient (Orbach, 1985); others use nursing care (Crisp, 1980; Russell, 1977), behavior modification (Blinder, Freeman, & Stunkard, 1970; Halmi, Powers, & Cunningham, 1975), or coercive techniques such as hyperalimentation (Maloney & Farrell, 1980). Some would not use coercive techniques under any circumstances, preferring to discharge the uncooperative patient (Crisp, 1980), while others use tube feeding on the resistant patient (Strober & Yager, 1985). It would appear that a restrictive behavior modification approach is no more effective than a lenient one. (Touyz, Beumont, & Glaun, 1984) or competent milieu care (Eckert, Goldberg, & Halmi, 1979). The clinician should develop an approach that can be used consistently and comfortably, bearing in mind that weight restoration is always a team effort and that the clinician's method of choice is not necessarily the perfect or most logical one. Thus input from other members of the team must be considered; otherwise treatment may be undermined.

There are many other unresolved issues regarding the diagnosis, treatment, and outcome of the eating disorders. Some may not be of immediate interest to the clinician (e.g., whether the eating disorders are one disorder or two) but others are (e.g., how to prevent relapse). Unfortunately, most of the opinions expressed by experts are based more on intuition, clinical experience, and preference than on painstakingly conducted research. In the following discussion on the treatment of the eating disorders, the author will attempt to give a balanced view while acknowledging the relative lack of research data.

GENERAL PRINCIPLES OF MANAGEMENT

The clinician must bear in mind that the eating disorders are usually long illnesses with many relapses. Treatment goals therefore may vary at different stages of the illness. Furthermore, different patients may have different needs; thus the treatment of a 13-year-old high school anorectic living at home may be very different from that of a 35-year-old divorced woman living alone. Treatment goals must always be clearly formulated and communicated to the patient and, when appropriate, to the family as well. The clinician must therefore be flexible and adept at different treatments or at least be able to work with another clinician specializing in the use of a different treatment approach. For instance, while antidepressants are sometimes remarkably effective in alleviating the urge to binge in bulimia nervosa, it is highly unlikely that a bulimic patient can be treated with medication alone without some form of dietary advice and psychotherapy being given at some stage of the treatment process.

The clinician must not overlook the patient-therapist interaction even when medication or a behavioral approach is used. Eating disordered patients are hypersensitive to the feelings of others and to demands, imagined or real, that are placed on them. They are also good at rationalizations and are outwardly very compliant. Initially, they may appear to improve quickly only to drop out of treatment suddenly if these hidden issues are not carefully explored.

For an adolescent patient, a detailed discussion of identity and sexual issues and family and peer relationships can rarely be avoided. This does not mean that the clinician must subscribe to the view that the treatment of the eating disorders, particularly of anorexia nervosa, is essentially a reorientation of the patient and the family to the normal vicissitudes of the adolescent process and crisis, as advocated by some authorities (e.g., Crisp, 1980; Strober & Yager, 1985). It does mean, however, that the management of a chronic illness in an adolescent necessarily involves the management of the developmental issues with which the patient is grappling.

Treatment is often carried out in a team, particularly for an inpatient unit. Team members usually consist of a psychiatrist, a psychologist, a therapist, a nurse, and a dietician. Several authors have described the qualities of a therapist (e.g., Strober & Yager, 1985), but they seem to be those of an ideal clinician. It is true that some clinicians are more likely to be locked in a battle of wills with the patient or family, so that each clinical issue becomes an impasse demanding to be resolved by rigid rules (e.g., how many cups of water a patient can drink at each meal). Certainly, some rules are necessary, but it is more important for the clinician to be flexible, sensitive, and willing to explore as well as to be firm and authoritative when necessary. It is unclear how a past history of an eating disorder or personal views on fatness and femininity affect a clinician's effectiveness. Needless to say, open communication between team members is essential, and much time and effort may be needed to achieve it.

Dietary Advice

The dietary pattern of the eating disordered patients are so abnormal that dietary advice seems to be a logical treatment approach. Some authorities, however, believe that an eating disturbance is a reflection of deeper disturbances and is best left for the patient to deal with by herself (e.g., Orbach, 1985). For others, dietary advice is an integral part of treatment (e.g., Strober & Yager, 1985; Beumont, O'Connor, Touyz, & Williams, 1987), but unfortunately, its efficacy has never been formally evaluated. Hall and Crisp (1987) found that dietary advice may be as effective as combined individual and family psychotherapy for anorectic patients. In general, dietary advice includes nutritional education, teaching techniques of meal planning, education on the dangers of diuretic/diet pill/emetic abuse, and instructions on healthy eating habits.

While most eating disordered patients are intensely interested in food and cooking, their ideas of what constitutes a balanced diet may be very distorted. Patients not uncommonly divide food into "good," and "bad," "healthy," and "unhealthy" categories based on entirely mistaken notions. They also have very little understanding of the effects of starvation. The help of an experienced dietician is usually valuable, and most patients will benefit from a few sessions to work out meal plans and be educated on the basic principles of nutrition. Some patients may consider themselves to be nutrition experts, and much persuasion may be needed before they will accept dietary advice.

All patients should be educated on the dangers of vomiting and laxative, diuretic, and diet pill abuse. The chief danger of purging and diuretic abuse is electrolyte imbalance, which may lead to cardiac or renal failure. Some patients take syrup of ipecac, which can poison skeletal muscles, including those of the heart, thus leading to acute cardiac failure. Diet pills are generally habit forming and have various other side effects depending on their particular type. The ineffectiveness of purging for weight control should be emphasized, along with its tendency to cause rebound weight increase through fluid retention.

The patient may need particular advice on how to purchase and prepare nutritious foods. The cooperation and understanding of the family should be secured beforehand. A few sessions of eating out in a restaurant with a dietician may help reduce the anxiety the patient commonly experiences in such environments. The patient who complains of feeling full after even a small meal should be reassured that the discomfort will decrease with time and is probably related to a decrease in the gastric emptying rate.

Self-recording of intake and the associated feelings may be valuable as a part of cognitive therapy for both anorectics and bulimics. This allows for self-monitoring of both the intake and the associated feelings. However, sometimes the patient will spend almost all her spare time on the food diary, and a time may come for leading her to discontinue it.

PHARMACOLOGICAL APPROACHES

Treatment of Anorexia Nervosa with Medication

Medication is used in anorexia nervosa to facilitate weight gain (e.g., Crisp, 1965) or to correct the hypothesized underlying neurotransmitter disturbance (e.g., Needleman & Waber, 1977). Overall, the results are disappointing. Controlled studies of medication in anorexia nervosa are uncommon, and practically all of them yielded results that were hard to interpret because of methodological flaws. Two tricyclic antidepressants have been studied, clomipramine, an agent not marketed in this country, and amitriptyline (Lacey & Crisp, 1980; Halmi, Eckert, LaDu & Cohen, 1986). Overall, the effects on weight gain were unimpressive. Cyproheptadine, a serotonin blocker, may have some weight-gain effect on the restricting anorectic (Halmi et al., 1986). By virtue of this serotonergic effect, cyproheptadine also may be useful as an antidepressant. The phenothiazines were more popular in the 1960s; two recent controlled trials found Pimozide and Sulpiride to have no effect on weight gain (Vandereycken & Pierlott, 1982; Vandereycken, 1984). However, the duration of these trials was brief and the cross-over design added to the problem of interpreting the findings. In one study, Lithium Carbonate seemed to promote weight gain (Gross, Ebert, & Fadden, 1981).

In sum, the medication studies in anorexia nervosa have concentrated on the short-term weight-gain effects. This strategy is misguided for three reasons. First, over 90% of anorectic patients gain weight satisfactorily once they are hospitalized; thus it would be hard to prove that medication may be of any additional benefit. Second, rapid weight gain is generally undesirable because it induces fear in the patient; hence it is pointless to prove that a medication may induce more rapid weight gain than nursing care or behavioral therapy. Third, short-term recovery does not guarantee long-term cure. Whether medication can prevent relapse has never been studied.

Clinical experience suggests that antidepressants may be useful for anorectics who are depressed (Morgan, Purgold, & Welbourne, 1983). The small proportion of those who develop a psychosis should be treated appropriately with phenothiazines and/or antidepressants (Hsu, Meltzer, & Crisp, 1981).

Treatment of Bulimia Nervosa with Medication

Medication has been used for bulimia nervosa to alleviate the urge to binge and to improve the concurrent dysphoria. Most bulimic patients are reluctant to take medication and are overly concerned about the side effects, particularly of any possible weight increase. Some may confuse an antidepressant with a "diet" pill. The prescription of any medication should therefore be preceded by a detailed discussion of the indications, the possible benefits, and the possible side effects. Patients should be reassured that the taking of an antidepressant for the treatment of bulimia is not usually associated with weight increase.

Several double-blind studies have found antidepressants to be useful in bulimia. Pope, Hudson, Jonas, and Yurgelun-Todd (1983) in a 6-week study of 22 bulimic patients found Imipramine at the usual dosage to be significantly better than placebo. Walsh, Stewart, Roose, Gladis, and Glassman (1984) found Phenelzine to be significantly better than placebo in a 6-week study of 20 bulimic women, with over 50% of those on phenelzine reaching total cessation of their binge/purge behavior. Unfortunately, the side effects were substantial. Hughes et al. (1986) found Desipramine to be vastly superior to placebo in a 6-week study of 22 patients, with over 50% of those on medication reaching total abstinence. Mitchell and Groat (1984) found Amitriptyline to be better than placebo in improving the patient's mood, but both the medication and placebo group improved significantly with respect to their binge/purge behavior. In sum, antidepressants at an adequate dosage are likely to benefit many bulimic patients, provided they can tolerate the side effects. Patients who improve usually indicate a decrease in the urges to binge and an improvement in their mood. It is unclear whether bulimic symptoms in the absence of a concurrent depression will also respond to antidepressant. The study by Hughes et al. (1986) seems to suggest that they do. Perhaps the antidepressants act by virtue by their action on neurotransmitters.

In general, for the medication treatment of bulimia nervosa, a tricyclic antidepressant should be tried first. The dosage may be gradually increased and the blood level monitored if necessary. Because of the need for dietary restrictions, the monoamine oxidase inhibitors should be used as a second-line treatment agent. The newer antidepressant, Trazadone, may also be beneficial as a second-line agent. A new antidepressant, Fluoxetine, appears to be promising but is not yet available for use in this country. Maintenance treatment at the effective dosage should probably continue for at least 6 months, although there are no maintenance studies.

PSYCHODYNAMIC AND
PSYCHOTHERAPEUTIC APPROACHES

Treatment of Anorexia Nervosa

The principles of the treatment of anorexia nervosa have not changed much in the last 25 years (Hsu, 1986). In an emaciated patient, the first task is for nutritional rehabilitation with attention given to the electrolyte disturbances and other possible physical complications. Intensive individual psychotherapy is usually given concurrently to change the patient's distorted view toward herself and her body. Family therapy has become popular and is usually based on the view that a supportive and understanding family may facilitate recovery, while an intrusive and overprotective one impedes it. The third goal of treatment is relapse prevention, but there is very little data on what is the most effective approach. Some of the general treatment issues have been discussed in the previous sections.

Recent writings on the psychotherapy of anorectic patients have emphasized the patient's inward emptiness, the denial and fear of personal needs, the sense of ineffectiveness, and the low self-esteem, even self-hatred. Cognitive therapists have described more specifically the anorectic's distorted beliefs and thinking processes, such as dichotomous reasoning, superstitious beliefs, unrealistic fears, and irrational convictions (e.g., Garner & Bemis, 1982). Feminist writers have drawn attention to the vicissitudes of the passage from girlhood to womanhood in Western society and the influence of contemporary Western ideas of femininity on an individual's self-image (e.g., Orbach, 1985). In addition to the analytical task of interpretation, current descriptions of the treatment process emphasize the role of the therapist to educate, to modulate, to support, to evoke, to discuss, to challenge, to negotiate, to encourage, and to role model. Besides dealing specifically with the target symptoms of distortion toward self and weight, some therapists also challenge the patient's passive acceptance of the obnoxious cultural values regarding shape, weight, and womanhood (e.g., Garner, Rockert, Olmsted, Johnson, & Coscina, 1985b). Some have employed more nonverbal techniques (e.g., Wooley & Wooley, 1985). All agree that individual psychotherapy of the anorectic is a long and arduous process.

Minuchin's conceptualization has continued to dominate the family treatment approach to anorexia nervosa. His structural model emphasizes hierarchy, subsystems, and boundaries. Minuchin and his coworkers (Minuchin, Rosman, & Baker, 1978) identified five predominant characteristics detrimental to the functioning of the anorectic family: enmeshment, overprotectiveness, rigidity, lack of conflict resolution, and involvement of the sick child in unresolved parental conflict. Recent writings avoided earlier claims that the family interaction pattern, at least in part, caused the illness. Minuchin and Fishman (1981) have described skillfully the techniques that are often helpful in the family therapy of the patient. These include techniques such as joining with the family, enactment of dysfunctional transactions, selective focusing on strategic issues, increasing the intensity of conflicts so that they are resolved, defining boundaries, delineating subsystems, unbalancing the dysfunctional hierarchy, establishing the complimentary of responsibility for problems, and prescribing change. Clinicians have found Minuchin's approach sometimes to be startlingly effective in helping an adolescent anorectic patient, particularly when buried feelings are shared or when the patient is freed from being trapped between parental conflicts. For older patients living away from home, family sessions may overcome an impasse in individual therapy.

Very little has been written about group therapy for anorectics. Hall (1985) discussed in detail the difficulties of group therapy for anorectics, namely the patient's rigidity, withdrawal, high anxiety and dysphoria, hypersensitivity to criticism, constant preoccupation with weight and food, difficulty in identifying and expressing feelings, and the tendency to escape by losing weight. With careful patient selection and attention to such difficulties, group therapy may provide a useful alternative or conjunctive form of treatment, although it seems difficult to establish definite indications for its use as the sole or primary treatment approach.

As already mentioned, inpatient treatment for the purpose of weight and nutritional restoration is successful in over 90% of cases. However, perhaps 50% of patients will relapse within 1 year of discharge from the hospital (Hsu, Crisp, & Harding, 1979). There are no studies published on relapse prevention, but common sense suggests that individual, group, and family therapy should continue for perhaps 6 months to a year. The proportion of outpatients successfully treated is unclear. Two studies (Hsu et al., 1979; Morgan et al., 1983) found their outcome to be more favorable than those treated as inpatients, perhaps because they were less severely ill to begin with.

A more uniform picture of the immediate term (4 to 10 years) outcome of anorexia nervosa has emerged in the past few years following the publication of several studies using similar methodology (Morgan & Russell, 1975; Hsu et al., 1979; Morgan et al., 1983; Hall, Slim, Hawker, & Salmond, 1984; Burns & Crisp, 1984). In brief, about one-half to two-thirds of the patients are at normal weight, and female patients are menstruating regularly; but chaotic eating and persistent weight phobia are common, with perhaps one-third of the patients qualifying for a diagnosis of bulimia nervosa. Dysthymic symptoms and social phobia are also common. Twenty percent of the patients remained at very low weight, and mortality varied between studies from 0 to 5%. A more recent 20-year follow-up study, however, found the mortality to be 18% (Theander, 1985), and this suggests that there is no room for optimism regarding the outcome of this disorder.

The Treatment of Bulimia Nervosa

Bulimic patients are more open and expressive and in general more motivated for treatment by the time they seek consultation. The immediate goals of treatment are the establishment of a regular eating pattern to prevent starvation and to control the bulimic behavior. Cognitive and interpersonal issues are also dealt with concurrently or after a more normal eating pattern has been established. Positive results have been obtained by the use of cognitive therapy, conducted either individually or in a group. Common elements of this approach are: educating the patient about the disorder, giving nutritional advice, discussing the functions of a binge, identifying and verbalizing feelings, making connections between thoughts and feelings and actions, identifying antecedents to binges, monitoring of food intake, monitoring of feelings, using self-instructions, developing alternative coping skills, and taking responsibility for change (for review, see Mitchell et al., 1985; Garner, Fairburn, & Davis, 1987).

Treatment should be intensive in the beginning to facilitate control of the bulimic behavior, and patients are seen two times or more a week at this stage (Fairburn, 1985; Mitchell et al., 1985). Treatment is usually time limited, with significant symptom remission occurring within a few months. Several treatment manuals have been published (e.g., Fairburn, 1985; Root, Fallon, & Friedrich, 1986), and readers may find them helpful.

The benefits of individual versus group therapy are unclear; perhaps that choice depends more on the preference of the therapist. Group therapy has the advantage of decreasing the patient's isolation and withdrawal and increasing her sense of sharing and purpose through the members' mutual encouragement and support. However, patients entering a group should be well prepared; otherwise, there may be a significant dropout (Garner et al., 1987). In general, perhaps it is best to begin with individual cognitive therapy alone or to combine it with group therapy. It usually is not advisable to mix bulimics with anorectics or males with females in a group. Such combinations may encourage competition and inhibit disclosure and sharing. If there is no significant improvement in the binge/purge behavior in 4 to 6 weeks, consideration must be given to medication.

Following the pioneering effort by Fairburn (1981), many studies have been published that use nutritional and cognitive behavioral principles in the treatment of bulimia nervosa. Garner et al. (1987) have reviewed a total of 19 studies of acceptable methodology published between 1981 and

1986 and found that, on average, there was a 79% reduction in binge-free frequency from pretreatment to posttreatment, with a range of 51% to 97%. At the end of treatment, which lasted from a few weeks to 1 year, between 20% and 80% of the patients were no longer binging or vomiting. Eight control studies have been published (Fairburn, Kirk, O'Connor, & Cooper, 1986; Freeman, Sinclair, Turnbull, & Annadale, 1985; Kirkley, Schneider, Agras, & Bachman, 1985; Lacey, 1983; Lee & Rush, 1986; Ordman & Kirshenbaum, 1985; Wilson, Rossiter, Kleifeld, & Lindholm, 1986; Wolchik, Weiss, & Katzman, 1986). Those that used a waiting list group as the controlled condition all found cognitive behavioral treatment to be vastly superior (Lacey, 1983; Lee and Rush, 1986; Ordman & Kirchenbaum, 1985; Wolchik et al., 1986). Cognitive treatment is somewhat more effective than short-term therapy (Fairburn et al., 1986) and nondirective therapy (Kirkley et al., 1985), while cognitive restructuring and exposure and vomit prevention is more effective than the former alone (Wilson et al., 1986). No good follow-up studies have been published, and the long-term outcome of the disorder is unknown. Experience suggests that relapse after a few years of apparent cure is not uncommon. There is no consensus on how to prevent relapse.

Support Groups

Support groups generally consist of patients at various stages of treatment and recovery and their families. The groups are usually led by a recovered patient and/or a parent of a patient, although sometimes professionals also are involved in a supportive capacity. The greatest benefit lies in the giving of information and peer support and in confronting and encouraging reluctant or resistant patients to begin or continue treatment. There is some concern among clinicians that patients may be thrust prematurely into a helping role and derive vicarious satisfaction from helping others. In general, the benefits probably outweigh the disadvantages.

SUMMARY

This chapter provides a review of the prevalence, etiology, diagnosis, and treatment of the eating disorders of anorexia nervosa and bulimia nervosa. The review is intended primarily for the clinician; research is discussed when it is clinically relevant, and review articles are cited for the interested reader to pursue. It is clear that the eating disorders will continue to be of concern for clinicians and researchers in several disciplines. They are intriguing because they display the complex interaction of the body, the mind, and various social cultural influences.

REFERENCES

American Psychiatric Association (1987). *Diagnostic and statistical manual of mental disorders* (3rd ed., revised). (DSM-III-R). Washington, DC: Author.

American Psychiatric Association (1980). *Diagnostic and statistical manual of mental disorders* (3rd ed.). (DSM-III). Washington, DC: Author.

Beumont, P., O'Connor, M., Touyz, S., & Williams, H. (1987). Nutritional counseling in the treatment of anorexia and bulimia nervosa. In P. Beumont, G. Burrows, & R. Casper (Eds.), *Handbook of eating disorders, part I* (pp. 349–360). Amsterdam: Elsevier.

Blinder, B. J., Freeman, D. M. A., & Stunkard, A. J. (1970). Behavior therapy of anorexia nervosa: Effectiveness of activity as a reinforcer of weight gain. *American Journal of Psychiatry, 126,* 1093–1098.

Bruch, H. (1985). Four decades of eating disorders. In D. M. Garner & P. E. Garfinkel (Eds.), *Handbook of psychotherapy for anorexia nervosa and bulimia* (pp. 7–18). New York: Guilford.

Buhrich, N. (1981). Frequency of presentation of anorexia in Malaysia. *Australian and New Zealand Journal of Psychiatry, 15,* 153–155.

Burns, T., & Crisp, A. H. (1984). Outcome of anorexia nervosa in males. *British Journal of Psychiatry, 145,* 391–325.

Button, E. J., & Whitehouse, A. (1981). Subclinical anorexia nervosa. *Psychological Medicine, II,* 509–516.

Casper, R. C. (1982). Treatment principles in anorexia nervosa. *Adolescent Psychiatry, 10,* 86–100.

Casper, R. C., Eckert, E. D., Halmi, K. A., Goldberg, S. C., & Davis, J. M. (1980). Bulimia: Its incidence and clinical importance in patients with anorexia nervosa. *Archives of General Psychiatry, 37,* 1030–1035.

Collins, M., Hodas, G. R., & Liebman, R. (1983). Interdisciplinary model for the inpatient treatment of adolescents with anorexia nervosa. *Journal of Adolescent Health Care, 4,* 3–8.

Crisp, A. H. (1965). A treatment regime for anorexia nervosa. *British Journal of Psychiatry, 112,* 505–512.

Crisp, A. H. (1980). *Anorexia nervosa: Let me be.* New York: Grune & Stratton, Inc.

Crisp, A. H., Palmer, R. L., & Kalucy, R. S. (1976). How common is anorexia nervosa? A prevalence study. *British Journal of Psychiatry, 128,* 549–554.

Druss, R. G., & Silverman, J. A. (1979). Body image and perfectionism of ballerinas. *General Hospital Psychiatry, 2,* 115–121.

Eckert, E. D., Goldberg, S. C., & Halmi, K. A. (1979). Behavior therapy in anorexia nervosa. *British Journal of Psychiatry, 134,* 55–59.

Fairburn, C. G. (1981). A cognitive behavioral approach to the management of bulimia. *Psychological Medicine, II,* 707–711.

Fairburn, C. G. (1985). Cognitive-behavioral treatment for bulimia. In D. M. Garner & P. E. Garfinkel (Eds.), *Handbook of psychotherapy for anorexia nervosa and bulimia* (pp. 391–430). New York: Guilford.

Fairburn, C. G., & Cooper, P. J. (1982). Self-induced vomiting and bulimia nervosa: An undetectable problem. *British Medical Journal, 1,* 1153–1155.

Fairburn, C. G., Kirk, J., O'Connor, M., & Cooper, P. J. (1986). A comparison of two psychological treatments for bulimia nervosa. *Behaviour Research and Therapy, 24,* 629–643.

Franklin, J. C., Schiele, B. C., Brozek, J., & Keys, A. (1948). Observations of human behavior in experimental semistarvation and rehabilitation. *Journal of Clinical Psychology, 4,* 28–45.

Freeman, C., Sinclair, F., Turnbull, J., & Annadale, A. (1985). Psychotherapy for bulimia: A controlled study. *Journal of Psychiatric Research, 19,* 473–478.

Frish, R. E., Wyshak, G., & Vincent, L. (1980). Delayed menarche and amenorrhea in ballet dancers. *New England Journal of Medicine, 303,* 17–19.

Garfinkel, P. E., & Garner, D. M. (1982). *Anorexia nervosa: A multidimensional perspective.* New York: Brunner/Mazel.

Garfinkel, P. E., Moldofsky, H., & Garner, D. M. (1980). The heterogeneity of anorexia nervosa: Bulimia as a distinct subgroup. *Archives of General Psychiatry, 37,* 1036–1040.

Garn, S. M., & Clark, D. C. (1975). Nutrition, growth, development, and maturation findings from the ten-state nutrition survey of 1968–1970. *Pediatrics, 56,* 306–319.

Garner, D. M., & Bemis, K. M. (1982). A cognitive-behavioral approach to anorexia nervosa. *Cognitive Therapy and Research, 6,* 123–150.

Garner, D. M., Fairburn, C. G., & Davis, R. (1987). Cognitive-behavioral treatment of bulimia nervosa. *Behavior Modification, II*(4), 398–431.

Garner, D. M., & Garfinkel, P. E. (1980). Social cultural factors in the development of anorexia nervosa. *Psychological Medicine, 10,* 647–656.

Garner, D. M., Garfinkel, P. E., & O'Shaughnessy, M. (1985a). Validity of the distinction between bulimia with and without anorexia nervosa. *American Journal of Psychiatry, 142,* 581–587.

Garner, D. M., Olmsted, M. P., Polivy, J., & Garfinkel, P. E. (1984). Comparison between weight-preoccupied women and anorexia nervosa. *Psychosomatic Medicine, 46,* 255–266.

Garner, D. M., Rockert, W., Olmsted, M. P., Johnson, C. L., & Coscina, D. V. (1985b). Psychoeducational principles in the treatment of bulimia and anorexia nervosa. In D. M. Garner & P. E. Garfinkel (Eds.), *Handbook of psychotherapy for anorexia nervosa and bulimia* (pp. 513–572). New York: Guilford.

Gershon, E. S., Schreiber, J. L., Hamovit, J. R., Dibble, E. D., Kaye, W., Nurnberger, J. I., Andersen, A. E., & Ebert, M. (1984). Clinical findings in patients with anorexia nervosa and affective illness and their relatives. *American Journal of Psychiatry, 141,* 1419–1422.

Gross, H. A., Ebert, M. H., Faden, V. B., (1981). A double-blind controlled trial of lithium carbonate in primary anorexia nervosa. *Journal of Clinical Psychopharmacology, 1,* 376–381.

Hall, A. (1985). Group psychotherapy for anorexia nervosa. In D. M. Garner & P. E. Garfinkel (Eds.), *Handbook of Psychotherapy for anorexia nervosa and bulimia* (pp. 213–238). New York: Guilford.

Hall, A., & Crisp, A. H. (1987). Brief psychotherapy in the treatment of anorexia nervosa: Outcome at one year. *British Journal of Psychiatry, 151,* 185–191.

Hall, A., Slim, E., Hawker, F., & Salmond, C. (1984). Anorexia nervosa: Long-term outcome in 50 female patients. *British Journal of Psychiatry, 145,* 407–413.

Halmi, K. A. (1983). Treatment of anorexia nervosa. *Journal of Adolescence Health Care, 4,* 47–50.

Halmi, K. A., Eckert, E., LaDu, T. J., & Cohen, J. (1986). Anorexia nervosa: Treatment efficacy of cyproheptadine and amitriptyline. *Archives of General Psychiatry, 43,* 177–181.

Halmi, K. A., Falk, J. R., & Schwartz, E. (1981). Binge-eating and vomiting: A survey of a college population. *Psychological Medicine, II,* 697–706.

Halmi, K. A., Powers, P., & Cunningham, S. (1975). Treatment of anorexia nervosa with behavior modification. *Archives of General Psychiatry, 32,* 93–96.

Healy, K., Conroy, R. M., & Walsh, N. (1985). The prevalence of binge-eating and bulimia in 1063 college students. *Journal of Psychiatric Research, 19,* 161–166.

Hoffman, L. W. (1974). Fear of success in males and females. *Journal of Consulting and Clinical Psychology, 42,* 353–358.

Holland, A. J., Hall, A., Murray, R., Russell, G. F. M., & Crisp, A. H. (1984). Anorexia nervosa: A study of 34 twin pairs. *British Journal of Psychiatry, 145,* 414–419.

Hsu, L. K. G. (1980). Outcome in anorexia nervosa: A review of the literature (1954–1978). *Archives of General Psychiatry, 37,* 1041–1046.

Hsu, L. K. G. (1982). Is there a disturbance of body image in anorexia nervosa? *Journal of Nervous and Mental Disease, 170,* 305–307.

Hsu, L. K. G. (1986). The treatment of anorexia nervosa. *American Journal of Psychiatry, 143*(5), 573–581.

Hsu, L. K. G. (1987). Are the eating disorders becoming more common in blacks? *International Journal of Eating Disorders, 6,* 113–123.

Hsu, L. K. G., Crisp, A. H., & Harding, B. (1979). Outcome of anorexia nervosa. *Lancet, 1,* 61–65.

Hsu, L. K. G., & Holder, D. (1986). Bulimia nervosa: Treatment and short-term outcome. *Psychological Medicine, 16,* 65–70.

Hsu, L. K. G., Meltzer, E. S., & Crisp, A. H. (1981). Schizophrenia and anorexia nervosa. *Journal of Nervous and Mental Disease, 169,* 273–276.

Hsu, L. K. G., Milliones, J., Friedman, L., Holder, D., & Klepper, T. (1982, October). A survey of eating attitudes and behavior in adolescents. Paper presented at the 25th Annual Meeting of the American Academy of Child Psychiatry, Washington, DC.

Huenemann, R. L., Shapiro, L. R., Hampton, M. C., & Mitchell, B. W. (1966). A longitudinal study of gross body composition and body conformation and their association with food and activity in a teenage population. *American Journal of Clinical Nutrition, 18,* 324–338.

Hughes, P. L., Wells, L. A., Cunningham, C. J., & Ilstrup, D. M. (1986). Treating bulimia with desipramine: a double-blind, placebo-controlled study. *Archives of General Psychiatry, 43,* 182–186.

Isaacs, A. J. (1979). *Endocrinology in anorexia nervosa.* In P. Dally, J. Gomey, & A. Isaacs (Eds.) *Anorexia Nervosa* (pp. 159–209). London: Heineman.

Johnson, C. L., Lewis, C., Love, S., Stuckey, M., & Lewis, L. (1983). A descriptive survey of dieting and bulimic behavior. In G.J. Bargman (Ed.), *Understanding anorexia nervosa and bulimia* (pp. 14–20). Ross Laboratories, Ohio: Fourth Ross Conference on Medical Research.

Johnson, C. L., Stuckey, M., Lewis, D., & Schwartz, D. M. (1982). Bulimia: A survey of 500 patients. In P. L. Darby, P. E. Garfinkel, D. M. Garner, & D. V. Coscina (Eds.), *Anorexia nervosa: Recent developments* (pp. 159–171). New York: Alan R. Liss.

Jones, D. J., Fox, M. M., Babigan, H. M., & Hutton, H. E. (1980). Epidemiology of anorexia nervosa in Monroe County, New York: 1960–1976. *Psychosomatic Medicine, 42,* 551–558.

Kandel, D. B., & Davies, M. (1982). The epidemiology of depressed mood in adolescents: An empirical study. *Archives of General Psychiatry, 39,* 1205–1212.

Kaye, W. H., Ebert, M. H., Gwirtsman, H. E., & Weiss, S. R. (1984). Differences in brain serotonergic metabolism between nonbulimic and bulimic patients with anorexia nervosa. *American Journal of Psychiatry, 141,* 1598–1601.

Kaye, W. H., Gwirtsman, H. E., George, D. T., Weiss, S. R., & Jimerson, D. C. (1986). Relationship of mood alterations to bingeing behavior in bulimia. *British Journal of Psychiatry, 149,* 479–485.

Kendell, R. E., Hall, D. J., Hailey, A., & Babigan, H. M. (1973). The epidemiology of anorexia nervosa. *Psychological Medicine, 3,* 200–203.

Keys, A., Brozek, J., Henschel, A., Michelson, O., & Taylor, H. L. (1950). *The Biology of Human Starvation: Vol I & II.* Minneapolis: University Press.

Kirkley, B. G., Schneider, J. A., Agras, W. S., & Bachman, J. A. (1985). Comparison of two group treatments for bulimia. *Journal of Consulting and Clinical Psychology, 53,* 43–48.

Lacey, J. H. (1983). Bulimia nervosa, binge eating, and psychogenic vomiting: A controlled treatment study and long-term outcome. *British Medical Journal, 1,* 1609–1613.

Lacey, J. H., & Crisp, A. H. (1980). Hunger, food intake and weight: The impact of clomipramine on a refeeding anorexia nervosa population. *Postgraduate Medical Journal, 56,* 79–85.

Lee, N. F., & Rush, P. A. J. (1986). Cognitive-behavioral group therapy for bulimia. *International Journal of Eating Disorders, 5,* 599–615.

Leibowitz, S. F., & Shor-Posner, G. (1986). Brain serotonin and eating behavior. *Appetite, 7,* Supplement, 1–14.

Maloney, M. J., & Farrell, M. K. (1980). Treatment of severe weight loss in anorexia nervosa with hyperalimentation and psychotherapy. *American Journal of Psychiatry, 137,* 310–314.

Marsha, J. E., & Friedman, M. L. (1970). Ego identity status in college women. *Journal of Personality, 38,* 249–263.

Mickalide, A. D., & Andersen, A. E. (1985). Subgroups of anorexia nervosa and bulimia: Validity and utility. *Journal of Psychiatric Research, 19,* 121–128.

Minuchin, S., & Fishman, H. C. (1981). *Family therapy techniques.* Cambridge: Harvard University Press.

Minuchin, S., Rosman, B. L., & Baker, L. (1978). *Psychosomatic families.* Cambridge: Harvard University Press.

Mitchell, J. E., & Groat, R. (1984). A placebo-controlled, double-blind trial of amitriptyline in bulimia. *Journal of Clinical Psychopharmacology, 4,* 186–193.

Mitchell, J. E., Hatsukami, D., Eckert, E. D., & Pyle, R. L. (1985). Characteristics of 275 patients with bulimia. *American Journal of Psychiatry, 142,* 482–485.

Mitchell, J. E., & Laine, D. C. (1985). Monitored binge-eating behavior in patients with bulimia. *International Journal of Eating Disorders, 4,* 177–183.

Miyai, K., Yamamoto, T., Azukizawa, M., Ishibashi, K., & Kumahara, Y. (1975). Serum thyroid hormones and thyrotropin in anorexia nervosa. *Journal of Clinical Endocrinology and Metabolism, 40,* 334–338.

Morgan, H. G., Purgold, J., & Welbourne, J. (1983). Management and outcome in anorexia nervosa: A standardized prognosis study. *British Journal of Psychiatry, 143,* 282–297.

Morgan, H. G., & Russell, G. F. M. (1975). Value of family background and clinical features as predictors of long-term outcome in anorexia nervosa: Four-year follow-up study of 41 patients. *Psychological Medicine, 5,* 355–371.

Needleman, H. L., & Waber, D. (1977). The use of amitriptyline in anorexia nervosa. In R. A. Vigersky (Ed.), *Anorexia nervosa.* New York: Raven.

Nogami, Y., & Yabana, F. (1977). On kibarashi-gui. *Folia Psychiat. Neurol. Japan, 31,* 159–166.

Nylander, I. (1971). The feeling of being fat and dieting in a school population. *Acta Sociomedica Scandinavica, 3,* 17–26.

Offer, D. (1969). *The psychological world of the teenager.* New York: Basic Books.

Orbach, S. (1985). Accepting the symptom: A feminist psychoanalytic treatment of anorexia nervosa. In D. M. Garner & P. E. Garfinkel (Eds.), *Handbook of psychotherapy for anorexia nervosa and bulimia* (pp. 83–106). New York: Guilford.

Ordman, A. M., & Kirschenbaum, D. S. (1985). Cognitive-behavioral therapy for bulimia: An initial outcome study. *Journal of Consulting and Clinical Psychology, 53,* 305–313.

Orlofsky, J. L. (1978). Identity formation, achievement, and fear of success in college men and women. *Journal of Youth and Adolescence, 7,* 49–62.

Pirke, K. M., Pahl, J., Schweiger, U., & Warnhoff, M. (1985). Metabolic and endocrine indices of starvation in bulimia: A comparison with anorexia nervosa. *Psychiatric Research, 15,* 33–40.

Pope, H. G., Hudson, J. I., Jonas, J. M., & Yurgelun-Todd, D. (1983). Bulimia treated with imipramine: A placebo-controlled, double-blind study. *American Journal of Psychiatry, 140,* 554–558.

Pope, H. G., Hudson, J. I., Yurgelun-Todd, D., & Hutton, M. S. (1984). Prevalence of anorexia nervosa and bulimia in three student populations. *International Journal of Eating Disorders, 3,* 45–51.

Pyle, R. L., Mitchell, J. E., & Eckert, E. E. (1983). The incidence of bulimia in freshman college students. *International Journal of Eating Disorders, 2,* 75–85.

Rivinus, T. M., Biederman, J., Herzog, D. B., Kemper, K., Harper, G. P., Harmatz, J. S., & Houseworth, S. (1984). Anorexia nervosa and affective disorders: A controlled family history study. *American Journal of Psychiatry, 141,* 1414–1418.

Root, M. P. P., Fallon, P., & Friedrich, W. N. (1986). *Bulimia: A systems approach to treatment.* New York: Norton.

Russell, G. F. M. (1977). The present status of anorexia nervosa. *Psychological Medicine, 7,* 353–367.

Russell, G. F. M. (1985). The changing nature of anorexia nervosa: An introduction to the conference. *Journal of Psychiatric Research, 19,* 101–109.

Russell, G. F. M., & Beumont, P. (1987). The endocrinology of anorexia nervosa. In P. Beumont, G. Burrows, & R. Casper (Eds.), *Handbook of eating disorders* (pp. 201–232). Amsterdam, Elselia.

Rutter, M., Graham, P., Chadwick, O. F. D., & Yule, W. (1976). Adolescent turmoil: Fact or fiction. *Journal of Child Psychology and Psychiatry, 17,* 35–56.

Schiele, B. C., & Brozek, J. (1948). Experimental neurosis resulting from semistarvation in man. *Psychosomatic Medicine, 10,* 31–50.

Shepherd, M., Oppenheim, B., & Mitchell, S. (1971). *Childhood behavior and mental health.* London: University of London Press.

Silverstone, T., & Goodall, E. (1986). Serotoninergic mechanisms in human feeling: The pharmacological evidence. *Appetite, 7,* Supplement, 85–97.

Simmons, R. G., & Rosenberg, F. (1975). Sex, sex roles, and self-image. *Journal of Youth and Adolescence, 4,* 229–258.

Strober, M., & Yager, J. (1985). A developmental perspective on the treatment of anorexia nervosa in adolescents. In D. M. Garner & P. E. Garfinkel (Eds.), *Handbook of psychotherapy for anorexia nervosa and bulimia* (pp. 363–390). New York: Guilford.

Szmukler, G. I. (1983). Weight and food preoccupation in a population of English schoolgirls. In G. J. Bargman (Ed.), *Understanding anorexia nervosa and bulimia* (pp. 21–27). Ross Laboratories, Ohio: Fourth Ross Conference on Medical Research.

Szmukler, G., McCance, C., McCrone, L., & Hunter, D. (1986). Anorexia nervosa: A psychiatric case register study from Aberdeen. *Psychological Medicine, 16,* 49–58.

Swift, W. J., Andrews, D., & Barklage, N. E. (1986). The relationship between affective disorder and eating disorders: A review of the literature. *American Journal of Psychiatry, 143,* 290–299.

Theander, S. (1970). Anorexia nervosa: A psychiatric investigation of 94 female patients. *Acta Psychiatrica Scandinavica,* Supplement 214.

Theander, S. (1985). Outcome and prognosis in anorexia nervosa and bulimia: Some results of previous investigations, compared with those of a Swedish long-term study. *Journal of Psychiatric Research, 19,* 493–508.

Touyz, S. W., Beumont, P. J. V., & Glaun, D. (1984). A comparison of lenient and strict operant conditioning programmes in refeeding patients with anorexia nervosa. *British Journal of Psychiatry, 144,* 517–520.

Vandereycken, W. (1984). Neuroleptics in the short-term treatment of anorexia nervosa: A double-blind placebo-controlled study with sulpiride. *British Journal of Psychiatry, 144,* 288–292.

Vandereycken, W., & Pierlott, R. (1982). Pimozide combined with behavior therapy in the short-term treatment of anorexia nervosa: A double-blind placebo-controlled cross-over study. *Acta Psychiatrica Scandinavica, 66,* 445–450.

Walsh, B. T., Stewart, J. W., Roose, S. P., Gladis, M., & Glassman, A. H. (1984). Treatment of bulimia with phenelzine: A double-blind, placebo-controlled study. *Archives of General Psychiatry, 41,* 1105–1109.

Willi, J., & Grossman, S. (1983). Epidemiology of anorexia nervosa in a defined region of Switzerland. *American Journal of Psychiatry, 140,* 564–567.

Wilson, G. T., Rossiter, E., Kleifeld, E. I., & Lindholm, L. (1986). Cognitive-behavioral treatment of bulimia nervosa: A controlled evaluation. *Behavior Research and Therapy, 24,* 277–288.

Wolchik, S. A., Weiss, L., & Katzman, M. A. (1986). An empirically validated, short-term psychoeducational group treatment program for bulimia. *International Journal of Eating Disorders, 5,* 21–34.

Wooley, S. C., & Wooley, O. W. (1985). Intensive outpatient and residential treatment for bulimia. In D. M. Garner & P. E. Garfinkel (Eds.), *Handbook of psychotherapy for anorexia nervosa and bulimia* (pp. 391–430). New York: Guilford.

Wurtman, R. J., & Wurtman, J. J. (1986). Carbohydrate craving, obesity and brain serotonin. *Appetite, 7,* Supplement, 99–103.

Author Index

Subject Index

434